The Cytokines of the Immune System

The Cytokines of the Immune System
THE ROLE OF CYTOKINES IN DISEASE RELATED TO IMMUNE RESPONSE

ZLATKO DEMBIC

Professor of Immunology, Cell Biology and Microbiology,
Department of Oral Biology, University of Oslo, Norway
and Visiting Professor of Medicine, Medical Faculty,
University of Rijeka, Croatia

Amsterdam • Boston • Heidelberg • London
New York • Oxford • Paris • San Diego
San Francisco • Singapore • Sydney • Tokyo
Academic Press is an imprint of Elsevier

Academic Press is an imprint of Elsevier
125 London Wall, London EC2Y 5AS, UK
525 B Street, Suite 1800, San Diego, CA 92101-4495, USA
225 Wyman Street, Waltham, MA 02451, USA
The Boulevard, Langford Lane, Kidlington, Oxford OX5 1GB, UK

Notices
Knowledge and best practice in this field are constantly changing. As new research and experience
broaden our understanding, changes in research methods, professional practices, or medical treatment
may become necessary.

Practitioners and researchers must always rely on their own experience and knowledge in evaluating
and using any information, methods, compounds, or experiments described herein. In using such
information or methods they should be mindful of their own safety and the safety of others, including
parties for whom they have a professional responsibility.

To the fullest extent of the law, neither the Publisher nor the authors, contributors, or editors, assume
any liability for any injury and/or damage to persons or property as a matter of products liability,
negligence or otherwise, or from any use or operation of any methods, products, instructions, or ideas
contained in the material herein.

Library of Congress Cataloging-in-Publication Data
A catalog record for this book is available from the Library of Congress

British Library Cataloguing-in-Publication Data
A catalogue record for this book is available from the British Library

ISBN: 978-0-12-419998-9

For information on all Academic Press publications
visit our website at http://store.elsevier.com/

  Working together
to grow libraries in
ELSEVIER Book Aid
International developing countries

www.elsevier.com • www.bookaid.org

Publisher: Mica Haley
Acquisition Editor: Linda Versteeg-Buschman
Editorial Project Manager: Halima William
Production Project Manager: Chris Wortley
Designer: Maria Inês Cruz

Typeset by TNQ Books and Journals
www.tnq.co.in

Printed and bound in the United States of America

CONTENTS

Foreword   *ix*

Acknowledgments   *xi*

1. **Introduction—Common Features About Cytokines**   **1**
   Division   3
   Structure   3
   Receptors   6
   Intracellular Signal Transduction   8
   Hormones and Cytokines   11
   Function   14

2. **The Immune System—Definition and Development of Immunity**   **17**
   Organization of the Immune System   19
   Humoral Innate (Nonspecific) Immunity   25
   Cellular Innate (Nonspecific) Immunity   30
   Adaptive Humoral (Specific) Immune System   39
   Cellular Adaptive (Specific) Immune System   42

3. **Activation of Cells of the Immune System**   **57**
   Activation of Immune Cells in the Periphery of the Immune System   57
   Specific Recognition   58
   Coreceptors of T Cells: CD4 and CD8   70
   Costimulation during T-Cell Activation   71
   Signal Transduction in T Cell   72
   Signal Transduction in the B Cell   80
   Signal Transduction in Mast Cells   81
   Further Development of Immune Cells Upon Activation   83
   T lymphocyte Homeostasis   93
   Repertoire and Tolerance   94

4. **The Role and Regulation of the Immune Responses**   **99**
   The Course of the Immune Response   99
   Regulation of Immunocyte Development after Activation   105
   Important Control Functions of Cytokines   106
   The Role of Th1-Type of Immune Response   114
   The Role of Th2-Type of Immune Response   115
   The Role of Th9 Subset   116

The Role of Th17 Subset   116
The Role of Th22 Subset   118
The Role of Th3, and Tr1 Cells   119
The Role of Regulatory CD4 T Lymphocytes—Tregs   119
The Role of the Tfh Subset   121

5. Cytokines of the Immune System: Interferons   **123**
Interferon-α/β   124
Interferon-γ (IFN-γ)   129
Interferon-λ (IFN-λ)   140
References   140
Further Reading   142

6. Cytokines of the Immune System: Interleukins   **143**
IL-1   143
IL-2   151
IL-3   160
IL-4   162
IL-5   166
IL-6   168
IL-7   175
IL-8   178
IL-9   179
IL-10   181
IL-11   184
IL-12   186
IL-13   190
IL-14 (IL-14 Does Not Exist in Databases)   193
IL-15   193
IL-16   197
IL-17   200
IL-18   202
IL-19   205
IL-20   207
IL-21   209
IL-22   212
IL-23   214
IL-24   216
IL-25   218
IL-26   219
IL-27   221

IL-28 and IL-29 (Type III Interferon, λ1–3)   224
IL-30   225
IL-31   225
IL-32   227
IL-33   228
IL-34   229
IL-35   230
IL-36   232
IL-37   233
IL-38   234
References   235
Further Reading   238

7. Cytokines of the Immune System: Chemokines   241
About Chemokines   241
The Role of Chemokines in the Immune System   246
CCL Chemokines (CCL1–CCL28)   248
CXCL Chemokines (1–16)   255
CX3CL Chemokine   259
XCL Chemokines (1–2)   260
Other Features of Chemokines   260

**8. Cytokines Important for Growth and/or Development of
Cells of the Immune System   263**
TNF-α/β   263
TGF-β   266
TSLP (Thymic Stromal Lymphopoietin)   269
KGF (Keratinocyte Growth Factor)   271
SCF (Stem Cell Factor) and Growth Factors (CSF, GM-CSF, M-CSF) of
    Hematopoietic Lines   271
LIF—Leukemia Inhibitory Factor   272
CNTF—Ciliary Neurotrophic Factor   274
OSM—Oncostatin M   276
A Short Description of Other Cytokines that Regulate Growth and
    Development of Various Tissues   277

9. Theories about the Function of the Immune System   283
About Scientific Theories   283
Self–Nonself Discrimination   285
The "Pathogen-Associated Molecular Pattern (PAMP) Recognition"
    Theory (Janeway)   288

Idiotypic Networks and Suppression (Jerne)   289
The "Danger" Model (Matzinger)   291
The "Integrity" Model (Dembic)   293
Other Theories About Immunity   299
References   301

Index   *303*

FOREWORD

The book is aimed at undergraduate and postgraduate training of physicians and dentists, but it can be used as a learning source for those interested in biology and biochemistry.

Over the last decade I have been motivated by the idea of writing a manual for physicians, dentists, and biologists that was also a textbook for those who want to enter the world of biomedical science. This book can serve as a guide for experienced medical specialists in their planned clinical investigations, or as a source of information in the field in which they are taking an interest because of professional or personal experience.

The first goal of this book is to explain the essential principles underlying immunology and its relationship to cytokines. With their diverse actions cytokines are an unavoidable part of the complex function of the immune system. They are described in a way that I hope will help in motivating research to find the simplest solution as to their physiological role in the body.

The encyclopedic display of cytokines helps in viewing the properties of each member as a combination of easily recognizable categories: structure, function, receptor, association with disease, and therapeutic options. Such easily accessible information can be used by physicians for differential diagnosis and in searching for possible new therapies, or by scientists in creating new projects and interpreting their data.

Another goal of the book is that it should allow motivated and interested readers to find possible links between cytokines and diseases. For this purpose I have presented the detailed structure of cytokines and their assumed roles: from homeostasis to defense, and this is supplemented by several selected pathophysiological conditions. The therapeutic part of clinical assessment of disease has not been covered. Cytokines that have been considered for therapeutic purposes are highlighted and only some are described in detail with references for further reading. The other references are accessible over the Internet from various databases, and this book should provide an incentive for further study. Many therapeutic small molecules (biological) including monoclonal antibodies modifying the function of certain cytokines are described, also. They seem to be an important component of potential novel therapies in many diseases, and numerous beneficial treatments are yet to be discovered in the field of cytokine-action modifiers.

Finally, an index of terms and phrases is given at the end of the book. It is used to aid in the search for items such as new antibodies against certain cytokines or receptors, or new biologicals. It also serves as a source of knowledge crosslinking different chapters.

Due to the rapid progress of research, this book will over time need an update. I hope that, regardless of this, the main message of this book will aid further understanding of the immune system, with cytokines as major communicators in the immune response, as well as various diseases with which they are, or might be, associated.

ACKNOWLEDGMENTS

I thank my fellow colleagues at the University of Oslo, Norway, for helping me in collecting material, pictures, figures, and information about various parts of this book. I am also indebted to Karl Schenck and Olav Schreurs at the Department of Oral Biology, for figures representing microscopic pictures of lymph nodes, tonsil, and spleen. I thank Ludvig A. Munthe for letting me have tens of his presentation figures, which made a starting point for many of my figures in the book. Most of the figures are derived from my own lectures, presentations, and talks that I have prepared for various forms of teaching over the last 25 years. Several figures were contributed by Maja Dembic, and I gratefully thank her. Many chapters were initially written in the Croatian language, and then translated, mostly by myself. I thank Zdravko Jotanovic who helped me with translating several important pages. I did the updating and finalizing of the book during the first part of 2014.

CHAPTER 1

Introduction—Common Features About Cytokines

Cytokines are cell-to-cell messengers similar to hormones with the strongest activity in the microenvironment of the cells that secrete them. The majority have an immunomodulating effect and this book focuses on them. The name cytokine derives from Greek *cyto* (cell) and *kinos* (movement), implying their role in cellular traffic (e.g., towards sites of infection). Differences between endocrine hormones and cytokines are mentioned later in the Introduction.

Structurally and genetically, cytokines are defined as polypeptides, proteins, and glycoproteins, unlike some other heralds in the microenvironment, such as prostaglandins, which have a different structure. The physiological role of cytokines, in general, is in tissue homeostasis and cellular activation, relocation and differentiation. The oldest described functions were in regulating the immune system's response to trauma, inflammation, and infection. However, the details about actions for the majority of cytokines are still largely unknown. Many diseases show aberrant communication between tissues and the immune system that involves cytokines. Research about the action of cytokines is therefore essential for the understanding of their pathophysiology. As this part of biomedical research is very dynamic, facts concerning the function of cytokines are increasingly accumulating in the scientific and clinical literature.

In a number of cases, abnormalities in cytokines' actions were found either as a cause or effect of a disease, and therefore responsible for all or part of the symptomatology. For this reason, this book lists current available knowledge about the link between various diseases and immunomodulating cytokines hoping to facilitate further research. In addition, it is expected that new knowledge about cytokine function will promote the advancement of medical diagnosis and therapy.

Cells within tissues with well-known architecture typically communicate with each other through direct contact using molecules (mostly glycoproteins) imbedded in their cellular membranes. Examples are inhibition of growth in differentiated solid tissues, or by electrochemical signals such as

The Cytokines of the Immune System
http://dx.doi.org/10.1016/B978-0-12-419998-9.00001-8

those in the heart, muscle, and brain. Cytokines, on the other hand, are generally produced as a consequence of cell activation. They serve as communicators for a variety of characteristic functions in specific tissues. They are important for local homeostasis including growth, differentiation, development, and interaction with other tissues and organs in the body. They act in most cases at shorter distances (with exceptions such as IL-1, IL-6, "insulin like growth factors" [IGF], TNF and a few more). However, cytokines penetrate most tissues, being delivered by migration of white blood cells of the hematopoietic tissue, which permeates virtually all other tissues in vertebrates. This delivery method is influenced by a specialized set of cytokines called chemokines. The latter are important not only for regulating white-blood-cells' traffic but also for the activation and coordination of certain immune reactions. Unfortunately, this latter area seems to be very complicated, because the regulation of the immune system is not completely understood. It is assumed that cytokines hold the "key" of the remaining unknowns in immune responses, as well as diseases related to disorders of immunity.

Therefore, in order to understand the function of cytokines one needs to have knowledge of the biology of cells of various tissues as well as of the functioning of the immune system, which is described in the first part of the book. The vast majority of cytokines are very important for growth, development, and mobilization of immune cells as well as for the creation and regulation of effector functions in the immune response to infections, organ transplants, and autoimmune diseases. Furthermore, the immune competent cells are one of the largest sources of cytokines that with their ability to migrate in almost all tissues of the body represent moving regulators of the local microenvironment.

Throughout history, functional principles in biology were learned and based on studies of diseases and their pathophysiological processes. Similarly, a large number of disorders, in which cytokines were a cause or a consequence of a disease, have been described. Most of them have an immunological sign.

Immunological disorders are divided into (a) congenital and acquired immunological deficiencies; (b) autoimmunity; (c) allergy (as a result of insufficient, incorrect, or exaggerated immune system reactions); and (d) the damage that is caused by secondary somatic primary disease or unknown cause (idiopathic). Of secondary disorders it is important to mention neoplasias of the immune system (lymphomas and leukemias) and primary diseases of various organs that result in failure of immunity. Malignant tumors of solid tissues, according to the theory of immune surveillance, develop as a result of impaired immunity or its lack. However, the sole emergence of cancer cells is a process in which the immune system probably does not have a direct impact. It is possible that in the process of cancer development (cellular transformation) caused by teratogenic viruses (or some yet unknown combination of microorganisms), a chronic immune response against such cancer cell can be a continuous stimulus for secretion of some cytokines. The latter might indirectly promote tumor development by the selection of more malignant mutations.

DIVISION

Cytokines are divided into several groups of molecules bearing different names that tend to illustrate their functions. However, many have retained older names that describe only a minor portion of their activities like tumor necrosis factor (TNF) or transforming factor. When their collection of activities were discovered they were not re-named, although their relatives bear names that are signs of a group like interferons, interleukins, chemokines, or factors that affect growth and development of various tissues. There is no unified agreement on how to categorize cytokines and this book might provide help in this matter. I kept the division of cytokines according to their group names, and only a minority are presented with their original name. Their belonging to a specific group is mentioned under the subsection about their function, and basically, we can distinguish cytokines that have effects on hematopoietic (blood forming) tissues from those that do not, but directed towards other somatic tissues.

STRUCTURE

Cytokines are products of one to several genes that appear as monomeric or polymeric polypeptides and proteins, which are usually glycosylated. The most common forms are dimers (homodimers or heterodimers) and trimers (homotrimers and heterotrimers).

Examples of structures are shown in the Figure 1-1. As the monomer, interleukin-1 (IL-1) is a typical representative of this group. There are antagonists of cytokines such as IL-1 receptor antagonist (IL-1Ra) and IL-18 binding protein (IL-18 BP) that prevent the binding of cytokine to their receptor. Some cytokines such as *transforming growth factor-β* (TGF-β) are secreted in the intercellular space in an inactive form. Their activation

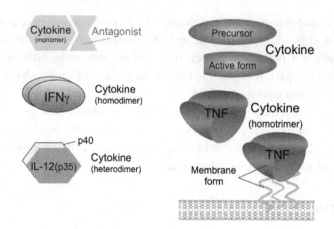

Figure 1-1 Schematic exemplars of various structures of cytokines.

involves an enzymatic process that produces an active part of the molecule. Since the TGF-β is everywhere in the body and constitutively secreted by many types of cells, the regulation of its activity is influenced by tissue-specific proteases.

Of dimers, a representative is interferon-γ (IFN-γ), which is a homodimer. The active form of IFN-γ has two molecules that are set in antiparallel position, according to the crystallographic studies. Heterodimers are mostly interleukins, of which the most interesting exemplars (regarding the structure) are IL-12, IL-23, IL-27, and IL-35, because they cross-share a part of their molecule. Each has two subunits encoded by different genes. However their composition varies, as each is a combination of different subunits. This increases a potential to exert specific effects in different locations (or tissues) through regulation of expression of each particular subunit. For example, IL-12 and IL-23 share a common heavy subunit (p40), while the lighter subunits p35 (of IL-12) and p19 (of IL-23) can be differently regulated. Furthermore, p40 subunit can form homodimers, and it is considered that such a cytokine (so far unnamed) has an antagonistic effect on both, IL-12 and IL-23 cytokines. Furthermore, IL-27 is also composed of two similar subunits, and shares one with IL-35 (the latter includes the IL-12 p35 subunit). The complexity in interleukin structure probably reflects their multi-faceted role in the regulation of immune responses.

The most representative trimer is the TNF. Its structure is a molecular triangle formed by three monomers. The first monomer binds with the N (amino)-terminal part to the C (COOH)-terminal part of the second monomer, which, in turn is linked to a third one, and the latter encloses the triangular space by binding to the C-part of the first monomer (Figure 1-1).

Although cytokines are mainly secreted, many are attached to the cell membrane. The membrane-bound cytokines are no different from the secreted ones, but some may also act as receptors (producing so-called reverse signaling), such as IL-15 cytokine. TNF has a membrane-bound form, but it is unknown whether it has a reverse signaling. Interestingly, the membrane form of TNF-α can be associated with another related cytokine (lymphotoxin-β) to make heterotrimers.

Extracellular portions of membrane-bound cytokines can be cleaved by metalloproteases called sheddases, and thus secreted. Sheddases are a group with a large number of members having different actions. Most act specifically, some promiscuously, and some bidirectionally. For example, in the Notch factor (affecting growth and development) that crosses the cell membrane, a sheddase cleaves the intracytoplasmic part of the molecule making the signal traveling also in reverse: namely, the cytoplasmic portion enters the nucleus, where it acts as a transcription factor. Extracellular portion (of the Notch factor) binds to the receptor on a neighboring cell, setting in motion the second part of the Notch action.

There are other names for sheddases: metallopeptidases (ADAM1-17); α-, β-, γ-secretases; aspartate protease; or TNF-α *converting enzyme* (TACE). In addition to cytokines, sheddases can act and release extracellular parts of other transmembrane proteins like adhesion molecules or some cytokine receptors. If the latter happens then the receptor and ligand can reverse their roles, in that the soluble receptor can now act as a cytokine, and a membrane form of the original cytokine as its *de facto* receptor. One such example is a soluble form of the IL-6 receptor subunit gp130 or IL-6 signal transducer (IL-6ST).

Cytokines (or their subunits) with homologous structures form groups and families. Figure 1-2 shows a group of IL-6 related cytokines. However, although structurally similar, a relatively small number of IL-6 related cytokines have similar functions, a fact obvious just by reading their names (Figure 1-2). Interestingly, two heterodimeric cytokines are formed by a mix of homologous and non-homologous subunits: IL-6 related subunits like IL-12 p35 and IL-23 p19 are associated with the non-IL-6 homologous p40 subunit. However, the latter is homologous to one of the IL-6 receptor subunits (IL-6Rα), suggesting a probable evolutionary link concerning their origins.

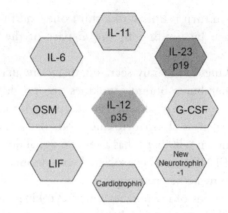

Figure 1-2 Schematic exemplar of a group of cytokines with homologous structure.

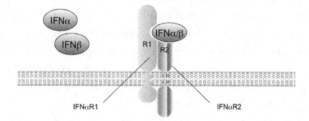

Figure 1-3 Cytokine receptors—schematic exemplar of a heterodimeric form.

RECEPTORS

Cytokine receptors are transmembrane glycoproteins commonly composed of several subunits. We distinguish receptors whose subunits cross the cell membrane once from those that cross it more than that (like, e.g., the chemokine receptor with seven transmembrane regions). Subunits vary in molecular weight and the ways in which they interconnect or bind the ligand. There are different types of cytokine receptors regarding the composition of subunits. We have monomeric and multimeric receptors, and the latter can be homo- or heteromultimeric. Binding of extracellular ligands to cell-surface receptors can recruit additional molecules in the ligand-receptor complex within the cell membrane and in the cytosol.

The ligand binding affinity is usually distributed unequally across the subunits of multimeric cytokine receptors.

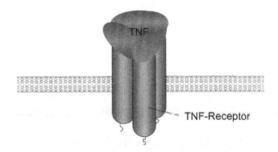

Figure 1-4 Cytokine receptors—schematic exemplar of a homotrimer.

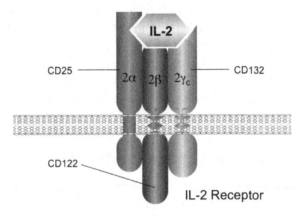

Figure 1-5 Cytokine receptors—schematic exemplar of a heterotrimer.

An example of a heterodimeric receptor is the IFNα/β receptor (Figure 1-3). It has a subunit with a higher affinity for the ligand and another chain that contributes to the overall affinity to a lesser degree. Ligand affinities can be measured by utilizing ligand and receptor in a soluble phase (i.e., only an extracellular portion of a receptor). Most cytokine receptors have affinity-interaction levels between 10^{-10} and 10^{-11} M, which are 10 to 100 times more powerful than the largest measured affinity between antibodies and antigens.

Examples for homotrimers are two TNF receptors (p55 and p75). Both resemble a structure depicted schematically in Figure 1-4.

A heterotrimeric receptor is, for example, the IL-2 receptor (IL-2R), which is shown in Figure 1-5. Interestingly, in some cells a part of it can also be a receptor. A heterodimer composed only of IL-2Rβ and IL-2Rγ subunits, which has a weaker affinity than the heterotrimeric IL-2R, can similarly signal inside the cell. Although each IL-2R subunit has also a weak affinity for the ligand, their interaction seems to be without functional effects.

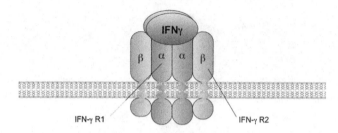

Figure 1-6 Cytokine receptors—schematic exemplar of a heterotetramer.

Thus, in general, an increase in a cytokine receptor's affinity for a ligand is often correlated with the higher likelihood of triggering that cytokine's action(s).

An example of a heterotetrameric receptor is the IFNγ receptor (Figure 1-6). Homodimeric ligand (IFNγ) can bind to the IFNγR1 homodimer, which can then recruit a pair of IFNγR2 chains to form the four-chain receptor complex.

INTRACELLULAR SIGNAL TRANSDUCTION

Signal transduction into the cell is caused by interaction of cytokines with their receptors. In general, receptors mostly span the cell membrane, unlike those of hormones that can have intracellular ones. Intracellular signaling progresses depending on the type of receptor a cytokine engages with.

Cytokines can cause either rapid or slow action of target cells. Slow action usually involves novel protein synthesis, whereas a slow one can have many direct consequences including ion mobilization and protein–protein interactions in the cytosol.

Chemotaxis is an example of a fast action that develops within a few seconds. It is controlled by cytokines called chemokines. (The action has a consequence of adaptation to the signal after a few minutes.) Such a signal degrades the actin skeleton of cells in one place and builds it elsewhere in the direction of the chemotactic signal. Thus, rapid signal transduction characterizes chemokine receptors (Figure 1-7). These in turn engage G (GTP-binding) proteins that open an ion channel. The latter is made by the chemokine receptor protein chain (bound to the ligand) with its seven transmembrane parts (that are usually not in contact with the ligand).

Slow action of cytokines is observed within a few minutes to a few hours (and even days). These actions occur by phosphorylation of intracellular

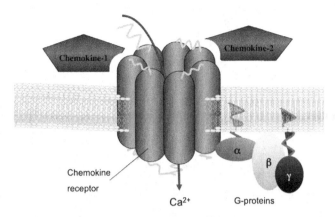

Figure 1-7 Cytokine receptors—schematic exemplar of a receptor with seven transmembrane regions and signal transduction in the cell.

messengers. There are various signal transduction molecules called kinases that become parts of the receptor complex or bind to the inner side of the membrane receptor. These molecules can further recruit additional polypeptide chains (called adapter proteins) that allow further signaling inside the cell. Phosphorylation of amino acids like tyrosines, serines, and threonines usually causes a change in polypeptide conformation. Conformational changes allow interactions with different molecular (usually polypeptide) partners leading to transfer of information by inducing changing the conformation of a new partner. Thus, if the second messenger is another kinase (causing phosphorylation) then a cascade of events follows, which consume time. Different cells have a different repertoire of intracellular messengers, but many are ubiquitous like NF-κB (nuclear factor kappa B), which can be activated by degradation of its inhibitor (I-κB). Activated factors that enter into the nucleus and bind to DNA, thereby allowing the beginning of transcriptional activity on certain genes, are called transcription factors.

Therefore, based on signaling, we can divide cytokine receptors into (a) G-protein coupled; (b) with intrinsic enzymatic (tyrosine kinase) activity; (c) with associated enzymatic activities like tyrosine kinase or serine-threonine kinase; and (d) the ones that involve interactions with other molecules in the cytosol.

Products of genes, as a result of the actions of some cytokines, are intracellular, membrane or secretory proteins. The synthesis of these proteins can endow cells to become responsive to other cytokines, or even bind the same one with a higher affinity, thus altering the initial effect. For example, creation of new intracellular molecules can promote survival (regulate growth

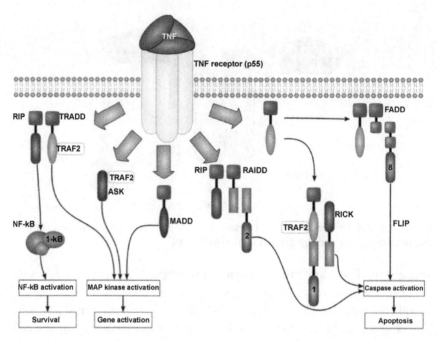

Figure 1-8 Cytokine receptors—schematic exemplar of signal transduction.

and development) or induce death (apoptosis, which is programmed by activation of specific proteases called caspases). Similarly, producing new transmembrane molecules provides cells to communicate with their environment differently. The complexity in signal transduction can also vary, and an illustrative example (Figure 1-8) shows that of the TNF receptor 1 (TNFR1, p55).

Molecules involved in signal transduction are also divided into several groups. First, we should mention molecules that bind intracellular portions of receptors and have associated tyrosine or serine-threonine kinase activities. The former are called *Janus* kinases (JAK) and STAT (*"signal transducer and activator of transcription"*) factors (mostly involved in signaling by interferons and interleukins). The latter comprise various proteins like SMAD system used by transforming growth factors (TGFs) and bone morphogenetic proteins (BMP), and mitogen–activated kinases (MAPK). Second, some receptors have intrinsic tyrosine kinase activity (EGF receptor, PDGF receptor) in their cytoplasmic parts, that can recruit cytosolic molecules named "adapters," as they can, in turn, bind to other signaling molecules in cytosol forming either a cascade of interactions, or a specific group of

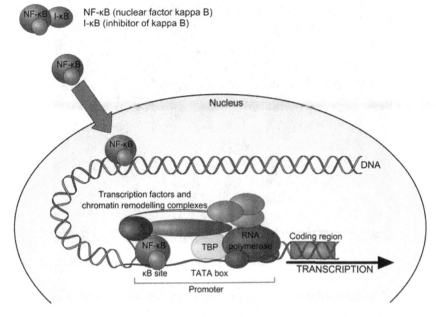

Figure 1-9 Schematic example of signal transduction and activation of genes.

molecules performing specific actions, all ending with activation of some nuclear factor. An example of nuclear factors is the NF-κB system (see TNF receptor, Figure 1-8).

Nuclear factors, upon entering the nucleus, can bind sequence specific elements in the DNA. Different DNA elements are found in promoters of genes, as well as in their enhancers and silencers. This means that a specific interplay of various nuclear factors plays a distinct role during the regulation of gene expression. For example, a typical eukaryotic promoter has a complex of over 30 proteins that together with RNA polymerase II regulates the initiation of transcription of messenger RNA (Figure 1-9). At other sites (i.e., other than promoter), nuclear factors also regulate gene expression, but they mainly exert that via modifying transcription characteristics (i.e., the speed of elongation or stability of transcripts).

HORMONES AND CYTOKINES

Cytokines are very similar to some endocrine hormones. Yet, in general, many aspects and characteristics seem different (Figure 1-10). However, these differences are slowly reduced, with each new result describing their molecular

Features	Hormones	Cytokines
Number of production sites	Small	Large
Amount of target cells	Large	Small
Biologic role	Homeostasis of an organism	Local, clonal - defence, growth, differentiation & tissue homeostasis
Biologic redundancy	Small	Large
Biologic pleiotropy	Low	High
Concentration in blood	High	Low
Sphere of action	Wide	Narrow (juxtacrine)
Induction of secretion	Phyisiologic variation	By external provocation

Figure 1-10 Differences between cytokines and endocrine hormones.

actions. No matter how hard we try to define the dissimilarities between hormones and cytokines, we will always find an exception to such rules. Perhaps the distinction between them is barely historical and semantic. Despite this, we can try to describe this difference. Cytokines are a group of cellular products with the following predominantly different characteristics:

The Number of Sources (Sites of Origin)

Sources of cytokines have a larger spread and can be found at various locations, whereas hormones are mostly produced by a dedicated gland or tissue. All nucleated cells in an organism are capable of producing IL-1, IL-6, and TNF. Furthermore, some cytokine producing cells are mobile and can be scattered throughout the body (like, e.g., a subset of activated T cells during infection).

The Number of Target Cells

Cytokines influence smaller numbers of target cells than hormones. They usually act in the microenvironment, whereas hormones act on almost all cells in the body. However, there are exceptions like TGF and TNF, which produce direct effects across the whole of the body. Similarly, fever is an indirect influence by IL-1 and TNF on the whole organism.

Biological Role

Cytokines are cell-to-cell messengers that contribute to immune responses and incite movement to sites of trauma, inflammation, and infection.

Hormones control the organism as a whole by regulating homeostasis of the internal *milieu* like, for example, growth hormone. Cytokines usually have a single biologically relevant function (i.e., pro-inflammatory, chemotactic, anti-inflammatory, differentiating, or the like) and generally act on fewer specific cell types or developmental stages of tissues. Exceptions are FGF-23 and FGF-21, both with two known roles. The former regulates calcium excretion independently of PTH, and the latter increases the entry of glucose into adipocytes independently of insulin, in addition to being connective tissue growth factors (for fibroblasts). Additional exceptions are some chemokines that cause migration and activation of attracted cells. Lastly, exceptions are interleukins IL-1 and IL-6, which have multiple functions throughout the body.

Redundancy (Sufficiency Without Necessity, or Replaceability)

Many cytokines have overlapping actions on cells, implying that an action of a single cytokine is less unique. Thus, cytokines have higher redundancy in their activities than hormones. It means that the lack of one cytokine can usually be substituted by the actions of others and might not affect survival (unless under extreme selective pressure, as in a rare infection). The examples are chemokines and some interleukins (IL-2, IL-4). Absence of a particular hormone, in comparison, is not replaceable, and always leads to a known clinical syndrome. The exception is the cytokine IFN-γ (whose hereditary lack of its receptor leads to rare lethal syndrome in children that are vaccinated with BCG)

Breadth of Actions (Pleiotropy)

By exerting systemic, developmental and local effects, cytokines seem to have wider action width than hormones.

Occurrence in Blood Circulation

Because cytokines act in the microenvironment, circulation is not a physiological means of transmission to the target tissue, as it is for the hormones. For example, elevated production of cytokines at the site of infection or trauma can cause their occurrence in the circulation. This might represent a spillover into the blood and lymph vessels, in which case a thousand-fold increase in their (otherwise picomolar) blood concentration can be detected. The exceptions are IL-1 and TNF, as they cause fever by elevating the set point of *thermostat* cells (neurons that can increase body temperature) in hypothalamus.

Sphere of Influence

Cytokines' effect is diluted with distance and concentration. Therefore, they usually influence neighboring cells. This is called juxtacrine or paracrine action, and if they affect cells that have produced them, autocrine. The exceptions to the rule are: (a) FGF-21, a member of the *fibroblast growth factors* that is produced in the liver and acts on adipocytes; and (b) IL-6, which operates at remote sites throughout the body, but it is mainly produced by inflammatory cells focused at the site of infection. Hormones generally operate in almost all tissues.

Mode of Action

Their secretion is not continuous, because production is usually triggered by events like trauma and infection. In general, induction of cytokine secretion follows an external provocation. This includes activation by soluble factors, stress or direct signal from neighboring cells. Although some cytokines are secreted constitutively, they exist in a non-active form, and the production of active forms is provoked by proteases (that in turn need to be induced and activated). An exemplar of such a cytokine is *transforming growth factor beta 1* (TGF-β1). Some cytokines can have a simple negative feedback mechanism that would regulate their secretion, but the regulation has not been completely understood. It would be logical to assume that in some pathophysiological conditions these regulations might be destroyed. Usually, it is assumed that cytokines' effect would cease when their (production and) concentration falls below the levels that can activate receptors on target cells.

Hormones, on the other hand, have usually regular secretion patterns, and their concentration in body fluids may vary less than an order of magnitude (i.e., 10-fold variations are rare). The change in their physiologic action usually depends on their concentration, which is subject to internal negative feedback loops. Thus, the reduction of a product of hormonal action causes an increase in secretion of that hormone, leading in turn to an increase in the concentration of the product. This increase reduces the production of hormones and thereby maintains physiological levels of their secretion.

FUNCTION

Biological function of cytokines can be roughly divided into five groups (A–E):

Defense Against Viruses and Regulation of Immunity

Holders of these functions are interferons. There are three types of interferons: type I—IFN-α1-21/β/τ/ω, type II—IFN-γ, and type III interferons—IFN-λ (lambda) (Interleukin-28A, -28B, -29), which exert their effects via specific membrane receptors.

Inter-Cellular Communication Between Leukocytes Defines the Cytokines that are Called Interleukins

The main feature of such signals is in the regulation of immunity, and a small but essential part lies in the development and growth of cells of hematopoietic tissues. Representatives are cytokines IL-1 to IL-38 with the exception of IL-8, which is a chemokine. All act through specific cell-membrane bound receptors.

Migration of Cells

Cytokines that have chemotactic properties are called chemokines. Most chemokines can act by binding specific cell-membrane receptors. Each receptor can bind more than one ligand and are hence called promiscuous. There are four families of receptors (R). They are divided according to presence of two cysteines in their primary structure and the distance between them: XCR, CCR, CXCR, and CX_3CR (X stands for any amino acid; C denotes cysteine; and R is receptor). Chemokine receptors are also ion channels that have a characteristic tertiary structure. Chemokines comprise 50 factors, which are separated into four groups according to the ability to bind a defined group of promiscuous receptors like XCL, CCL, CXCL, and CX_3CL (L stands for ligand). Adding a number after their group name forms individual names for chemokines as well as for receptors.

Regulation of Growth and Development (of Particular Tissues in the Embryo and Adults)

In this function we include tissue regeneration (the growth and development of stem cells of a tissue) and homeostatic cell division (maintenance of a fixed number of cells in a particular tissue without their differentiation). Here we can divide cytokines according to their breadth of influence. Thus, we have those that influence only single line of cells, specific tissues, or across all of the body. Cytokines of this family influence the following:

(i) Germ line stem cells and cells of hematopoietic tissues, such as *erythropoietin* (EPO), *Stem Cell Factor* (SCF), *Colony Stimulating Factor* (CSF), *Granulocyte-CSF* (G-CSF), *Macrophage-CSF* (M-CSF), *Granulocyte macrophage-CSF* (GM-CSF, CSF-2), *Leukemia inhibiting factor* (LIF), *Oncostatin M* (OSM), and *ciliary neurotrophic factor* (CNTF). The last three have overlapping functions with the next group.

(ii) Specific tissues (except blood-forming), as, for example, a growth factor of liver cells *Hepatocyte Growth Factor* (HGF), *Fibroblast Growth Factors* (FGF), *Epidermal Growth Factors* (EGF), *Platelet Derived Growth Factor* (PDGF), *Insulin-Like Growth Factors* (IGF), *Vascular Endothelial Growth Factors* (VEGF), Endothelin, *Nerve Growth Factors* (NGF), *Neural Differentiation Factor* (NDF), *Ciliary Neurotrophic Factor* (CNTF), and *Bone Morphogenetic Proteins* (BMP). For embryonic development, the important factors in this group are *Wnt* and *Hedgehog*.

(iii) All tissues. Usually such pan-specific cytokines have a typical mosaic function, which depends on the state of the target cells. These include TNF-α and TNF-β as representatives of the TNF superfamily (TNFSF) and TGF-β, from the TGF family of cytokines.

Other Functions (Metabolism, Ion Balance, etc.)

This group includes the remaining factors, the effects of which cannot be classified in the above, even if the name and structure may belong to above-mentioned groups or superfamilies. As an example, we list the regulation of calcium excretion independently of PTH with cytokine FGF-23.

CHAPTER 2

The Immune System—Definition and Development of Immunity

There are three barriers that stop the entry of microorganisms in the tissues of the body: physical, chemical, and biological. Physical barriers are the skin and mucous membranes. The horny part of the skin is a tough fibrous material consisting mainly of keratin, and provides a very effective defense against the penetration of microorganisms. The mucus is a natural defense, sometimes supported by other physical factors (like specialized epithelia such as the ciliary respiratory system for the removal of small particles) or chemical (e.g., low or high pH of the stomach or duodenum, respectively). Chemical defense, furthermore, comprises the secretion of inorganic and other small molecules that kill microorganisms or just slow down their reproduction. Of biological factors that are already engaged in battle with microorganisms outside the body, we should mention defensins (short peptidic natural antibiotics) and enzymes (lysozyme) in the mouth. If microorganisms venture into the tissues, they will encounter another barrier—the immune system. Thus the immune system can help physical and chemical barriers with biologic mediators whose part can already be excreted in the mucosa.

Vertebrates are protected from attacks from harmful viruses, bacteria, and parasites by the immune system as a last line of defense. It is usually very effective, because it can completely destroy the intruders. However, many microorganisms that live on the skin or mucous membranes (and have ten times higher number [10^{-14}] than that of body cells [10^{-13}]) are generally not harmful. Only occasionally or under certain conditions do we encounter microorganisms that pose a threat to our lives or the survival of the species.

The main issue that remained unclear in immunology is the way that the immune system distinguishes the action of microorganisms in the body. Lacking a definitive answer, conventional wisdom is that the immune system is used for the defense of the organism. The immune system can do this because it can discriminate *self* from *nonself*—and then reject the latter. Others think that the immune system distinguishes the *dangerous* from the *harmless,* and the third—that the immune system communicates between its parts (like "reflecting") before performing defensive or additional actions like

The Cytokines of the Immune System
http://dx.doi.org/10.1016/B978-0-12-419998-9.00002-X

tolerating commensals and (actively) protecting the integrity of tissues. According to the latter hypothesis, the immune system can analyze the effects of penetration of microorganisms, and these might postpone the rejection (or even actively inhibit it) in order to perform selection of the *useful* microorganisms and distinguish them from both, the *harmful* or the *harmless* ones. Thereby, the immune system can protect beneficial microbes. The latter would not be "understood" as potentially dangerous. According to this hypothesis (*the Integrity Model*) the main function of the immune system is maintaining the structural and functional integrity of tissues. This allows for the notion that some microorganisms can be *useful* and even *necessary* (like, e.g., commensal bacteria in the digestive system that produce vitamin K), although they are by definition *nonself* that by conventional standard theory should be rejected. The screening and searching for *useful* would be conducted on the principle that *nonself* is *useful* until proven *dangerous*, and therefore it should be tolerated (neither rejected nor attacked by the immune response). A special program would protect *useful*, or in other words, there are *cells* that would guard the *useful* from rejection by the immune response (which usually destroys *dangerous* or *nonself*). At the molecular level, it is likely these philosophical notes can be translated into the language of membrane molecules and cytokines as a "conversation" between cells of hematopoietic origin including macrophages, dendritic, lymphoid, and natural killer (NK) cells and those in their microenvironment. Hematopoietic cells, however, are the main protagonists of the immune response. The reason why there are many interactions between them and the stromal cells at each particular location is the existence of a large number of their subspecies (and developmental stages) that are still insufficiently clarified. Deciphering their messages is only possible if we assume that cytokines have a role in cellular "conversation" (cross-talk). That is why some think that cytokines are the most important factors that determine the fate of microorganisms in the tissues. However, we must not forget the fact that cell membrane proteins are very important too, because they start the cross-talk. In order to better understand the interaction of such cells, it is necessary to explain firstly the roles of cell-membrane molecules, and then upgrade such knowledge to that of the effects of cytokines. During normal embryonic development of each individual, conceptually, similar cytokine-dependent interactions between developing tissues occur, only the cellular types are different. Concerning the immune system, there is a combination of cytokine developmental signals on precursor (or stem) cells that are interwoven with cytokine action effects on differentiated counterparts of immunocytes.

ORGANIZATION OF THE IMMUNE SYSTEM

Physiological participants of the immune system consist of (a) hematopoietic tissue and lymphoid organs; (b) various types of cells in the blood and lymphatics; and (c) the freely circulating molecules in body fluids.

The organs of the immune system are divided into central and peripheral. The first lead to the formation and development of immune cells, such as bone marrow and thymus in adult mammals. Peripheral organs (and tissues) of the immune system are the spleen, lymph nodes, clusters of lymphoid cells in somatic organs, and the vascular system of lymph and blood. During the embryonic development of mammals, the spleen and the liver have similar functions as the bone marrow. In birds there is a separate organ for the development of B lymphocytes called the *bursa* of *Fabricius*.

Definition of Antigen

Antigens are macromolecules that can induce specific immune response (hence, they are called immunogenic). Smaller molecules and chemical compounds (haptens) and some metal ions are immunogenic only if they are covalently bonded to a carrier molecule such as a protein.

Those antigens that cannot induce the immune response are assumed to be tolerogenic (causing unresponsiveness) or immunosuppressive (causing "regulation" of the immune response in a different direction than as defined above with immunogenic antigens).

Classification of Immunity

The immune system can be divided in different ways with respect to following characteristics:

  (i) Type of recognition of antigens (specific–nonspecific);
 (ii) Developmental, hereditary features (innate–adaptive); or
(iii) Functional aspects (autonomous–centralized) of its factors and cells.

The relationship between the divisions is shown in Figure 2-1. Today, the preferred division is the usage of innate (inborn, inherited) and adaptive (not inherited in a functional state, but as pieces, then acquired and implemented in adults) immunity from the older division into specific and nonspecific. The third division of the autonomic and centralized immunity is listed to understand immunity through the perspective of the *Integrity* hypothesis (Dembic, 1996; see Chapter 9).

Innate immunity is preserved across many species and is largely nonspecific. If compared to the nervous system, it would represent a defensive

Divisions of immunity

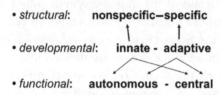

Figure 2-1 Principles for divisions of the immune system.

Table 2-1 Innate and adaptive parts of the immune system

	Cellular	Humoral
Innate immunity	Dendritic cells Macrophages, granulocytes, and mast cells NK (and NKT) cells	Complement system Cytokines (and interferons) Extracellular enzymes Other small molecules
Adaptive immunity	B lymphocytes αβ T lymphocytes γδ T lymphocytes	Antibodies

"reflex" against microorganisms. Adaptive or acquired immunity is largely specific. It is implemented during ontogeny and is different in each individual of the same species in higher animals. It can be fine-tuned for better defense against invading microorganisms, and it seems that it can predict (anticipate) unknown molecular forms of potential attackers. This is possible due to clonally distributed repertoire of responses, with which the immune system can recognize millions of different molecules. At the first meeting with the intruder, successful specific immunity takes approximately two to three weeks to respond to the challenge. Each subsequent encounter with the same intruder (antigen) takes shorter time, usually about a week or two. If we continue conceptual comparison with the nervous system, the specific part of the immune system might resemble some subconscious higher functions of the nervous system.

The main factors and cells of the immune system are shown in Table 2-1 and Figure 2-2, according to division in innate and adaptive immunity. In a typical innate response to microorganisms, an inflammation develops. This is caused by distress of a tissue and production of proinflammatory factors by stressed cells including macrophages, granulocytes, mast cells, and NK cells. Inflammation is a complex process that can begin even as aseptic tissue injury, for example, during physical stress or myocardial ischemia.

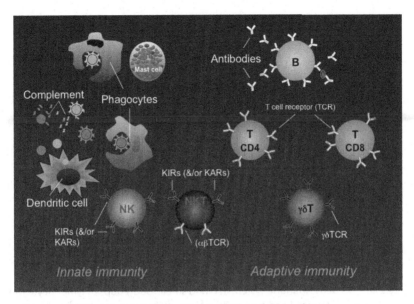

Figure 2-2 Cells and factors of the immune system.

In a typical adaptive (specific) immune response, contact with the antigen (protein or polysaccharide part of pathogens) stimulates naïve T cells to proliferate and differentiate into effector (decision-making) cells. Effector T cells are divided into (1) helper (CD4), which, for example, can help B cells to multiply and develop into effector cells (plasma); and (2) cytotoxic (CD8) cells, which, for example, can kill virally infected cells in the tissue. Once the pathogen is destroyed, most effectors are destroyed, but some cells survive and become memory cells. It is unclear whether effector cells have a limited lifespan or they are downregulated actively (as a negative feedback loop) to normal-repertoire-concentration levels.

Microscopic analysis of blood smears (Figure 2-3) shows that cells of the immune system are difficult to discern visually. Lymphocytes seem like small cells with little cytoplasm; monocytes are bigger, with larger nuclei and more cytoplasm, whereas granulocytes have grainy nuclei, with each subset having its own kind of granules (neutrophilic, eosinophilic, and basophilic). More accurate detection of these cells requires analyses either by specific immunohistochemical staining methods or by functional analyses of their cell surface markers by flow cytometry. For the scientific results that might shake-up and eventually change our current understanding of the immune system in the future, new knowledge will be obtained from studying sorted clusters of cells or even single cells by employing next generation methods like primary

Resting lymphocytes

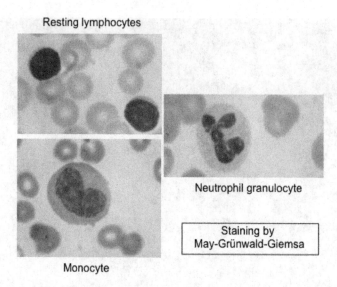

Neutrophil granulocyte

Staining by
May-Grünwald-Giemsa

Monocyte

Figure 2-3 Cells of the immune system in blood smear. Subgroups of lymphocytes and other cells can be detected and differentiated by specific markers using flow cytometry (and immunohistochemistry in tissue sections).

structure (sequence) determination, gene expression, genomic variability, epigenetic and proteomic analyses of their constituents.

The functional division of immunity follows the above description of events during the immune response and defines cells that are capable of rapid responses as "autonomous immunity" that includes (among other mediators of innate immunity) NK cells and most γδ T lymphocytes. In contrast to the innate–adaptive division concept, dendritic cells (DCs) are listed as a part of the central immunity (Figure 2-4), since they are messengers that bring information about intruders and distress to the centers of immunity (lymph nodes). Namely, by migrating from tissues to lymph nodes, where they interact with T lymphocytes, DCs set in motion a response that results with T and B effectors to migrate back into tissues, where the effectors perform a function acquired in the centers of immunity (Figure 2-5).

Definition of the Immune Response

Definition and description of the immune response comes from experimental experience. Because the mouse immune system is very similar to the human, we can infer from experiments with mice how the human immune system would work.

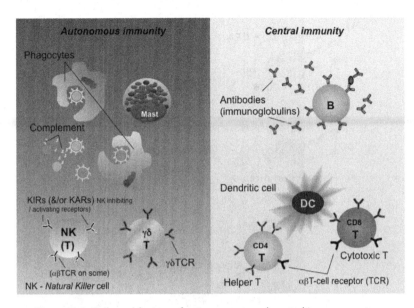

Figure 2-4 Cells and factors of autonomous and central immune system.

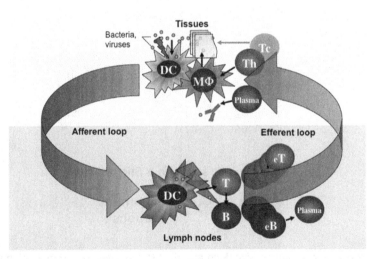

Figure 2-5 Schematic representation of cellular interactions and outcomes during the immune response. DC—dendritic cell; MΦ—macrophage; eT/eB—effector T/B cells; Th—helper T cell; Tc—cytotoxic T cell.

The immune response was defined as a proliferative response of lymphocytes after immunization with an antigen that results in defensive effect (formation of antibodies and defending cells). This is the basis of vaccination against various infections. A proof that lymphocytes are involved in the

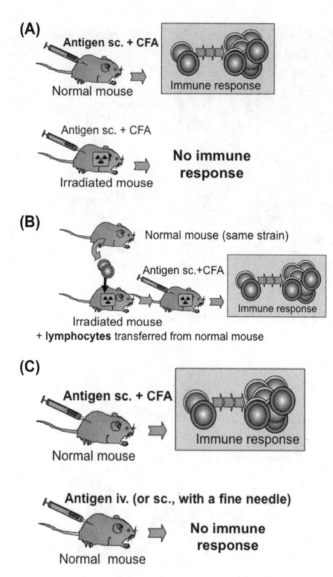

Figure 2-6 Biologic features of antigen injection: (A) Consequence of irradiation with γ-rays. (B) Transfer of lymphocytes from normal into irradiated mouse (of the same strain) rescues the immune response. (C) Role of complete Freund's adjuvant (CFA) and route of injection (s.c., i.v.) for the immune response.

immune response comes from findings that irradiation of mice with gamma rays abrogates immune responses (Figure 2-6A). Of course, the radiation must be so fine-tuned that all (and only) leukocytes and lymphocytes are destroyed.

If in such irradiated mice we add (transfer by injection) cells from non-irradiated mouse of the same strain, the reappearance of the immune response to the antigen occurs (Figure 2-6B). The Figures 2-6A, 2-6B, and 2-6C represent schematically these experiments. CFA (*complete Freund's adjuvant*) is a mixture of dead and decomposing bacteria that causes inflammation at a site of injection (humans should not be injected, as it would create a wound). Immunization with an antigen therefore includes coincident injection of an adjuvant—CFA at the same location; otherwise it would not result with the immune response (Figure 2-6C). A similar absence of the immune response occurs when antigen is injected intravenously (without adjuvants) (Figure 2-6C). This is actually one of the paradoxical facts in immunology that was continually suppressed as irrelevant (until recently). According to the self–nonself discrimination theory (which is still very respected), specific lymphocyte response should occur when the immune system meets foreign antigen even without adjuvant. To explain that it is nearly always necessary to have an adjuvant in order to elicit the immune response, the proponents of this theory resorted to complicated explanations, and this is where immunology came to fame as such. So, an expression of "immune tolerance" has developed to describe the lack of the immune response following antigen's intravenous injection (without adjuvant). Its mechanisms are partially known, however, the explanations seem still complicated. In recent years, with novel theories about the function of the immune system, explanations became somewhat simplified, and the need for an adjuvant received a significant place in them (see *Theories about the function of the immune system*, Chapter 9). A more detailed description of the immune response and the role of its cytokines can be found in the following section: *Cellular adaptive (specific) immune system*, p. 42.

HUMORAL INNATE (NONSPECIFIC) IMMUNITY

Innate immunity of the humoral type involves soluble factors outside and inside the body.

The Factors Secreted in Mucosal Surface

Those that are outside (and secreted in the oral mucosa by salivary glands) consist of enzymes, proteases, and factors that are combating intruding microorganisms, aiming to prevent their entry into the organism. These include (in mucosal surfaces of the oral cavity) lysozyme, LPO-SCN, various mucins, histatins, human beta-defensin (HBD) (β-defensins), lactoferrin, and cystatins. Together with humoral adaptive factors (soluble immunoglobulin type

A—sIgA, and soluble immunoglobulin type M—sIgM) they are the first barrier that basically excludes most of the microbes and parasites, which might try to penetrate the oral cavity mucosa. Those microbes that are eaten are confronted by the next set of defensive factors, which are not strictly considered innate immunity, but definitely contribute to the elimination of potential pathogens. Namely, the set comprises the stomach acid and digestive enzymes of the gastrointestinal tract.

If the microbes penetrate the organism through epithelial barriers they face humoral and cellular immune system. The humoral innate immunity located inside the body is called complement.

Complement

The easiest way to understand the function of the complement is to imagine that it helps immune cells to "eat" bacteria or viruses, which have penetrated the physical barrier floating around in blood, tissues, and body fluids. Complement, for example, is for macrophages what, for some people, is butter spread on bread—an appetizer.

Complement comprises cascades of interactions including over 30 proteins that can protect the host from microscopic intruders. All microorganisms that are either killed or wrapped by complement derivatives are engulfed and digested by phagocytes (phagocytosed). Some parts of the complement system have roles in the control of cellular interactions within the immune system (i.e., opsonins), as well as attracting cells to sites of intrusion (chemotactic factors). In addition, some factors are hypersensitivity mediators called anaphylatoxins.

Explanation of Figure 2-7A (and a more detailed description of Figure 2-7B): There are three pathways of complement activation: classic, lectin, and alternative.

Classic Pathway

The classic pathway (at the top, on the left) begins when natural antibodies or immune-response produced antibodies bind to antigen. To their tails binds complement factor C1q, which in turn activates serine proteases C1r and C1s. Together they break down (activate) C4 to C4b. C4b has a specific binding site for C2. C1s then decomposes C2 such that it can join C4b. The resulting complex is C4b2a, which is also called C3 convertase. C4b2a converts C3, resulting with C3a and C3b. C3b binds C3 convertase (C4b2a) and thus creates C5 convertase (C4b2a3b), which is the last step in the enzymatic cascade. The assembled enzyme converts C5 into two factors

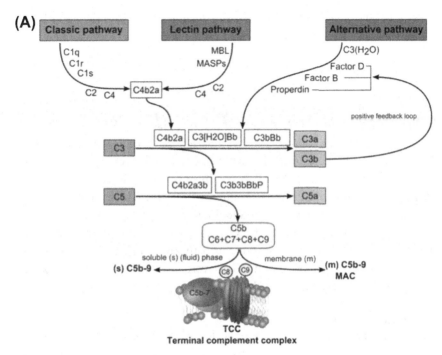

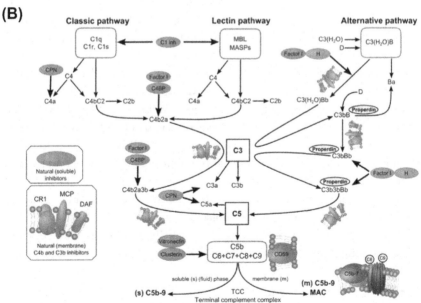

Figure 2-7 (A) Innate immunity. Complement cascade, in short. MAC: membrane attack complex. (B) Complement cascade, in detail.

C5a and C5b: the former is a very strong anaphylatoxin and the latter binds C6 starting the assembly of a terminal complex (C5b,6,7,8,9).

Lectin Pathway

The lectin pathway (at the top, in the middle): activation of complement via the lectin pathway is mediated by pattern recognition proteins (PRPs). There are five distinct PRPs: mannan-binding lectin (MBL), collectin-11 (CL-11), ficolin-1, ficolin-2, and ficolin-3. Each of them complexes with MBL-associated serine proteases (MASPs), of which there are three forms (MASP1, MASP2, and MASP3) and non-enzymatic proteins (MAP1 and sMAP). Activation, for example, begins with MBL, which binds mannose on bacteria with the help of immunoglobulin A (IgA) and damaged endothelium. MBL is homologous to C1q and starts a cascade with help of MASPs. In further reactions, the lectin pathway is almost identical to the classic pathway to create C3 and C5 convertases. There are indications that MASPs in some cases can directly activate C3.

Alternative Pathway

The alternative pathway (at the top, on the right) is different from the classic and lectin pathways and it has an enhancer (a positive feedback loop). It is activated by IgA immune complexes and bacterial membranes and cell wall components (polysaccharides or endotoxins). In physiological conditions C3 molecules have, to a lesser extent, spontaneous hydrolysis of intramolecular thiol ester. This causes them to bind factor B, which is then decomposed into Ba and Bb by factor D. The outcome leaves Bb bound to C3 creating a C3 convertase (C3[H$_2$O]Bb). This enzyme then converts C3 to C3a and C3b. The latter binds factor B, which breaks down the factor D and thereby creates a second (alternate-pathway-specific) C3 convertase C3bBb. The properdin (Pr) promotes association of C3b to factor B by stabilizing the C3bBb complex, and is the only known regulator that increases complement activation. This is called amplification or positive feedback loop (see Figure 2-7B). The latter molecule (C3bBb) breaks down another C3 molecule, binds additional part of it—C3b, ending in making the C5 convertase (C3b3bBbPr). This enzyme degrades C5 in the similar way as those found in the classical or lectin pathways.

Completion of the Cascade

Completion of the cascade or terminal pathway (at the bottom, in the center) uses the same mediators regardless of the initial activation pathway. In short, C5b associates with factors C6 and C7 forming lipophilic complex, which can be inserted into lipid membranes. There, the complex (C5b-7) can acquire a single C8 molecule, which acts as a precipitating event that makes a membrane attack complex (MAC). MAC is formed by adding one or more C9 molecules to the C5b-8 constituting a physical pore in the membrane C5b-9(m). This leads to the release of cellular components through the membrane that causes activation of cells or, in rare instances, cell lysis (bottom right). If the complement activation forms in the fluid phase without the presence of lipid membranes, C5b-7 complexes can bind to vitronectin and clusterin (which controls the terminal pathway in fluid phase), thus maintaining the hydrophilic properties. Binding of C5b-7 with C8 and C9 makes the final form of soluble (S) terminal complement complex C5b-9 (SC5b-9) (*the terminal complement complex;* TCC).

Complement Regulation

Activation of the complement is strictly regulated by the inhibitory proteins (Figure 2-7B).

Soluble Phase

In the soluble (fluid) phase of complement activation, C1-inhibitor (C1INH) controls C1r, C1s, and MASPs, while carboxypeptidase N (CPN) inactivates anaphylatoxins C5a, C3a, and C4a by detaching their terminal arginines.

Factor I degrades and inactivates C4b and C3b. It uses C4b-binding protein (C4BP) as a co-factor in the classical/lectin pathway, and factor H in the alternative pathway.

Membrane Phase

Membrane phase regulators are complement receptor 1 (CR1, CD35), membrane co-factor protein (MCP, CD46), and decay accelerating factor (DAF, CD55). They regulate the complement activation by acting as co-factors for the degradation of C4b and C3b (CR1 and MCP) that is mediated by factor I, or by accelerating the destruction of C3 and C5 convertases (CR1 and DAF).

CD59 is also a membrane regulator that prevents the binding of C9 to C5b-8 complex in the terminal pathway. CR1 and MCP are transmembrane proteins, whereas DAF and CD59 bind to the cell membrane via glycosyl—phosphatidylinositol anchors.

Many biological effects of complement activation are mediated by membrane receptors for C3a (C3aR), C5a (C5aR), and C3b (CR3, CD11b/CD18). Activated complement is considered a double-edged sword—that is, one that can have adverse effects in many clinical circumstances.

Nevertheless, knowledge about complement activation has led to many reagents with potential beneficent therapeutic effects.

CELLULAR INNATE (NONSPECIFIC) IMMUNITY

Cellular part of innate immunity comprises DCs, macrophages, monocytes, granulocytes, innate helper type 2 cells, and NK cells.

Dendritic Cells (DC)

DCs are heterogeneous population of cells that can be divided by differentiation (from lymphoid or myeloid precursor), localization (skin, mucosa, connective tissues, other organs), migratory properties (tissue vs lymphoid secondary tissue like lymph nodes, spleen, or Peyer's patches) and their maturation stage (immature vs mature). These subpopulations have been described to affect functions of T cells differently. For example, mature DCs stimulate defensive immune responses (important for infection, anti-cancer immunity, or if gone awry, autoimmunity), whereas immature DCs can stimulate regulatory T cells that can establish development of T cell tolerance (one mechanism of self-tolerance, but if deregulated, it can inhibit anti-tumor [anti-cancer] immune responses and thus allow development of cancers).

DCs can develop from myeloid or lymphoid precursors. DCs are found in almost all tissues and are important in that they are the strongest initiators of the immune responses. Langerhans cells in the skin (epidermis) are one type of such cells developing from monocytes. DCs, according to the Integrity model, are envoys of the destruction of tissue integrity. When such damage occurs, skin DCs should receive signals about (or *feel*) the lack of connections with other cells in a tissue (cytokines and unknown factors) detecting *Integrity-associated molecular patterns,* or IAMPs. Together with other factors of the microenvironment that tissue cells produce under distress or necrotic death (called *Danger-associated molecular patterns,* or DAMPs) and intruder-related factors such as bacterial products or viruses (called Pathogen-associated molecular patterns, or PAMPs) immature DCs are activated and become mature. During the first few hours after the activation, DCs intensively phagocytose various substances (including antigens) in their neighborhood. After that, they pull up their dendrites, migrate toward lymph vessels and begin to secrete some chemokines and cytokines. They find their way through the lymph to the nearest lymph node. In the lymph node they home in specific areas near T lymphocytes.

In secondary lymphoid tissues (lymph nodes, spleen) DCs begin to present antigens picked up from the place where they came from. During this time, ingested (phagocytosed and endocytosed) substances became proteolytically degraded in lysosomes, which melt with endosomes containing *de novo* synthesized glycoproteins called the Major Histocompatibility Complex (MHC) class II molecules. In the newly combined endosomes there is a large number of various peptides, the remains of a combination of proteins having foreign (nonself) and own (self) origin. These peptides are transferred into the grooves of two α-helical domains of class II MHC molecules. Following these events, endosomes reach the cell membrane, and by melting with it expose to the outside of a cell an antigen-presenting structure made up of a complex between a particular peptide imbedded in the cleft of the MHC-II molecule (peptide/MHC; p/MHC). The p/MHC molecular complex serves as a ligand for the "first signal" (which is an activating one) to T lymphocytes that are docked nearby.

This is the most important function of the DCs, which belong to a small group of cells in the body called antigen presenting cells (APC). CD4 T cells can recognize various peptide/MHC ligands on APCs with specific receptors called T-cell receptors (TCR) (Figure 2-8). APCs are also B cells and macrophages.

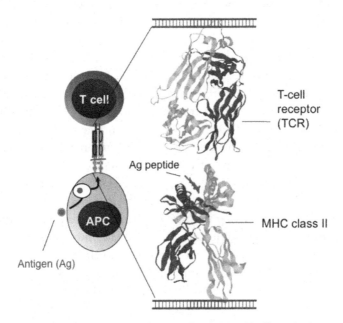

Figure 2-8 Adaptive immunity: Presentation of antigen to T cells on APCs.

In addition to these events with the DCs, it is also important to mention the expression of B7 molecules (CD80 and CD86) on the cell surface of DC after maturation. Both molecules, CD80 and CD86 bind to the CD28 molecule on T cells and thus give them a "second signal" for activation (also called costimulatory signal). These two signals are necessary and sufficient for the beginning of a specific immune response to T-dependent antigens. (T-dependent antigens are those that cannot elicit antibody response without the help of T cells). There are several other cell-surface molecules on APCs, which can interact with their binding partners on T cells that can regulate the immune response, but they will be described later.

Furthermore, DCs can regulate the type of the immune response by secreting cytokines. Types of the immune response are characterized by their varied outcome regarding function in defense or balancing their relative strength in it (regulation). The whole process of mounting an immune response usually involves various kinds of stimulator as well as effector cells, molecules including cytokines. These will be described in more detail in the later sections. By now, there are over eight different types known. However, this is also one of the most controversial parts of immunology. Namely, some believe that there are just a few major types of the response; some think there are several types; and a minority believes that there are many more. The gist of the argument centers on the ability of the immune response to survive and win the fight against microorganisms, while the latter is under constant selection pressure too. Historically, the first two identified types were type I response as the answer to secreted IL-12 (by DC1 type), and a type II response, generated by IL-4 (produced by almost all T cells in minute quantities, perhaps DC2 or the like cells). In addition to these two types of DCs there are plasmocytoid DC (PDC), which have, as a marker, IL-3 receptor (CD123) on the cell surface, and secrete IFN-α. PDC cells have still incompletely explained immunoregulatory effects, and perhaps create a unique type of the immune response (or precede some other types). Probably there are more types of DCs. *In vitro,* they can be grown with GM-CSF and IL-4 cytokines from monocytes (or myeloid precursors) and differentiating into DC1. Further incubation with different cytokines can probably additionally modulate the immune response with regard to size, outcomes and time it would take to alter it.

The research on DCs is interesting and promising. DCs were discovered relatively late (20 years after T and B lymphocytes), because they were for a long time thought to be macrophages. Their research is expected to yield many more new insights, which may possibly lead to fundamental changes in understanding the function of the immune system. Furthermore, DCs are major constituents or at least a part of many *in vitro* immunotherapy protocols for almost all types of cancer. In fact, despite recent relative disappointing results of clinical trials, some DC-based vaccine adjuvant cancer therapies are in advanced state of clinical trials. There are two DC-vaccination therapies (for prostate cancer, *Provenge*; and melanoma) that have been approved by the FDA.

Other Features

DCs can be distinguished by their differentiation profile, cell-surface marker profiles, and by their secreted cytokine profiles.

Differentiation Profiles

DCs can be developed in culture from monocytes by supplementing the growth media (of peripheral blood mononuclear cells) with GM-CSF and IL-4. These cytokines give rise to immature DCs, which can be then further matured by various treatments that are still not completely understood. For example, treatment with IFN-γ can lead to DC maturation, or incubation with particular monoclonal antibodies directed at specific cell markers (albeit yet without completely clear understanding of the processes they induce). Most importantly, it has been recently established, that if DCs maintain the expression of the cell marker CD31, they would remain immature (and thus be important for T cell tolerance), but when they downregulate the CD31, they become mature and lead to prototypic defensive (anti-infectious agent) immune response.

Cell Marker Profiles

The list of CD antigens expressed by various subpopulations of DCs are numerous and the most important include: CD1a (dermal DCs), CD8 (in mouse, CD141 in humans), CD11c, CD14 (dermal, not LC DCs), CD80, CD83, CD86, CD103 (mucosal DCs), CD184 (CXCR4), CD197 (CCR7), CD215 (IL-15R), CD282 (TLR2 and TLR4), and CD286 (TLR6). PDCs have additionally CD123 (IL-3R), TLR7 and TLR9 markers. Other subpopulations probably have a range of other pattern recognition receptor sets (TLRs, NLRs, etc.).

Secreted Cytokine Profiles

The list of cytokines expressed and secreted by various subpopulations of DCs are for DC-1 like: IL-12, IL-1α, IL-1β, IL-6, TNF-α, M-CSF,

GM-CSF, IL-8, IL-15, IL-18, IL-23, IL-27, CCL5 (RANTES); for PDCs: IFN-α, IFN-β; for immature DCs: IL-10, TGF-β; and in rare occasions IFN-γ.

Macrophages

Macrophages are cells of myeloid origin, and they were thought to be generated in connective tissues after extravasation and activation of monocytes. However, recent studies show that they can be generated by their own specific tissue precursor, which is different from monocytes and probably presents a macrophage-lineage stem cell. This is likely to occur when monocytes meet bacteria or some of their products. Bacterial molecules such as lipopolysaccharide or peptidoglycan can be bound by Toll-like receptors or other receptors that allow cells to recognize molecular phylogenetic patterns of evolutionarily older organisms like prokaryotes. Macrophages have many features. In most tissues they are activated by the IFN-γ, which is a product of effector T-helper type 1 (Th1) lymphocytes and a major activator of macrophages (for details, see Chapter 5, *Interferon-γ (IFN-γ)*) Recently, a cytokine IL-17, which is a product of effector CD4 Th17 lymphocytes, was also found to be their activator. Once activated, macrophages secrete oxidative radicals in their microenvironment, which can kill bacteria and destroy viruses. In addition, these radicals damage host's own tissues (as killing microorganisms is nonspecific). Macrophages are best described as cells with major role in cleaning and restoring damaged tissues (wounds). They can phagocytose not only live or dead bacteria and viruses, but also cellular debris of one's own tissues, as well as the intercellular matrix. They further help the renewal of tissue integrity (wound healing) by secreting various cytokines and chemokines. Killing of bacteria can also take place intracellularly, after macrophages become activated with IFN-γ (because some bacteria can live inside cells, such as those belonging to *mycobacteria, salmonella,* or *leishmania*). Macrophages secrete pro-inflammatory cytokines (IL-1β and TNF-α), chemotactic cytokines (chemokines such as IL-8 = CXCL8), regulatory cytokines including proinflammatory IL-1, IL-6, IL-12 and TNF-α, when activated (Figure 5-5), but also anti-inflammatory cytokines, such as IL-10 and TGF-β in non-activated state. However, the role in the generation of specific immune responses is one of macrophages' most important functions. Following their activation by sensing microorganisms in combination with tissue damage, distress or cell death in the neighborhood, they engulf, digest, and process the proteins in their whereabouts. Then they present bacterial, viral, and host tissue peptides in a complex with various

MHC molecules, and at the same time express costimulatory CD86 molecules on the cell surface, similarly to the DCs. However, since they do not migrate, they stay in tissues and when the effector cells wander in, they communicate with them. For example, they have the ability to trigger effector CD4$^+$T cells. Unlike DCs, macrophages remain in the tissues, and therefore cannot stimulate naïve or resting T cells. This means that macrophages cannot start an immune response under physiological conditions (the primary immune response), but they can only reinforce it, and perhaps start a secondary response (after re-encounter with antigen).

Other Features

Macrophages are heterogeneous populations of cells. Their differentiation profile, cell-surface marker profiles, and their secreted cytokine profiles are very similar to that of tissue DCs. Apart from the differentiation (they can be induced from PBMCs by FLT3L, GM-CSF, and M-CSF), almost the sole difference between DCs (in immature stage) is the functional evidence that DCs can become migratory (i.e., by switching the expression of CCR5 with CCR7), and the macrophages remain CCR5 positive. Additionally, CD31 can distinguish macrophage lineage from DCs, as immature DCs express it uniquely (and mature immunogenic DCs downregulate it).

Monocytes

Monocytes develop from myeloid precursors in the bone marrow, circulate in blood, and migrate and home in various tissues residing there as mononuclear cells or differentiating into tissue resident macrophage-like cells such as microglia, bone osteoclasts, epidermal Langerhans cells (one type of DCs), and liver Kupfer cells. They are not APCs in the proper sense (*in strictu senso*) as they do not have MHC class II expression.

Granulocytes

Granulocytes are polymorphonuclear (PMN) cells that comprise neutrophils, basophils, and eosinophils, of which neutrophils are the most frequent type found in blood. All have the possibility of endocytosis. Although neutrophils cannot phagocytose large particles as macrophages, they have some properties similar to them. It seems that they cannot stimulate specific immune responses, as they cannot present antigens. Thus they are not APCs under physiological conditions. Granulocytes can secrete many different cytokines and change the type of the immune response. They are effector cells, and a cytokine, secreted after activation of another type of white blood cell—T cell helper 17 (Th17)—can regulate their distribution and function in tissues. This cytokine is IL-17. It has an important role in the recruitment of granulocytes at sites of inflammation in various tissues. Furthermore, some granulocytes secrete a little bit of histamine, and its production can be boosted 50 times in particular circumstances (allergy, anaphylaxis), and even become larger than those of mast cells.

PMN cells express CD11b, CD66b, CD16, and CD32 that can be measured by flow cytometry, whereas PMN production of myeloperoxidase, IL-17, and TNF can be measured with ELISA (enzyme-linked immunosorbent assay).

CCL11 and CCL24 are eosinophil chemoattractants.

Mast Cells

Progenitors of mast cells develop in the bone marrow, circulate in the blood and home into different tissues. The main factor important for development of mast cells is a stem cell factor (SCF), which binds to c-Kit receptor. Mice deficient in SCF or c-kit gene have a lack of mast cells (along with other defects in hematopoiesis and gametogenesis).

Their distinguishing quality is that they can attach a specific class of immunoglobulins (IgE) thereby "weaponizing" themselves. Igs give them specificity, and the possibility to be rapidly activated to perform their function (for details see *Cellular adaptive (specific) immune system* (p. 42), and *Signal transduction in mast cells* (Chapter 3, p. 81). Activation results in rapid degranulation and the secretion of histamine and IL-4 cytokine. Histamine causes atopic and allergic changes in the tissues where the mast cells home. IL-4 helps to create a class of immunoglobulin (Igε [epsilon]; IgE). IgE can bind with the opposite (from antigen-binding) part of the molecule (the Fc portion) to the mast cells (through the interaction with the Fc receptor). Mast cells are among cells of the first line of (biologic) defense against microorganisms. However, in syndromes with the disorder of their function, they often cause hyperactivity, anaphylaxis, or allergies. Antihistaminic preparations are standard therapy for such syndromes and symptoms. There are already several generations of drugs that act quickly and effectively.

Natural Killer Cells

NK cells are naturally occurring cytotoxic cells of innate (nonspecific) immunity that develop from the lymphoid precursors. NK cells are observed in the form of *large granular lymphocytes* (or LGL cells) in the blood. They can be activated by cytokines or (and) by NK receptors. Activated NK cells can kill virus-infected cells by recognizing target cells (not by recognizing virus presence, but indirectly). They can also assist in the destruction of tumor cells in the body. Many activated NK cells secrete a multitude of cytokines that can regulate specific (adaptive) immunity.

It is well known that the lack of a single allele of MHC molecules on target cells can lead to killing by NK cells. However, conversely, the expression of certain alleles of MHC molecules, which are normally not expressed in normal conditions, can also lead to killing targets. Recognition is made by NK receptors that exist in two kinds: inhibitory receptors or KIRs (*killer inhibiting receptors*) and activating receptors KARs (*killer activating receptors*). In humans, CD56 (high and low levels) as well as combinations of KIRs and KARs characterize subsets of NK cells, whereas in mouse, CD49b and Ly49 family members distinguish them.

NK cells selectively kill target cells without expression of particular MHC class I molecules on the cell surface. This usually happens in diseases like viral infections or cancers (by downregulating MHC molecules, probably to avoid antigen presentation and to evade the immune response). Highly likely, NK cells activation is a result of two processes being integrated. Namely, signals received through inhibiting and (or) activating receptors can reach the threshold for activation, and trigger NK cell degranulation. This causes inoculation of granzymes (serine proteases) via perforin-made pores in the cell membrane. Another mechanism involves Fas ligand (FasL) or TRAIL mechanism (similar to CD8 T cells—see section on cytotoxic CD8 T lymphocytes, Chapter 3, p. 85–87).

Cytokines such as IL-2, IL-12, IL-15, IL-18, IL-21, IFN-α, and IFN-β activate resting NK cells (or, perhaps, lowering the overall signal thresholds across different KIRs and KARs). Cytokine IL-15 is an important factor for development of NK cells, because mice without the IL15 gene have almost no NK cells.

In humans, NK cells can be distinguished from other lymphocytes by being CD3-negative and CD56^{+}. The frequency of NK cells among leukocytes in the blood is 10–15%. It is interesting that the frequency rises up to 30% in the liver sinusoid. It is important to note that NK cells are found in the red pulp of the spleen, lymph nodes (small but significant), and in uterus. NK cells can be further divided into subgroups with respect to the expression of CD56 and CD16 markers (by flow cytometry and immunohistochemistry). Most NK cells (90%) are cytotoxic while the rest are not. Despite that, they are important due to production of cytokines that can regulate local immunity. For example, many activated NK cells are major sources of

IFN-γ (type II interferon), which can further regulate the type I immune response (see *Definition of the immune response,* p. 22).

Natural Killer T Cells

Beside the major $CD3^-CD56^+$ type, there are NK cells expressing $CD3^+$ molecules. The $CD3^+CD56^+$ NK cells define a separate group of cytotoxic cells called NKT cells, because they have additionally a TCR (see *Specific receptors for antigen (BCR and TCR),* Chapter 3, p. 59). Their role in immunity is less clear, but we hope that their function will be more clarified in the future.

Research revealed the existence of many NK cell receptors that regulate their activation. While the inhibitory receptors (KIRs) were mainly classified into two families of proteins—one with the c-lectin domain, and the other with the immunoglobulin domain in the primary structure of the molecule—the activating NK receptors (KARs) belong to many diverse protein families. Activating NK receptors (such as CD2, NKGD, etc.) shows synergy or cooperation between themselves, if they are expressed on the same NK cell. This is usually observed as the activation with two or more sub-optimal stimuli (e.g., a single sub-optimal stimulus would be insufficient, while two would suffice). Furthermore, the activation of NK cells can be elicited with either monoclonal antibodies that are activating agonists of KARs, or antagonists to KIRs. It is believed that antibodies *Herceptin* and *Retuximab*, which are used in the treatment of various cancers, probably act through NK cells in this way.

These findings might show the way for potential new cancer therapies, such as the transfer of allogeneic or autologous NK cells into recipients, after employing short-term NK cell culture with or without additional factors that could enhance the cytotoxic function. In the presence of IL-2, NK cells can kill multiple target cells and thus become so called LAK (*"lymphokine activated killer"*) cells. LAK cells were tested in some malignant tumors as immunotherapy with autologous leukocytes, but their effect was not encouraging, and the therapy was abandoned because of the unpleasant side effects of the IL-2. Nevertheless, anti-tumor therapy with transplantation of NK cells is still in its infancy.

In autoimmune diseases, NK cells could have a dual role, either disease promoting or disease inhibitory. Recent studies indicate that the NK cells might play a disease-inhibitory role in autoimmune diseases such as multiple sclerosis and systemic lupus erythematosus. They were also implicated in having a beneficial role in inhibiting graft-versus-host disease in animal models.

The Innate Helper Type 2 Cells

These cells are those that can steer the Th2 type response. They include natural helper cells (NHC) and multi-potent progenitor (MPP) also called innate helper type 2 (Ih2) cells and basically can, under influence of IL-25 and IL-31, produce IL-13, which, in turn, can facilitate secretion of IL-4 from basophils, mast cells, and macrophages (M2 type).

ADAPTIVE HUMORAL (SPECIFIC) IMMUNE SYSTEM

Soluble mediators called antibodies represent humoral immunity. They are part of γ-globulin or immunoglobulin (Ig) protein fraction of the blood. They are the secreted product of plasma cells, which represent the final stage of B-lymphocyte lineage differentiation. Antibody molecule binds to macromolecules called antigens. Antigen is any macromolecule capable of eliciting the immune response. The most common antigens are glycosylated proteins derived from microorganisms or eukaryotic tissues, and polysaccharides usually from bacterial cell walls or membranes. Glycolipids can also stimulate some immunocytes (see γδT cells). Small molecular weight compounds or metal ions can bind to a larger molecule like protein and become immunogenic. Small molecules are called haptens, while their larger helping counterparts—carriers.

Immunoglobulins

Antibodies are glycoproteins with a similar basic molecular structure stemming from a pair of heavy and light chains (Figure 2-9). Each antibody has two heavy chains linked to each other by disulfide bridges at one end (closer to the C-terminal). Another disulfide bridge brings association with light chains. Light chains are divided into two types (*kappa* and *lambda*). It is important to mention that these types were never observed mixed in a single antibody molecule. The same is true for the heavy chains. Antibodies are defined according to the presence of heavy chains in the molecules. Heavy chains are organized into five classes (μ, δ, γ, α, and ε) and several subclasses. Thus, μ (*mu*) heavy chains with either κ (*kappa*) or λ (*lambda*) light chains represent IgM class of antibodies. Similarly, δ chains that associate with light chains form IgD class; γ chains form IgG (there are subclasses: $\gamma1$, $\gamma2a$ and $2b$, $\gamma3$ and $\gamma4$); α chains make IgA class, and finally ε (*epsilon*) heavy chains define the IgE. A common feature among both heavy and light chains are regions called variable (V) and constant (C). V regions of heavy and light chains are located at the N-terminal, oriented in parallel with each other, and can therefore enter simultaneously into the molecular interaction

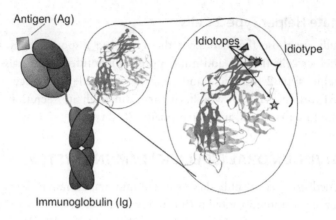

Figure 2-9 Adaptive Immunity: The structure of antibody molecule (immunoglobulin) predicted by crystallographic analysis.

with antigen. Since the basic unit of antibodies is composed of identical pairs of light and heavy chains, there are two binding sites for antigen (Figure 2-9). With them, antibodies can either bind two identical antigens or two binding sites on the same molecule (if the antigen is a polymer-like polysaccharide). At the primary structure, Ig domain looks like a stretch of about 100 amino acids in length that has a C-C (cysteine) disulfide bond between the two cysteines, one at the start and the other at the end of the domain. The structure in–between them is shaped in a characteristic two beta-plated sheets with several anti-parallel strips of amino acids.

Binding sites for antigen (called idiotopes) are conformationally different between individual antibodies. Each antibody has a set of markers called idiotype. Constant regions determine the class of heavy chains and the type of light chains.

In addition to the basic structure, IgM and IgA have a superstructure. Specifically, IgM are pentamers, while IgA are dimers. The possibility of association of identical molecules is provided with *joining* (J) chain (which has no resemblance to J genetic segment of the Ig gene). Joining chain connects the constant parts of Ig molecules. By adding another protein called the secretory chain, IgA molecules can be secreted across the epithelium (into breast milk, in digestive tract, and over other mucous membranes).

The Great Diversity of Variable Parts of Antibody Molecules

The diversity of antibodies is generated by somatic recombination of the immunoglobulin genes (called gene rearrangements) during the development

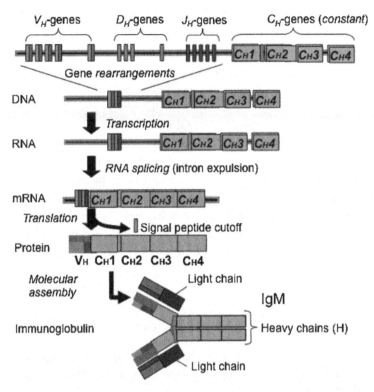

Figure 2-10 Generation of diversity in immunoglobulins. Schematic representation of the heavy chain gene rearrangements of the Ig (BCR) in higher vertebrates.

of B lymphocytes. Antibodies have similar structure to B-cell receptors (BCR). In fact, Ig gene rearrangements occur in the BCR genes and the same gene segments encode both Ig and BCR molecules. To better understand the origin of diversity, we should first explain the structure and organization of Ig genes. Variable and constant parts of the heavy chain gene are encoded by different genetic segments that are far apart on the same chromosome. The variable region of mature heavy chain gene is further separated into three sections (that are more apparent in precursors of B lymphocytes) called variable (V), diversity (D), and joining (J) gene segments. D and J gene segments are located 5' upstream (in front) of constant parts of Ig genes in DNA. Antibody of the IgM class is coded for by a single constant region gene segment that has four domains (Figure 2-10). Constant gene parts of other Ig classes of heavy chains are encoded in a row 3' downstream (behind) of the constant M gene. Every variable region can be rearranged (somatically recombined) to each D or J, and every D can join each J region, thus, by random association during the development of B cells, such process can create a large variability in the repertoire of antigen recognition by Igs and BCRs.

Genes of Ig light chains have similar structure to those of the heavy chains, but with a smaller number of V segments and a single C gene for *kappa* chains, or a few V regions and several C genes for *lambda* chains. In the progenitor B cells during the development, different VJ gene rearrangements of light chain genes occur by chance. Additionally, random pairing of heavy and light chains contributes even more greatly to the diversity of antibodies. Light chain genes are being rearranged after the heavy chain counterparts. Birds and amphibians have different classes of heavy chains (IGY and IGX).

This organization has the ability to produce about 10^{16} different molecules (after selection during B-cell development to exclude those that would harm self) that constitute the repertoire of diversity by which antibodies can fight harmful microorganisms.

Summary
A. Antibodies (Igs) are built from two identical pairs of heavy and light chains.
B. Each chain has a variable and a constant part.
C. There are different classes of antibodies. Antibody class (isotype) depends on the difference in the constant parts of the heavy chains (IgM class, IgD, IgG, IgA, and IgE).
D. Enormous variation of V regions of antibodies is based on their polygenic organization and somatic recombination (rearrangement) during development of B cells.

CELLULAR ADAPTIVE (SPECIFIC) IMMUNE SYSTEM

T, NKT, and B lymphocytes are cells of adaptive immunity. T cells are either αβT or γδT.

αβT lymphocytes are further divided into
- helper (CD4$^+$) and
- cytotoxic (CD8$^+$).

CD4 cells can be subdivided into subgroups (like Th1, Th2, Th9, Th17, and Th22), and regulatory Treg cells (CD4$^+$).

Tregs have a combination of activation markers (CD25$^+$FoxP3$^+$) and production of immunosuppressive cytokines (TGF-β) as the specific designation of the population. On the other hand, γδT cells have a narrow specificity and are divided by the expression of their V regions of the γδT-cell receptor. B lymphocytes are divided into classes (IgM/IgD, IgG, IgA, and IgE) according to expression of their BCR heavy chain gene constant regions (that determine the isotype). There are B1, B2, and Breg cells.

Clonal Distribution

Clone of cells is a population that has identical genetic and phenotypic features with its precursors. As for the B or T lymphocytes, clone refers to a group of cells with the identical receptor recognition of antigen and peptide/MHC ligand, respectively, while all other features are ignored that may be different. Therefore, we categorize lymphocytes into clones of naïve, activated, effector, and memory cells. All of the above cell clones are generated by the division of a single predecessor cell (such as naïve T or B lymphocytes) through several generations. Thus, each clone of T or B cells has essentially monospecific TCR or BCR, respectively. In humans, there are about 5-30% exceptions, because it has been found that αβ T cells can have two different TCRs, which gives them the ability to have dual specificity of recognition.

Summary

For B and T cells, a clone means belonging to a group of cells that have identical antigen (BCR) or peptide/MHC ligand (TCR) recognition molecules, respectively.

Common Precursor of B and T Lymphocytes

B and T lymphocytes arise from a common ancestral cell—lymphoid progenitor or common lymphoid precursor-2 (CLP-2). The common B- and T-cell progenitor can be found in the bone marrow. During the development of T- and B-cell lines in the organs of the central immune system (thymus and bone marrow) they begin to express various cell surface markers. The distinctive mark is primarily specific receptor for antigen. For T cells, TCR molecule is structurally similar to Ig, but smaller in size. TCR belongs to the Ig superfamily of molecules, having the Ig domain for the basic primary structure. Unlike antibodies, which are heterotetrameric, TCR is a heterodimeric molecule. During development in thymus, T cells acquire expression of CD4 or CD8 molecules. The latter are helpful in identifying the differentiation stage of T-cell development. CD4 and CD8 serve as additional receptors (coreceptors) in the recognition of antigens, for which the main receptor is the (αβ)TCR molecule (found on 95% of T cells in human blood), which can

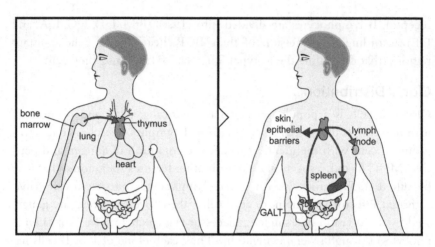

Figure 2-11 Stages in T-cell development. Migration of precursors from bone marrow to the thymus. Emigration of mature T cells from thymus to the periphery of the immune system. Central lymphatic organs: bone marrow and thymus, and peripheral immune system: spleen, lymph nodes, and epithelial barriers like skin and mucosa (GALT—gastrointestinal-associated lymphoid tissue).

bind an antigenic peptide in the clefts (alpha helices) of the MHC molecules (on the surface of APCs). The coreceptor CD4 can bind to the non–polymorphic part of the class II MHC molecule (a part without the antigenic peptides), and the CD8 coreceptor can bind a portion of the class I MHC molecule (also without antigenic peptides).

T-Cell Development

For development in the thymus, CLP-2 migrates from the bone marrow in the thymus cortex (Figure 2-11). (The identifiable markers on CLP-2 cells are CD34 with a very low expression of CD4 molecules, which is immediately lost in the next stage of development). In the thymus cortex, immature T cells develop over 4 developmental stages (DN1–DN4) of double negative (DN) thymocytes (Figure 2-12), named so because of the lack of both CD4 and CD8 coreceptors.

The stages of the development can be monitored by examining the expression of CD25, CD44, and IL-7R molecules on the cell surface. During the early stages δTCR genes are first to begin rearranging. In DN2 stage the rearrangements of the β-chain TCR genes also start (Figure 2-13). IL-7 is a co-factor in the rearrangement of TCR β chains during this stage. The β-chain TCR is expressed on the cell surface together with the precursor of the α-chain

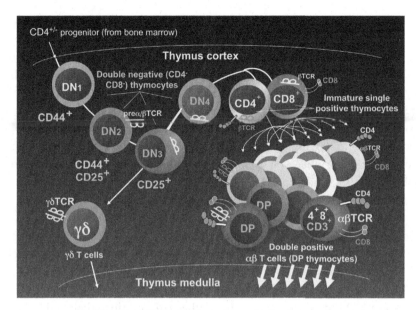

Figure 2-12 T-cell development in the thymus.

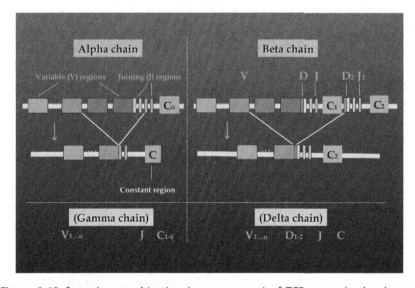

Figure 2-13 Somatic recombination (rearrangement) of TCR genes in the thymus. V—variable regions; D—*diversity* segments; J—*joining* regions; and C—constant regions of the TCR genes.

TCR called pre-α chain (which is encoded by a single gene that does not rear-range). Pre-α and β chains form heterodimeric receptors called pre-TCR.

Signaling through the pre-TCR is important for further development of αβT and γδT cells (Figure 2-12). Several subgroups of γδT cells develop in the thymus, though many γδT cells can develop outside. It seems that signaling via the pre-TCR and Notch system decides whether αβ or γδ T lymphocytes would develop. Namely, the creation of further stages of development (DN3 and DN4) of αβT lymphocytes is dependent on synergy between Notch and pre-TCR signals, while γδT can develop without the Notch signal (utilizing only pre-TCR). In addition, IL-7 action must stop, as IL-7 inhibits transcription factors that are essential for transition into the next stages of development.

If the αβT cells pathway is engaged, pre-α chain becomes shut off, causing β-chain to remain inside the thymocytes, because it alone cannot be expressed on the cell surface. Further development of the αβ T lymphocytes, which constitute the majority of cells within the thymus, includes a short period called immature single-positive stage (ISP). In detail, during this stage the CD4 and CD8 molecules start to be synthesized, and since their production is slightly unsynchronized, cells pass through this stage for a short period of time. After several hours, such ISP thymocytes become double positive (DP) ones. DP thymocytes begin to proliferate, and at the same time they rearrange α chains of the TCR (Figures 2-12 and 2-13). Since there is already a β-chain TCR in the cytoplasm, as soon as DP cells successfully rearrange one (or both) allele(s) of the α chain, the αβTCR can be expressed on the surface of thymocytes. In doing so, they receive help from accompanying molecules such as the CD3 complex that bonds the TCR chains together in the membrane, and serves as the signal transduction system.

Thymic Checkpoints

In the thymic cortex, thymocytes need to pass several checkpoints in their development for further differentiation:

1. The first checkpoint occurs at the stage of the pre-TCR expression. The development will continue only if the rearrangement of the β-chain genes is successful (and thus expressed on the surface with the pre-α).

2. The second checkpoint is at the DN2 stage. Notch/pre-TCR system signaling balance decides on the type of receptor to be expressed (αβ or γδ). Hence, if γδT would be selected, the γδT cells rearrange γ-chain genes, express the TCR on the surface, and migrate out of the thymus into mucosal sites or skin.

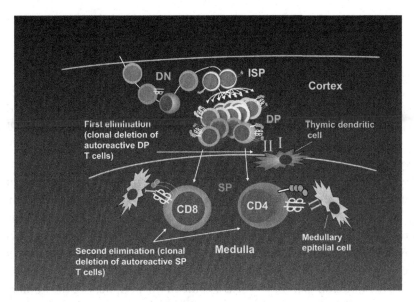

Figure 2-14 T lymphocyte development in the thymus. CD4 or CD8 coreceptor expression identify double negative (DN), immature single positive (ISP), double positive (DP), and single positive (SP) T lymphocytes during their differentiation and migration from cortex to medulla.

3. The next checkpoint concerns the expression of CD1 recognition ability at the DP stage. Such cells also have αβTCR, and are exported from the thymus as NKT cells (and continue to be DP).

4. The fourth checkpoint is at the DP stage and involves the αβTCR expression. Here, three selection processes occur because of the αβTCR binding to ligands on thymic epithelial cells. Based on the affinity of the αβTCR, the DP cells are either neglected, positively selected, or eliminated (negatively selected).

The mechanism of selection is still debated, but consensus has been that the most important factor is the affinity of the αβTCR for self-peptides in the clefts of the MHC molecules. Thus, clones of thymocytes that cannot bind any available self-peptide/MHC ligands would die out of neglect. Those that can bind with high affinity would die by apoptosis (Figure 2-14). Only those with the intermediary affinity would be allowed to pass into the next stage of development (and they represent barely a few percentages of all thymocytes at that stage). This process can generate αβT-cell repertoire capable of recognizing about 10^{14} different molecules being essential for the immune defense. This is calculated with a principle that, in general, a single clone represents a single specificity. We now know, that 5–30% of T cells in the blood can have two functional TCRs (due to imperfect gene rearrangement mechanism), and these clones can increase the breadth of the repertoire.

At the selection stage in the thymus, coreceptors CD4 and CD8 also contribute in the recognition of self-peptide/MHC ligand (by binding constant portions of the MHC molecules). The joint affinity of TCR with that of the CD4/CD8 coreceptors is called avidity. The function of T cells depends on a combination of TCR and coreceptor expression. If the TCR can recognize a self-peptide ligand in the groove of class I MHC molecule, the CD8 coreceptor would be also engaged (during positive selection) in binding to the same molecule that presents the antigenic peptide, and the CD4 molecules is lost in the next stage of development. On the other hand, if the TCR binds to self-peptide in the cleft of class II MHC molecule, then the CD4 molecules will remain expressed, while the CD8 would be lost in the next stage. The selection of the coreceptor molecules at this stage influences the function that these T cells acquire in the periphery of the immune system as effector cells. Namely, CD4 T cells develop mostly into helper cells, whereas CD8 T cells become cytotoxic.

However, there is an exception with respect to CD4 thymocytes that show the highest avidity for the self-peptide/MHC class II ligand in the thymic cortex. If they receive help from the DN2 stage of developing thymocytes, they can avoid death, and proceed further in the next stage, becoming natural regulatory CD4 T cells—nTregs, expressing CTLA4 and Foxp3 markers (see *Development of Treg cells* below).

Positively selected thymocytes will become single positive (SP) and move into the core (medulla) of the thymus. There SP thymocytes become mature after about two weeks (in the mouse), when they become ready to exit and seed peripheral lymphoid organs. During the maturation in the thymic core, another negative selection on auto-antigens (Figure 2-14) takes place. Namely, the thymic core (medullary) epithelial cells can express almost any self-antigen encoded in the genome by the special mechanism that includes expression of a gene called the autoimmune regulator (AIRE). AIRE is a transcriptional regulator that promotes activation of thousands genes in medullary epithelial cells. AIRE controls transcription in elongation stage by releasing stalled RNA polymerase. Smaller RNAs can be translated and give rise to a variety of self-encoded peptides that can be presented in the grooves of MHC class I and class II molecules. Despite many ideas, the mechanism of action of AIRE is not completely understood. However, it is quite clear that brain-specific or muscle-specific proteins can be synthesized there, and even insulin can be expressed in minute quantities. It is assumed, that for example, insulin expression in thymic medullary epithelial cells has a different function than that in the pancreas, namely, it is used only for the purpose of selecting the T-cell repertoire (in this case negatively).

It is important to mention that one of the main cytokines that supports the thymic microenvironment is RANK (with its RANK Ligand), which is likely to play an important role in mTEC maturation and thus regulate the induction of central tolerance.

Thus, the negative selection is done by clonal deletion of auto-reactive clones of SP T cells (with nTregs being an exception, *see later*). The process involves processing of self-antigens and presentation (in the form of peptides) in clefts of MHC molecules to αβT SP thymocytes. Those SP T cells that can recognize self-peptide in the context of self-MHC molecules would die by apoptosis. The αβT cells that survive negative selection leave the thymus. Emigrants are just a few percent of those cells generated on a daily basis. Early thymic emigrants are still not reactive regarding the immune response. They become responsive after they home in the paracortex of lymph nodes or white pulp of spleen (Figure 2-11).

Development of Treg Cells

Treg precursors are developed between the DN1 and DN2 stages by transconditioning of DN1 cells by particular DP ones. In doing so, DP cells create two populations of DN2. Most become large, as they are blasts (DN2-L), while a minority remains small (DN2-S). DN2-L cells are further developed as previously described, following the αβT-cell development pathway including DP and mature SP (CD4 or CD8) stages. DN2-S cells also develop into DP cells and have a similar positive selection. However, they undergo somewhat different negative selection than those DPs of the DN2-L line. Particularly, the DN2-S derived DP cells with high affinity are clonally deleted, but those with the highest affinity for the self-peptide/MHC are positively selected, and they develop into natural Treg cells (nTregs). There are also induced Tregs in the periphery, which are different from nTregs (and will be discussed later).

For the development of nTregs, an important soluble factor is a cytokine called thymic stromal lymphopoetin. Secreted by Hassall's bodies, it activates thymic dendritic cells (TDC) to express large amounts of CD80 and CD86 (B7) molecules. Thymic DCs can stimulate the expression of Foxp3 nuclear factor in $CD4^+CD25^+$ population of thymocytes (derived from DN2-S line) to become $CD4^+CD25^+Foxp3^+$ –nTreg cells. This transition requires a cytokine IL-2 and two molecular interactions between the nTreg and TDC and: (**1**)

TCR with peptide/MHC ligand; and (2) B7 (CD80 and CD86) with CTLA-4 (*Cytotoxic T lymphocyte antigen-4,* CD152) molecule. Therefore, nTreg clones are auto reactive with a strong affinity for self-antigens (see *T-cell recognition repertoire*). DN2-S derived clones with moderate affinity to self-ligands (so-called partial agonists) also develop in SP thymocytes, and the latter do not differ from most SP T cells (derived from DN2-L cells). Thus, they become indistinguishable from induced Tregs (iTregs) in the periphery. Induced Tregs in the periphery are defined as CD4 T cell clones with any αβTCR that upon activation can secrete cytokines characteristic for Tregs (IL-10 and TGF-β) and have direct inhibitory action on other (neighboring) T-cell clone that is on the way to become activated by some antigen (during, e.g., infection).

After leaving the thymus, Tregs can be activated in a specific way (different from the "normal" αβT cells). Namely, if they encounter antigen instead of the proliferation, they become inactive and do not multiply (or rather poorly). Instead, they have the ability to inhibit the already (or just being) activated T cells (which are found in the vicinity) and prevent their peripheral development after activation. Because they can induce tolerance to antigens, they are called regulatory T lymphocytes. It is believed that they can have a role in defending self tissues from the attack by autoreactive T cells (i.e., those that passed through negative selection by mistake), and in maintenance of bacterial flora (commensals). Their importance stems from evidence that mice made artificially deficient for the Foxp3 gene develop lethal autoimmune syndrome. Transfer of T cells that are positive for the Foxp3 factor cures the syndrome.

Tregs are characterized by the expression of CD4, CD25, and Foxp3 in naïve conditions. Furthermore, *Helios* can be used as a marker for distinguishing thymic derived Tregs (tTregs or nTregs) from peripherally induced Tregs (pTregs or iTregs).

However, although Tregs exist, we still have no clear physiologically relevant biological role for them according to prevalent self–nonself discrimination theory. Perhaps they are just "stray" cells or inactivated CD4 lymphocytes under pathological conditions, which sometimes might have beneficial (preventing autoimmunity) or disadvantageous features (allowing development of infections or cancer). In particular, Tregs still have no specific population marker—just a combination of them, which can only rarely be found in other T cell populations, like for example activated CD4 T helper cell subpopulation that also displays CD25 and some transiently express Foxp3. This is the case for almost all naïve cells in mice, as well as for some CD4 T subsets in humans. Furthermore, there is a contradiction about Treg function in relationship with the proclaimed defensive function of the immune system (see *Self–nonself discrimination* theory in Chapter 9, p. 285 on *Theories about the function of the immune system)*. Namely, if the repertoire of Treg cells is similar to those of CD4 and CD8 αβT cells (that is if Tregs recognize any microbe simultaneously as other T cells), then the question remains, how does the antigen stimulate the immune response at all if both can run in parallel? Likewise, how does antigen inhibit the immune response? What determines the defensive immune response, and what causes tolerance of bacteria or viruses? It seems that the specificity of TCR (and the generation of T-cell repertoire) to recognize nonself (as a consequence of T-cell development in the thymus) is not a sufficient parameter in itself to explain the above-mentioned problem. Namely, we still wonder when, how, and why the immune response would occur, and when, how, and why it would not. The current S–NS view involves explanations that the strength and duration of receptor–ligand interactions (in T-cell synapse with APC) and/or the dose of antigen (in interaction with B cell) modulates the type of the immune response, or, in other words, they might distinguish response from tolerance (see further discussion on immunological theories in Chapter 9).

The Homing of T Cells in the Secondary Lymphatic Tissue (Immunologic Periphery)

After leaving the thymus, early thymic emigrant αβT cells rapidly mature and become naïve T cells. The latter can be activated by immunogenic stimuli and thus initiate the immune response (with the exception of Tregs, see previous section). Naïve T cells migrate by blood and exit in lymph nodes by extravasation over high-endothelial venules. (Figures 2-11, 3-14, and 4-4). They home in the T cell zones of the paracortex. Some believe that T cells can continuously recirculate from the blood into the lymph. Such T cells probably exist at a later stage of their development and they are resting—not in terms of movements, but growth. The lymph node naïve T cells wait to be activated. Tissue dendritic cells, for example, can notify them about harmful intruders. In that sense, we could envisage T cells as cells with ability to "observe" tissue integrity (in communication with tissue dendritic cells). If the intruder is benign (not-harmful), theoretically, it should be tolerated (e.g., Treg would help in suppressing those T cell clones that would react against non-harmful but useful intruders, like commensals).

B-Cell Development

There are two types of B cells: B1 is a minor subset and B2 is the major subgroup. Thus, throughout the book, all references to B cells actually refer to the B2 compartment, unless specifically addressed. B1 reside mostly in places such as peritoneal cavity, whereas B2 cells seed hematopoietic tissues and recirculate

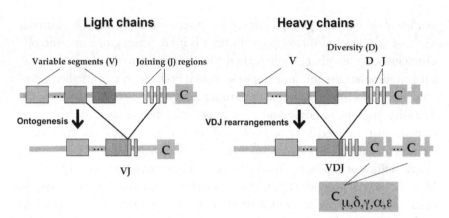

Figure 2-15 Somatic recombination of BCR genes during B-cell development in bone marrow. V—variable region; D—*diversity* segments; J—*joining* parts; and C—constant portions of the BCR genes.

in blood as follicular B cells having a CD23 marker. In secondary lymphoid organs (lymph nodes and splenic white pulp in germinal follicles) B cells can respond to antigens (that they have either picked up in circulation or detected on resident population of stromal cells, called follicular dendritic cells, FDCs) by developing into plasma cells that then secrete their BCR as antibodies. Some B cells need help of T cells in this process, but some do not. Therefore, the immune responses are divided into T-dependent and T-independent ones. The independent ones are the reason why there are so-called natural antibodies in the blood and tissues. They are antibodies with intermediate to low affinity to antigens that we found in our natural surroundings. Usually, they are of the IgM (or IgD) class. Most B1 cells are of this kind.

A significant fraction of B cells in the peripheral repertoire expresses self-reactivity, and many of these B cells belong to innate-like subsets such as the marginal zone (MZ) B cells. The MZ B cells are classical APCs. They can be found in secondary lymphoid tissues (spleen and lymph nodes in primary follicles) (see histologic examples of LNs and spleen in Figures 3-14 to 3-16). Their specificity for self antigens can be one of the reasons why (yet unknown and possibly aberrant) activation may break T cell tolerance. The latter could then help follicular B cells in the production of pathogenic autoantibodies.

B2 lymphocytes can belong to T-independent and T-dependent types of the immune responses. Lymphoid progenitor of B2 cells remains mainly in the bone marrow where through a series of developmental stages produces mature naïve B cells. Naïve B cells have membrane IgM (and IgD) as a receptor for antigen (B-cell receptor or BCR). BCR is made by Ig gene rearrangements (Figure 2-15) similarly to TCR genes (see the section on antibodies).

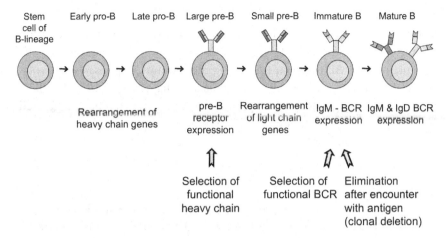

Figure 2-16 B-cell development in bone marrow and selection.

Differences between the Ig heavy chain genes and those from the TCR genes are in the larger amount of V, D, and J gene regions of the former. There are more constant regions (C) too, and they are located downstream of the J gene segments. They fall into several subgroups denoted by Greek alphabet letters *mu* (μ), *delta* (δ), *gamma* (γ), *alpha* (α), and *epsilon* (ε). Some subgroups have more members than the other. These gene segments encode Ig isotypes, which are used to divide Igs into classes. Thus, we have classes IgM, IgD, IgG, IgA, and IgE.

During the B-cell development, clones that carry BCR are selected in several stages (Figure 2-16) with the help of cytokine IL-7. First selection allows further development of clones that successfully assemble heavy chain genes. The second selection provides survival to those with successfully rearranged light chain genes, and ultimately a selection that checks the auto-reactivity of the BCR. All clones that can bind self-antigens attached to cell membranes succumb to apoptosis (negative selection). On the other hand, the auto-reactive clones that recognize soluble self-antigens develop clonal anergy. In the mature stage, naïve B cells can undergo further development after the activation by antigen, and replace the constant region of the heavy chain that they initially express with another C region thus making an isotype switch.

Also, the development into plasma cell involves transition of their membrane bound antibody molecule (BCR) into secretory form by genetic exclusion of transmembrane regions and intracellular portions in all isotype heavy chain genes. Thus, antibodies have the same specificity as BCRs, but plasma cells do not have BCRs anymore on the cell surface.

This is different from the mechanism by which cytokines are released if expressed as a membrane-bound form. Namely, metalloproteinases (sheddases) cleave off extracellular part of membrane-bound cytokines, whereas a genomic recombination event excludes membrane-anchoring coding sequence from the Ig genes during transition from activated B cell into plasma cell. All this happens during the immune response (see *Regulation of immunocyte development after activation*, Chapter 4, p. 105). Furthermore, there is a regulatory B cell population (Bregs) that has been suggested by some researchers that could regulate immune responses. The phenotype of this population is CD19+CD20+ and CD24^{hi}CD38^{hi}.

Summary

A. T lymphocytes develop in the thymus, and B cells in the bone marrow in adults.

B. During development, B or T cells express receptors (BCR = Ig or TCR, respectively) on the cell surface. Receptors can bind foreign antigen (BCR) or complex ligand made of antigenic peptide in the cleft of the MHC molecule (TCR).

C. There are three kinds of T cells that exit the thymus. The majority of them are αβT cells (95%). There are also γδT cells (3–4% in the blood), and NKT cells (up to 1%).

D. The αβT cells that leave the thymus carry only a single coreceptor—either CD4 or CD8, being the predecessors of helper or killer T cells, respectively. Coreceptors can bind to non-polymorphic parts of MHC molecules (CD4—class II, CD8—class I).

E. After B- and T-cell development in the central organs of the immune system, the exit is allowed only to those that have passed positive and negative selective process for their receptor specificity. They were tested for the ability to respond to body's own (self) antigens.

F. In the thymus, most αβT cells undergo apoptosis because of negative selection or neglect, provided they were too much or too little auto-reactive, respectively. Exceptions are thymocytes with medium and very strong auto-reactivity, which eventually become regulatory T cells (Treg).

G. Positive and negative selections endow a host organism with a functional immune defense repertoire that should not be auto-destructive. Since no biologic process is flawless, B or T cell clones that avoid negative selection (by mistake; so-called forbidden clones) and become activated in the periphery (i.e., during infection) can cause autoimmune syndromes or diseases.

H. T regulatory (Treg) cells guard self-antigen tolerance in case some forbidden T cell clones escape the negative selection in the thymus. They can probably tone down the immune responses after the elimination of a microorganism. Tregs might endow the host organism with tolerance to commensals' antigens.

I. Auto-reactive B cells during development in the bone marrow either die by apoptosis (negative selection) or become anergic, depending on the phase of antigen they recognize (cell membrane bound or soluble, respectively). The B-regulatory cells (Breg) have been suggested to exist.

T Lymphocytes with γδTCR (γδT Cells)

For γδT cells, it is believed that they play a role similar to NK cells, which is the primary line of defense against invasive microorganisms or parasites. However, since the genes of their receptor (γδTCR) rearrange like those of αβTCR, they have the ability to generate a diverse repertoire for recognition. Thus they belong to the adaptive immune system.

It is known that γδT cells can recognize stress (shock) proteins that belong to the heat shock protein groups in mammals and bacteria, as well as some non-classical MHC molecules. Unlike αβTCR (which bind peptides in grooves of classical MHC molecules), γδTCR bind ligands, which consist of lipid molecules in clefts of non-conventional MHC molecules such as CD1. It is thought that γδT cells can recognize shocked cells of self tissues (i.e., injured, distressed, or infected) and perform at least two main functions. The first is to inform other immunocytes of the specific (central, adaptive) immune system about the presence of damaged tissue integrity, and the second is to take action (perhaps under particular circumstances that are not quite clear yet) and kill the infected cell (and the virus in it).

In humans, Vγ9Vδ2 is the predominant subset of γδT cells. Furthermore, Vγ9Vδ2 represents one of the major subgroups of T cells in the blood (up to 1/20 of the lymphocytes in the periphery of the immune system). They have broad reactivity against microbes and tumors. Diversity of their repertoire depends only on D and J regions of the TCR. Despite this constraint their repertoire is as wide as those of the αβT cells. However, such focused diversity is just appropriate to recognize small organic compounds in the clefts of non-conventional MHC molecules. The γδT cells recognize microbial metabolites (intermediate products of non-mevalonate pathway during the biosynthesis of isoprenoids) and endogenous metabolites of the mevalonate pathway, whose production increases during cell stress.

Vγ9Vδ2 T cells recognize so-called phosphoantigens (pAgs), which are small molecules usually found as intermediates of the microbial and eukaryotic isoprenoid biosynthesis pathway. While bacterial pAgs can stimulate γδT cells at pico- or nanomolar concentrations, eukaryotic pAgs (like isopentyl pyrophosphate, IPP) require micromolar concentrations to do the same. Normally, IPP concentration is never produced that high as to activate γδT cells, but it is thought that prolonged cellular stress might lead to accumulation of IPP due to dysregulated mevalonate pathway. Such cellular transformation can be sensed by molecules such as BTN3A1 (CD277), which is probably an extracellular or intracellular receptor of pAgs. Although CD277s role is still investigated, its signaling could then lead to activation of γδT cells.

Most γδT cells express NKG2D (Natural Killer Group 2 Member D) receptors, which are NK activating molecules that recognize MHC-like molecules including stress-induced *Major Histocompatibility Complex (MHC) class I chain*-related antigen A/B (MICA/B). Many tumor cells express MICA/B and γδT cells can be cytotoxic toward them.

On the other hand, neutrophils can inhibit γδT cell activation by production and secretion of azurophile-granule-stored serine proteases: proteinase 3, neutrophil elastase, and cathepsin G. The likely mediator of inhibition is the degradation of IL-2 and down regulation of CD277 expression.

From the functional viewpoint, Vγ9Vδ2 cells can produce IFN-γ, TNF-α, and also IL-4 and IL-17. However, they are not able to produce IL-2, which is needed for their growth and division. They thus require exogenous or CD4 T-cell produced IL-2 for proliferation. In addition, they display a variety of regulatory and antigen-presenting abilities showing a rather large functional plasticity.

CHAPTER 3

Activation of Cells of the Immune System

ACTIVATION OF IMMUNE CELLS IN THE PERIPHERY OF THE IMMUNE SYSTEM

Naïve cells are mature lymphocytes in the periphery (outside the thymus and bone marrow) that have never encountered foreign (nonself) antigen. For CD8 T cells, there is also a term "precursors of cytotoxic T cells," and for naïve B, a phrase "virgin B cells" can also be found in the literature. Under normal circumstances, naïve immunocytes can divide and differentiate only after the activation process (for division of such cells in *lymphopenia*, see "*T lymphocyte homeostasis*" (p. 93). The activation of $\alpha\beta$T lymphocytes, for example, occurs as a result of the destroyed tissue integrity (characterized by damage, distress, and necrosis) and the appearance of novel peptides (parts of foreign or hidden self-antigens) on the dendritic cells (DCs) in the form of peptide/major histocompatibility complex (MHC) ligands at a specific location (lymph node or spleen). The immunocytes that can be activated are as follows:

(a) Naïve CD4$^+$ T helper (Th) cells (and their clonally identical resting memory Th cells).

(b) Precursors of CD8$^+$ T lymphocytes (and their clonally identical resting memory cytotoxic T cells, Tc).

(c) Naïve (virgin) B cells (and their clonally equal resting memory B cells).

Activation of immunocytes starts when a complex process of antigen recognition by these cells is supplemented by additional stimuli. Most of these events have been largely known; however, particular details are not yet completely elucidated for all listed. For simplicity, we can transform this usually analog biological process into a digital, and divide it into three signals. The first signal is specific recognition of antigen or peptide/MHC ligand through BCR/TCR, respectively. The second signal could be costimulatory signals to T cells, and for B lymphocytes, help by effector CD4$^+$ T helper cells. The third signal might be cytokines and some other interactions between immunocytes with tissues that are not completely clear yet. Generally, there will be no activation of naïve or resting

The Cytokines of the Immune System
http://dx.doi.org/10.1016/B978-0-12-419998-9.00003-1

immunocytes (with consequent defensive immune response) if the second and/or third signals are lacking.

Therefore, this process results in *activated* CD4, CD8, or B cells, or, in other words, these cells become *effectors* (with a relatively short lifespan). A very small portion of these cells will survive and create a memory cell that is sometimes difficult to differentiate from naïve when it is dormant or in the resting state (in terms of growth). Thus, despite called "resting," they can recirculate from lymphoid organs to tissues and back via blood and lymphatics. The resting (memory) cells also need activation signals; however, they might be different from those of naïve cells.

Naïve cells can also divide by a homeostatic mechanism when their numbers are scarce as in lymphopenia. This is a division without the presence of stimulating antigen, and cytokine IL-7 is a necessary component of this process.

SPECIFIC RECOGNITION

The activation stimulus leads to the immune response. It is called specific, because recognition molecules should ideally be specific for a single ligand. However, due to a large diversity of ligands in nature, it is now known that each receptor (BCR as well as TCR) can have more than one ligand, despite the fact that this would happen only rarely during the life of an individual under normal circumstances. This was the main reason why the older division of immunity into specific–nonspecific kinds was abandoned. A more appropriate description of immune recognition would therefore be "oligo-specific" (for cells like B and T cells) or polyspecific (for cells like DCs and macrophages). For simplicity (and to stress the very narrow recognition spectrum) we will continue to use the term *specific* instead of *oligospecific*.

Therefore, specific recognition of ligands will deliver the first signal to immunocytes. Recognition begins with binding of antigen (or peptide/MHC ligand) to specific receptors. In the specific recognition, there are fundamental differences between T and B lymphocytes.

Immunoglobulin receptors (Figure 2-9) and circulating antibodies can bind a part of an antigen. Binding site on the antigen must be on the outer side of globular macromolecules. They can have different shapes (conformations). For example, protein antigens are usually different combinations of α-helices alone or with β-plated sheets; various polysaccharides can have diverse polymer conformations, and hapten can associate with many carriers or even be without them.

In contrast, αβT cells can recognize ligand consisting of antigenic peptides in the clefts of *major histocompatibility complex* (MHC) molecules by TCR (peptide/MHC ligand). γδT cells can recognize parts of glycolipids or lipopeptides in the context of MHC-related proteins such as CD1 or other nonconventional MHC molecules (Tla, Q in mice, or human leukocyte antigen (HLA) E, G, F and E in humans).

Specific Receptors for Antigen (BCR and TCR)

Antigen receptors of B lymphocytes, or BCRs, are mainly molecules of IgM and IgD classes (Figure 2-9), which, unlike secreted Ig, have an *anchor*-like sequence at the end of the (constant region of the immunoglobulin) molecule with which they are embedded into the cell membrane. After encounter with antigen and consequent activation, B cells can switch the isotype of their BCR into IgG, IgA, and IgE. This can occur in germinal centers (in, e.g., the cortex of lymph nodes). During switching, another process also takes place in germinal centers with the result that B cells can mutate their V regions of the BCR, and end up with higher affinity for the same antigen. This mechanism is called somatic hypermutation (see "*Germinal center B cells*," p. 87–89).

T cell receptor—TCR—comprises two disulfide-linked chains with immunoglobulin-domain basic structure. The heterodimeric molecule is slightly less in size than Ig. Distinct TCR genes encode each chain. There are four genes: α, β, γ, and δ, that make up two TCR molecules: αβTCR and γδTCR. Both TCRs consists of a constant and a variable part a molecule (Figure 3-1).

Genes of the TCR are assembled (rearranged) during development in the thymus similarly to rearrangement of immunoglobulin genes in developing B cells (see *Development of B and T lymphocytes,* Chapter 2, pp. 44–54).

MHC Molecules

During APC–T cell interaction, TCR is in contact with a molecular structure consisting of antigenic peptide and two alpha helical polypeptide chains supported by a beta-plated sheet. This configuration is a typical conformation of the first two domains of classical MHC molecules and their look-a-likes (nonconventional MHC) (Figures 3-2 and 3-3).

The two helices leave between themselves a cleft into which it can accommodate a single peptide of 6–8 amino acids in length (for class I molecules; Figure 3-2), or 13–17 amino acids (for class II molecules; Figure 3-3). Each peptide makes contact only with a few critical amino acids of the

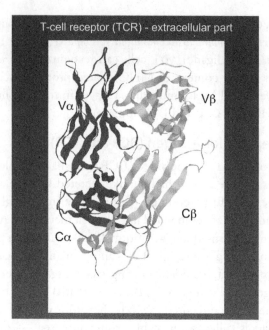

Figure 3-1 Structure of TCR molecule (schematic representation of C atom positions in molecular skeleton).

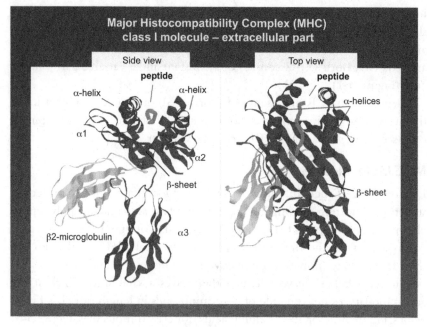

Figure 3-2 MHC class I molecule. Schematic representation of C-atom positions.

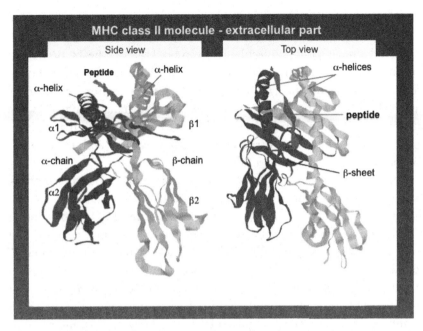

Figure 3-3 MHC class II molecule. Scheme of C-atom positions.

groove (including the bottom of the cleft made of a β-plated sheet). There are many peptides that can fit into such a molecular crevice. However, their number is finite and depends on the position of critical amino acids within the groove that they can come in contact with. In fact every MHC molecule has its own individual constellation (position map) of critical amino acids that restrict the selection of fitting peptides. The MHC molecule is therefore a receptor for a relatively narrow range of peptides that share a similar backbone structure.

Peptides that fit into the clefts of MHC molecules are derived from antigen processing in the liposomal compartment or from newly synthesized proteins in the endoplasmic reticulum and subsequently degraded in proteasomes. Peptides usually anchor themselves in the β-plated sheet of MHC molecules and with the remaining amino acids contact α-helices of the MHC molecules and the TCR. Logically, the wider range of peptide presentation would be possible only by having more such molecules. Research showed that MHC molecules are polygenic and highly polymorphic in higher vertebrates. It suggests that the greater the diversity of MHC molecules of a species, the wider the spectrum of presented peptides for immune recognition. This would lead to better defense and be of advantage for species survival. There are differences in the structure of MHC molecules among species, genera, and families of vertebrates. Yet their function is conserved, similar to the molecules that can bind them—the TCR. We can conclude that the specific recognition of a particular antigenic [peptide/MHC] ligand is individually distributed in higher vertebrates. This happens by the already described mechanism of (somatic) rearrangements of TCRs, and by a novel mechanism (to be described in the next section) that involves co-dominant hereditary distribution of MHC alleles and their gene-conversion type of variability in the progeny.

Peptides lying between the two helices of the MHC molecules, if originating from viruses, microorganisms, parasites, or transplanted tissue, are recognized as being "foreign" (nonself). That is, if the TCR of the resting T cell binds to them and the whole process leads to its activation and sequential immune response. The TCR binding site stretches over "foreign" peptide and α-helices of the MHC molecules, thus "nonself" is seen together with "self" molecules (Figure 3-4). Another interesting feature of T-cell recognition is that peptide need not necessarily be on the surface of an antigen in order to be recognized by T lymphocytes. It is important to mention that a single chain of the TCR—alone—does not bind only

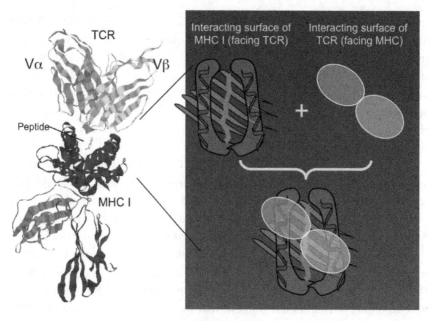

Figure 3-4 Interaction of peptide/MHC ligand and TCR. Map of C-atom positions (left) and interacting surfaces of the peptide, MHC class I, and α/βTCR molecules (right).

antigenic peptide (nonself), or just a part of MHC molecule (self). According to the crystal structure of the TCR–MHC interaction, each TCR chain is in contact with a combination made of a part of peptide and a part of the MHC molecule (Figure 3-4). Furthermore, both α-helices of the MHC molecules show mirror symmetry and are similar to each other. Analyses from animal studies, so far, showed few associations, but in general no clear cut correlation between TCR V region usage and alleles of the MHC molecules that have been recognized. However, this issue is still being debated. This is understandable because experiments with mouse MHC congenic strains point to some skewing of V TCR region usage with certain MHC haplotypes, and can thus be used as an argument to evolutionary conservation in species specific TCR–MHC pairing.

HLA Complex, Tissue Typing and Organ Transplantation

Every individual of a species of higher vertebrates has of set of genes called *MHC*. They are divided into several classes, with the function in T-cell recognition and activation. The proteins previously described in Figures 3-2 and 3-3 are called class I and class II MHC molecules, each class encoded by a separate locus. Human MHC is called *human leukocyte antigen* (*HLA*) complex, whose products are glycoproteins encoded on chromosome 6 (Figure 3-5).

MHC (HLA) molecules resemble each other in general tertiary (conformation) structure. However, they are dissimilar mostly in the finer

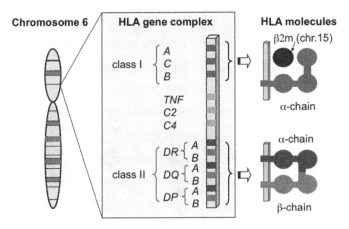

Figure 3-5 The genes encoding MHC molecules in humans (HLA complex). The expression MHC class I and II molecules on the cell surface (schematic).

structural forms usually focused around the first two N-terminal Ig-like domains of the class I MHC molecules, or the first N-terminal domains of the class II MHC proteins. The first two regions of class I molecule form a conformation that has two alpha helices lying on a beta-plated sheet. This conformation is supported from the side by the β2-microglobulin, which is a small globular protein encoded by a separate gene on a different chromosome. MHC class II molecules have similar double-α-helical and β-plated sheet structure. However, here, the heterodimer made of α and β MHC class II molecules have their first N-terminal domains intertwined so that this typical two–helix structure is made. The axes of the helices are slightly bent (curved) towards each other, which makes a gap between them. This cleft can accommodate peptides of distinct sizes (6–8 aa for class I, and over 12, up to 18, for class II molecules). The presence of a peptide in a cleft on the MHC molecules expressed on the cell surface is called presentation, and the whole structure a peptide/MHC ligand. This is a conformation to which a TCR can bind.

MHC class I molecules are expressed on all cells with a nucleus. In contrast, MHC class II molecules are mainly expressed on "professional" antigen-presenting cells (APCs)—DCs, B lymphocytes, and macrophages. In pathological conditions, they may be expressed in other tissues.

MHC molecules are polygenic and polymorphic. Polygenism describes multiplicity of MHC genes in an individual (Figure 3-5), and polymorphism describes observation that in a single species there is a large number of alleles at each genetic locus (Figure 3-6). In humans, MHC class I genes

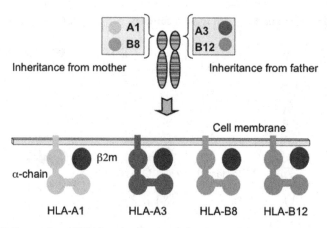

Figure 3-6 Expression of MHC molecules is co-dominant. Schematic representation of MHC class I molecules expression on all nucleated cells.

are divided into three classical genes (A, B, and C), and they have more than 500 alleles spread over various populations. The human MHC (HLA) class II genetic region has several genes (DR, DQ, DP, DO, DM) with altogether over 300 allelic variants. All MHC alleles have co-dominant inheritance (Figures 3-6 and 3-7). The numbers of MHC allelic variants surpass all other genetic loci in most genomes of higher vertebrates. Therefore, each individual human being has a unique set of MHC alleles (which is why it has been used for identification purposes). Because of polygenism and enormous polymorphism, it is almost impossible to find the equal match in the present human population. However, for organ or tissue transplantation, people are typed only for main MHC genes and their alleles, and their match suffices to avoid the acute rejection of transplanted tissue. Nevertheless, rejection can happen at a later stage, and therefore many if not all patients have to use immunosuppressants.

Immunological reasons for the graft rejection are, in principle, similar to those when fighting infection. The events during the destruction of an intruding microorganism are similar to the rejection mechanism of transplanted tissue. However, there might be few differences, which are also a matter of debate. The donor MHC alleles in the graft are recognized by (several) clones of host T lymphocytes (because each individual has a different set of MHC alleles, and the recipient is only tolerant to his/her own kind). T-cell clones specific for the MHC alleles (of individuals of the same species) are also known as allo-specific clones. It means that an allo-specific T cell can recognize (and be activated) by the MHC of another individual (let us call this MHC, allo-MHC). The issue for debate remains, whether or

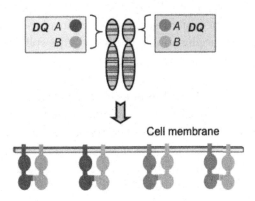

Figure 3-7 Generation of diversity in MHC molecules. Combinatorial expression of MHC class II molecules on antigen-presenting cells.

not allo-MHC has peptides in their clefts? It is highly likely that it does, as the MHC molecules have not been found empty on the cell surface, except under duress, as in some special experimental conditions. Therefore, are the peptides of donor or recipient origin? Which cells present allo-MHC molecules (to host T cells)? Can graft rejection happen if recipients' DCs (with self-MHC) present allo-derived peptides to host T cells? Are there DCs of donor origin that by migrating into recipients' lymph nodes would activate host T cell clones? It seems that these are all possible events that can lead to graft rejection, and this could be different from person to person, possibly due to the host's T cell repertoire of activities, and the specifics of the MHC match (perhaps some donor cells or antigens can interact with host Tregs— under yet unknown conditions—and then the graft might not be rejected). Thus, in conclusion, all these events can lead to host T-cell activation, which causes a sequence of reactions that can result in the rejection of the graft.

Almost every known protein antigen has one or more peptides that can bind to at least one MHC molecule in an individual. On the other hand, some antigens might have a peptide that can fit only to particular allele of a MHC molecule. A person that does not have that particular MHC allele will end up lacking T-cell response against that peptide. However, the immune response against the whole antigen probably would not be affected, because there will be other peptides that could fit into that MHC molecule (or perhaps other ones of the same class).

Transplantation of organs and tissues requires match in classical HLA molecules (class I and class II) between donor and host (recipient) in order to avoid immunologic rejection. After the transplantation of organs, the success of the operation can be measured in terms of time until rejection occurs. Several clinical phrases describe its intensity: hyperacute, acute, and chronic rejection. Hyperacute rejection is a rapid non-immunologic one, whose reasons are pathophysiologic and sometimes still not clear enough (necrosis of the transplant, etc.). The acute and chronic rejections usually have immunologic components. The acute rejection can start after several days, if not treated properly with immunosuppressants.

How does the acute graft rejection begin? Some believe that DCs from the graft migrate to the lymph nodes and trigger allo-specific T cells (CD4 and CD8), which start the rejection processes (killing graft cells) that also include B cells and antibodies. If we analyze deeper the molecular difference between the donor and recipient we can see that main variability lies in their MHC molecules. It might be counterintuitive, but let us analyze the facts first. For example, donor antigens like enzymes or cellular housekeeping proteins (and their peptides) may be almost indistinguishable between the donor and recipient. Indeed, some enzymes might have allelic variants and be special just for a particular person or a group of individuals. In comparison to the allelic variability of MHC molecules, the variability of non-MHC (or so-called house-keeping) alleles is very much lower not only in humans but in almost every species of mammals. Therefore, the recognition of the antigenic peptide does not play the most important role during the immuno logic rejection of the transplanted graft; however the MHC difference does. We have already called the MHC of another individual an allo-MHC. Similarly, a donor-derived graft is called allograft. Autologous graft is a transplanted tissue from host to host, and it will not be immunologically rejected, as it is an iso-graft. The reason is simple; all auto-reactive (iso-specific) T cells (and B cells) have been clonally removed from the repertoire of the host. This is not the case with allo-reactive T and B cells. They are still present, and can mount the immune response to transplanted allo-graft (or foreign tissue, or organ).

At the molecular level, let us consider the difference recognized by allo-specific TCRs. There is a multitude of allo-derived peptides that have a very low affinity for the contact surface with the (allo-reactive) TCR. The highest TCR affinity is towards the structures on allo-MHC (α-helices) molecules to which the (allo-specific) TCR binds.

Therefore, acute graft rejection can be avoided if the differences between donor and recipient MHC alleles are reduced to a minimum. Although this is theoretically essential, it is almost impossible to completely accomplish in practice. For organ and tissue transplantation, the practical goal is to find a match of a limited number of the major types of the MHC genes (for class I: HLA-A, -B, and -C, and for class II: HLA-DQ, -DR, -DP). Chronic graft rejection is a result of this imperfect practical consensus. Several MHC differences can give a long-term rejection symptoms; however, some might be nearly undetectable.

There is a worldwide organization with national institutions for tissue typing that communicates and publishes lists of potential donors and recipients of organs through their own networks. Its role is to quickly find suitable organs for transplantation with the lowest risk of rejection. In practice, it is difficult to find a perfect match or even fairly well HLA-matched organs. There is a high demand for donated organs. The organization has therefore lowered the match criteria to a minimum requirement. For ethical reasons, over the past decades, organ transplantations were made where the donor and recipient were less than 100% of the minimum of matching MHC alleles. Some of the observed postoperative courses of mismatched transplanted combinations were surprising, because the results turned out better than expected (grafts stayed longer), although it is still not known why. Most likely the reason for it lies in the intricacies of the immune system function. Nevertheless, these results have improved the existing criteria for transplantation of both solid organs and bone marrow.

Although matching histocompatibility (MHC) genes is important for avoiding the rejection of transplanted organs, it is believed that we would find better anti-rejection treatments in the future. Nowadays, general immunosuppressive therapy after transplantation is commonly in use (like, e.g., drugs such as cyclosporine, corticosteroids) alone, or in combination with living in isolation from microorganisms. We need a better knowledge about the regulation of the immune system at the molecular and cellular (communication) levels, as well as how to make specific tolerance to graft. These are the challenges for the development of new pharmacologic agents against graft rejection in the future.

MHC Associations with Diseases

MHC genes have been associated with almost all autoimmune diseases, which have as a pathologic feature the generation of autoantibodies against self-antigens, causing symptoms in relation to affected tissues that express such antigens. MHC genes are in linkage disequilibrium with each other, which means that they are inherited as a block of alleles on a single chromosome, which we call a haplotype. Thus, for example, DR3 haplotype denotes a specific set of class II alleles that are inherited as a block (DR3 = DRB1-03 allele linked with DQB1-02 and with DQA1-0501 alleles). On the other hand, DR4 is a haplotype that contains DRB1-04 allele together with the DQB1-0302 and DQA1-0301 alleles. Furthermore, DR7 haplotype contains the DRB1-07 allele linked with DQB1-02 and with DQA1-02 alleles. The DRB1-DQB1-DQA1 gene block has in HLA haplotypes "DR14" and "DR15" the following alleles (14-06-0102) and (15-06-01), respectively. Lastly, DQ2 and DQ8 are descriptions of single alleles, namely DQ2 = DQB1-0201 and DQ8 = DQB1-0302.

The HLA alleles and haplotypes associated with autoimmunity are as follows (some alleles can be protective and some predisposing to disease).

Predisposing Haplotypes and Alleles

Addison's disease—HLA-DR3;

Ankylosing spondylitis—HLA-B27 (B-2701, B-2704, B-2705);

Coeliac disease—HLA-DQ2 and -DQ8;

Diabetes mellitus type 1—HLA-DR3 and -DR4, and HLA-B (B-39, B-18) and HLA-A (A-24);
Graves' disease—HLA-DR3 (DRB1-08), HLA-C (C-07), and HLA-B8 (B-08);
Hemochromatosis—HLA-A3;
Hashimoto's thyroiditis—HLA-DR4 (and -DR3);
Multiple sclerosis—HLA-DR15, HLA-C (C-05, and C-15);
Myasthenia gravis—HLA-DR3;
Rheumatoid arthritis—HLA-alleles as follows: DRB1-0101, -0102, -0401, -0404, -0405, -0408, -1001, -1402);
Systemic lupus erythematosus—HLA-DR3, -DR8, and -DR15.

Protecting Haplotypes and Alleles
Addison's disease—none;
Ankylosing spondylitis—HLA-B27(B-2706, B-2709);
Coeliac disease—none;
Diabetes mellitus type 1—HLA-DR14 and -DR15, and HLA-A (A-01, A-11, A-31);
Graves' disease—HLA-DR7, HLA-C16, HLA-C03 and HLA-B44;
Hemochromatosis—HLA-A3;
Hashimoto's thyroiditis—HLA-DR7;
Multiple sclerosis—HLA-DR14, HLA-C (C-01);
Myasthenia gravis—none;
Rheumatoid arthritis—HLA-DR3 (DRB1-0103, -07, -1201, -1301, -1501);
Systemic lupus erythematosus—none.

The research is narrowing on finding additional associations that can either protect from disease or predispose to, and on detailing the nature of such interactions. For the latter, the peptide epitopes that are associated (or embedded) in the clefts of the associated alleles with particular diseases have been carefully analyzed. As an example, in RA, the associated haplotypes are (MHC class II) DR3 and DR4. In them, a particular HLA-DRB1 (-0401) allele might harbor some citrullinated peptides derived from self-proteins (e.g., *enolase*).

In other autoimmune diseases that show association with the HLA haplotypes, a different type of peptides (i.e., modified by transglutaminase, like in celiac disease, or any other putative peptide-modifying enzyme) could be the culprit for breaking the T cell tolerance, and thus be perhaps responsible for the onset of the disease.

Such knowledge is important for developing novel treatments of auto-immune diseases, as well as providing an understanding about their causes. If we can comprehend the rules of the mechanism by which these cells oper-ate in the body and what controls them, then we might devise a strategy to combat not only autoimmunity, or help acceptance of transplanted tissues and organs, but also to fight cancer, if we could turn the strategy around.

Nonconventional MHC Molecules

Nonconventional MHC (HLA-E, F, G etc.) and other related molecules (like CD-1) are transmembrane glycoproteins that have very similar confor-mation to the classic ones (HLA-A,-B,-C or HLA-DR,-DP,-DQ), but there are some important differences. One that has an important functional relevance (for recognition) is in the spacing between two α-helices (facing outward of the cell) as well as their length and position on the β-plated sheet. Because of that, there is not much space for fitting in peptides, and thus their clefts are empty. On the other hand, several like CD1 molecules have clefts into which smaller molecules such as lipids can fit. Some of these nonconventional MHC molecules can bind γδTCR much like the αβTCR can to classical MHC molecules.

In addition it is important to mention MICA/MICB MHC class-I like molecule that is induced by stress on epithelial cell line. It does not associate with β-2 microglobulin, and does not bind antigenic peptides. It might be involved in recognition of danger, or stressed cells.

CORECEPTORS OF T CELLS: CD4 AND CD8

CD4 T cells recognize MHC class II molecules (on APCs) by double bind-ing event: (1) with its TCR receptor to peptide/MHC ligand and (2) with the CD4 molecule that binds to a different site (than TCR) on the class II molecule. Analogously, CD8 T cells utilize CD8 molecules that bind to class I molecules. The coreceptor binding sites on MHC proteins are located near the TCR binding site, usually on the same MHC molecule, but a little closer to the cell membrane of APCs. CD4 and CD8 are called coreceptors, because they nonspecifically bind all allelic forms of MHC molecules. CD4 molecule binds class II, and CD8 binds class I MHC molecules. Moreover, they support specific T-cell recognition by increasing the strength of adhe-sion with APCs (Figure 3-8).

Phagocytosed (endocytosed, engulfed) antigen and its processed peptide is usually presented by class II (MHC) molecules (on APCs). On the other

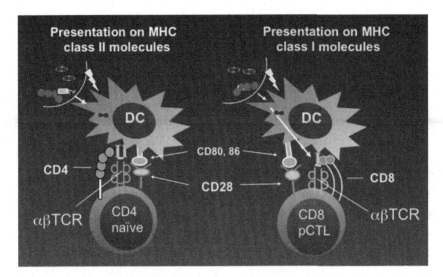

Figure 3-8 Activation of T cells: Antigen presentation on antigen-presenting cells. For MHC I molecules, presentation of internalized antigens is called *cross-presentation*.

hand, protein synthesized within the cell (self or viral) is degraded after some time, and its peptides presented, as the rule, by the class I (MHC) molecules. However, an exception to this rule is called cross–presentation, and it also occurs when MHC class I molecules present endocytosed antigen (Figure 3-8). The latter happens mostly in professional APCs like DCs (that migrate from tissues to lymph nodes or spleen) and very rarely in macrophages or B cells.

COSTIMULATION DURING T-CELL ACTIVATION

Costimulatory molecules on APCs are CD80 and CD86 (B7 is the older name). There are a number of molecules with similar function (including PD-1, CTLA-4), but their cellular distribution is narrow and the physiological role is still incompletely understood. Both costimulatory molecules CD80/86 bind to the CD28 molecule—which is their receptor on resting T cells (Figure 3-8). It is interesting to note that during the subsequent phases of activation, CD28 is no longer expressed, and some T cells begin to express CTLA-4 (CD152). CD152 also binds CD80/86 costimulatory molecules (and with higher affinity). At this stage, CD152/CD28 interaction acts as a brake for proliferation of activated CD4 T lymphocytes. Furthermore, it is important to mention the CD40 molecules on presenting cells such as DCs. They may increase the proliferation (stimulation) of

T cells; however, the interaction with CD40 is only possible when T cells express its ligand—CD40L (CD154)—on the cell surface. The expression starts as a result of activation of T cells. This usually happens after one day in experiments with cell cultures. Thus, the expression of CD152 and CD154 is one of the "conversation-like" events between APCs and T lymphocytes, and it is not a condition under which the quiescent T cells get activated.

SIGNAL TRANSDUCTION IN T CELL

Supramolecular Complexes and Immunologic Synapse

Binding to the peptide/MHC ligand on APCs' surface of a molecular complex that consists of TCR, CD3, and CD4 (or CD8) molecules on T-cell surface (Figure 3-9) collects the latter into lipid rafts called supramolecular

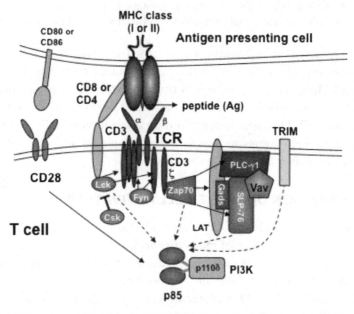

Figure 3-9 Signal transduction after T-cell activation. MHC (*major histocompatibility complex*); TCR (T-cell receptor); Ag (antigen); Lck (*lymphoid cell kinase*); Csk (*C-terminal Src kinase*); Fyn: tyrosin kinase of Src family; Zap70 (*zeta-associated protein of 70 kDa*); LAT (*linker for activation of T cells*); PLC-γ1 (phospholipase C-γ1); Gads (*Grb2 [growth factor receptor-bound protein 2]-related adapter downstream of Shc [SH2 domain-containing transforming protein]*); SLP-76 (*SH2 domain containing leukocyte specific phosphoprotein of 76 kDa*); Vav (exchange factor of Rho-family of GTP-ases); TRIM (*T cell receptor interacting molecule*); PI3K (*phosphatidyl-inositol-6-kinase*); p110δ: catalytic subunit of PI3K; p85: regulatory subunit of PI3K.

activation cluster (SMAC). The SMAC complex is surrounded by a circular strip of molecules important for an adhesive link between two interacting cells, called LFA-1 and ICAM-1. The contact area between the T cell and APC is also called immunological synapse. After a few minutes of interaction, the CD28 molecules on T cells (that is in contact with B7 molecules [CD80, CD86]) on the APC penetrate from the edge of the SMAC into the central parts of the synapse where they form a ring around the center (where TCR/CD3/CD4 is in contact with peptide/MHC ligand). Lipid rafts are parts of the cell membrane of T cells in the immune synapses with characteristic lipid (membrane that gives greater strength).

Signal transduction and transmission of the signal inside the cell is very complicated and many details are still unknown. Therefore, the simplified version of the intracellular signaling after the initiation event, which we call activation of resting T cell, will be described. The first change is usually registered within a few seconds and it manifests itself as rising of calcium ion concentration in the cytoplasm. The concentration of Ca^{2+} decreases after the peak values to a lower level and remains elevated during the period of activation. After a few hours, one can observe the *de novo* synthesis of proteins that regulate growth, development, and communication of activated T cells including cytokine production.

The first signaling events within the T cells (after binding of TCR and coreceptors to their respective targets on the APC) are molecular interactions involving the CD3 complex. CD3 consists of four different chains that associate with TCR, but do not form a covalent bond with it. The whole complex has two heterodimers, gamma-epsilon (γ ε) and delta-epsilon (δ ε), and one homodimer, zeta-zeta (ζ ζ). Although all are trans-membrane proteins, the bulk of CD3 chains are located within the cytosol. There are segments within the CD3 molecules that contain characteristic sequences around the key tyrosine amino acid called ITAM sequences. ITAMs are specifically recognized by the phosphokinase enzyme, which phosphorylates tyrosines at these sites. These events cause a change in conformation. The consequence is that CD3 acquires the ability to interact with some other intracellular protein messengers. ITAM phosphorylation can lower or increase the binding affinity for a potential molecular partner.

Initiation of the Activation Signal

Signal transduction from αβTCR on the cell surface (in SMACs) into the interior of the cells is shown in Figure 3-9. It is a simplified version of events that begins with tyrosine phosphorylation of zeta chain in the CD3 complex with Lck kinase, and continues with inclusion of a number of factors. The signaling is in balance with phosphatases that reverse the phosphorylation event on tyrosines. When the balance is set on "activate" (ON), then the cascade of signals runs towards the nucleus via numerous intermediaries. Here we include tyrosine kinases Lck and Fyn, phospholipase PLCγ, phosphatidyl–inositol–3–phosphate kinase (PI3K), mitogen–activated kinases (MAPK), adapters (Gads, LAT, SLP-76, Vav, TRIM, Carma1, BCL10, Malt1 etc.), and finally the transcription factors NFAT, AP-1 and NF-κB (Figures 3-9 and 3-10).

On the other hand, CD28 signaling activates the PI3K isoform p110delta (p110δ) that causes regulatory effects. Unfortunately, not all factors in the signal transduction are known, and all controlling, modulating or

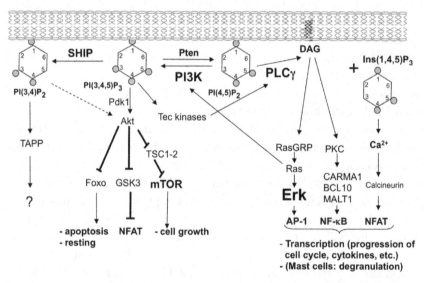

Figure 3-10 Actions of PLCγ (phospholipase Cγ) or PI3K (phosphatidylinositol-3 kinase) during signal transduction in T cell. Arrows denote activation, whereas stop lines, inhibition. **AP-1** (*activator protein-1*), **NFAT** (*nuclear factor of activating T cells*), and **NF-κB** (nuclear factor-κB) are transcription factors. **SHIP**: PIP3 phosphatase (*Src homology [SH2] domain-containing inositol phosphatase*); **Pten**: PIP3 phosphatase (*phosphatase and tensin homolog deleted on chromosome ten*); **DAG**: diacylglycerol; **PI(3,4,5)P3**: phosphatidylinositol-triphosphate; **PI(x,y)P2**: phosphatidylinositol-diphosphate; **Ins(1,4,5)P3**: inositol-triphosphate; Akt: protein kinase; PKC: protein kinase C; Ras: (*rat sarcoma*); Erk: (*extracellular signal-regulated kinase*) mitogen activated protein kinase (MAPK); CARMA1 (caspase recruitment domain membrane-associated guanylate kinase 1) adapter; BCL 10 (B cell chronic lymphocytic leukemia/lymphoma 10) adapter; MALT1 (mucosa-associated lymphoid tissue 1) adapter.

regulatory signals are also not completely understood. For example, the regulation of Lck kinase involves tyrosine kinase CSK (C-terminal Src kinase), which inhibits the Lck enzymatic activity. CSK can be induced by signals that generate cAMP in T cells. It is also important to mention staurosporine, which inhibits Fyn tyrosine kinase.

The functions of signaling molecules can be understood by studying their mutations. So, for example, mutation in LAT (*linker for activation of T cells*) gene, which inactivates the amino acid where phosphorylation takes place during the signal transduction, prevents recruitment of other factors listed in Figure 3-9 in lipid rafts. So signal transduction via LAT prevents activation of T cells (that has started through TCRs). Mice deficient in LAT gene have a complete block in thymic development of T lymphocytes at the DN (double negative) stage (see *T cell development,* Chapter 2, p. 44).

The Role of Phosphatidyl-Inositol Triphosphate Derivatives

Further signal transduction involves activation of phospholipase PLCγ1, which creates di-acyl-glycerol (DAG) and inositol triphosphate (IP3 or Ins[1,4,5]P_3). DAG and IP3 have important effects in the signal transduction (right side of Figure 3-10), and we will mention the most important details of their signaling pathways.

DAG activates protein kinase C (PKC, of which there are 13 known isoforms—their occurrence depends probably on the stage of development and the microenvironment) resulting in (through the activation of several other factors) the activation of nuclear factor-κB (NF-κB). In addition, DAG activates a cascade of mitogen-activated protein kinases (MAPK), such as Erk (*extracellular signal-regulated kinase*) through Ras factor (Rat sarcoma factor, which is encoded by a gene of the retrovirus that causes cancer in rats), and this path of signaling ends with activation of the AP-1 (*activator protein-1; fos/jun*) nuclear factor. Unlike DAG, the IP3 releases Ca^{2+} from internal cellular storages. Calcium ions activate a phosphatase *calcineurin*, which in turn activates NFAT (*nuclear factor of activating T cells*). NFAT, AP-1, and NF-κB factors enter into the nucleus where they activate genes that have binding sites for them in the promoters.

The joint action of these factors causes cell-cycle progression and cytokine synthesis (Figure 3-10) among which the most notable are IL-2, IFN-γ, and IL-4. There are other cytokines that activated T cells can produce. There are several subsets of T helper cells that can be distinguished by the production of particular pattern of cytokines and these include IL-3, IL-4, IL-5, IL-10, and IL-13 for $T_{helper2}$ (Th2) subset, IL-9 for Th9 subset, IL-17 and IL-22 for Th17 and Th22 subsets, respectively, whereas IL-10 and TGF-β cytokines are shared by at least two different kinds of regulatory CD4 T cells. It is further important to note that the described signaling induces production and cell surface expression of the alpha chain of the IL-2 receptor (CD25), together with markers of early T-cell activation, such as CD40 ligand (CD154, CD40L), CD44, and CD69, and creates smaller isoforms of the CD45RA phosphatase in the cell membrane (a transition from CD45-RA into the CD45-RB or -RC forms). CD45RA phosphatase has a function that allows repeated TCR signaling. Namely, it can de-phosphorylate CD3-zeta chain within the TCR-CD3 complex, and thus allow the reuse of the same molecules for signaling.

PTEN (*phosphatase and tensin homologue deleted on chromosome ten*) phosphatase activity converts phosphatidyl-inositol triphosphate (PIP3) into PIP2, and the latter is a substrate for phosphatidyl-inositol 3 kinase (PI3K). PI3K catalyzes reactions that counter the activity of PTEN (left side of the Figure 3-10). On the other hand, PIP3 acts through Akt factor (and many other mediators of which it is important to mention Foxo, GSK3, and mTOR) whose balance further makes T cell either to remain in a resting phase or grow and divide. In particular, mTOR (target of Rapamycin) factor is thereby inhibited as well as the growth of cells. Another PIP3 phosphatase—SHIP (*Src [Rous sarcoma virus] homology [SH2] domain-containing and inositol phosphatase*) enzyme catalyzes the formation of PIP2 isoforms, whose many actions and significance are still not completely known. PIP3 levels are strictly regulated in the cell, because the disturbance of the amount of either PTEN or SHIP creates immunopathology in experimental mice. In particular, heterozygous lack of either PTEN or SHIP phosphatases (or both) can create a progressive lympho-proliferative syndrome, hyper-gammaglobulinemia, and autoimmune symptoms.

PI3K and Treg Cells

PI3K is also involved in the activation of T cells. P110 isoform δ is considered important for the action of Treg cells (in the induction of immune suppression). Particularly, in mice, poor functional allele of PI3K p110δ causes (autoimmune?) colitis similar to that with the lack of TCR, the symptoms of which are lost after injection of Treg cells with a fully functional allele of this kinase.

However, an alternative explanation is that Tregs are nonexistent as a physiologic entity, but one of the stages of further development of T lymphocytes upon activation. In such a context, PI3K p110δ would participate in a hypothetical negative feedback upon activation of T cells (activation that subsequently would cause a halt of the same). According to this idea, activated T cells after reaching maximum activation (in a few hours or days) would accumulate enough PI3K p110δ enzymes to overcome the effect of PLCγ1 signaling pathway (Figures 3-9 and 3-10). The result would be accumulation of PIP3, and that would have an assumed effect on the cell to enter one of three possible pathways deciding on its fate: to reach the resting phase, or to die by apoptosis, or to become a memory cell (see *"Further development of immune cells upon activation,"* p. 83). It is not excluded that some other factors in the microenvironment might tip the balance in the choice between these three outcomes (like, e.g., inactivation of Tec kinases; Figure 3-10). Thus, the Tregs might hypothetically be formed during activation of normal peripheral T cells if they revert to resting state too early. Such ("half-activated") T cells would no longer be able to help the growth and development of neighboring cells, but would, on the contrary, suppress them (by direct contact and/or secretion of inhibitory factors), and that would be similar to the definition of Tregs. Many assume that such a scenario is happening and the cells are called induced Treg (iTreg), which are different from natural counterparts (nTregs). This idea also agrees with the observation that mice with low functional allele encoding PI3K p110δ fail to secrete IL-10 by T cells (for the function of IL-10, see section: *Important control functions of cytokines*, Chapter 4, p. 106). In conclusion, the alternative hypothesis for the development of Treg-like cells is that the activation of T lymphocytes can create intracellular negative feedback in signaling, the one that would be transformed in the extracellular positive feedback mechanism (*vicious circle*). The result would be the inhibition (suppression) of immunity to, for example, a range of antigens carried by some microorganisms or self-tissues that need to be tolerated or to escape autoimmunity, respectively.

Transcription Factors NFAT, NF-κB, Fos, Rel, and Jun

Inhibition of the NFAT signaling pathway creates a general immunosuppression, which is different from the pathways described above. Cyclosporine binds to calcineurin phosphatase (Figure 3-10) and prevents its activation by calcium. The consequence is a suppression of NFAT factor that in turn cannot exert its action; that is, it does not bind to sites in various gene promoters, like for example that in the IL-2 gene. This general immunosuppression prevents all T-cell activation and thus also B cell immunity to T-dependent antigens. Cyclosporines and similar pharmacologic compounds (FK506) are used as standard therapy that requires strong inhibition of T-cell immunity, such as after organ transplants.

NF-κB is a group of heterodimeric factors with a role in cell survival (Figure 3-10). They can be grouped according to the size of smaller subunits into two groups. Thus, NF-κB$_1$ has p50, whereas NF-κB$_2$ has the p52 subunit. The larger subunit has one of three proteins called RelA, RelB, and c-Rel. All are of the same size of 65 kDa (p65). Thus NF-κB$_1$ has three members, whose differences in function are not yet clear. In contrast, the NF-κB$_2$ has one member (RelA, p52), which is formed by the activation of Treg cells (CD25$^+$, Foxp3$^+$).

Master Regulators of Differentiation T-bet, GATA-3, RORyt, Bcl6, IRF4, FoxP3

T-Bet

Nuclear factor T-bet is increased in activated T cells of Th1-type responses, by the action of Th1-type cytokines such as IFN-γ. T-bet binds to the promoter of a gene encoding the IL-12 receptor B2 (IL12RB2).

GATA-3

On the other hand, GATA-3 is a nuclear factor that is induced (after activation in naïve T lymphocytes) by Th2-type cytokines (such as IL-4, IL-13, IL-19, IL-20, and IL-22) and guides development of Th2 type response.

RORγt

RORγt nuclear factor is a master regulator of differentiation of Th17 cells. The Th17 cells are responsive to IL-1R1 and IL-23R signaling.

Bcl6

Bcl6 is a nuclear factor that is master regulator of differentiation of T follicular helper cells. These are T cells found in edges of the B cell zones in secondary lymphoid tissues (germinal centers), and are important for the generation of antigen-specific effector and memory B cells. IL-6 and IL-21 are important for the induction of Tfh cells. CXCL13 is the chemokine that attracts Tfh to this location.

IRF4 (and PU.1)

The IRF4 is a candidate for master regulator of differentiation of Th9 cells together with PU.1.

FoxP3

This master regulation of differentiation is important in the generation of Treg cells. IL-2 cytokine is supporting the development of nTregs in the thymus, and maintains peripheral homeostasis of Tregs by signaling through IL-2Rβ (CD122). TGF-β induces FoxP3 expression in Th0 cells.

Communication Molecules CD28, CD152 (CTLA-4), ICOS, CD40L, and PD1

TRIM (Figure 3-9) has a role of a chaperone in attracting CTLA-4 (*cytotoxic T lymphocyte antigen-4*, CD152) molecule to the surface of cells (from the trans-Golgi network). CTLA-4 binds CD80 and CD86 with greater affinity than CD28 and thereby expels CD28 from the synapse. CTLA-4, when activated by binding CD80/86, strongly inhibits the response of T-cells. It seems that the arrival of CTLA-4 on the cell membrane creates a prerequisite for termination of T-cell activation (or inhibition of the next phases). CTLA-4 signaling seems to decrease IL-2 production and inhibits differentiation of Th1 and Th2 cells, whereas it induces iTreg generation.

In addition, the B7-H2 molecule (also called an inducible costimulator [ICOS]-ligand, which is a CD28-homolog) are shown to co-stimulate generation of Th2 cells, and probably also influence differentiation of Th1 or Th17 cells. ICOS molecules are found on activated T cells, but not on resting ones. B7-H2 molecules are expressed on classical APCs (DCs, macrophages, B cells) and many epithelial cells.

Crosslinking ICOS induces CD40L on activated T cells. The CD40L is upregulated by IL-2 and inhibited by IL-4. CD40 ligand (CD40L, CD154) on T cells can interact with APCs (DC, MΦ or B cells) by binding to CD40, which, for example, can prolong the life of interacting DCs in the lymph nodes for 3–5 days (superinduction), thus strengthening the immune response. Linking CD40 on B cells, follicular Tfh cells stimulate the growth and survival of B cells in the germinal centers. It should be noted, however, that immunization with a low dose antigen fails to induce CD40L during the T-cell stimulation that results with the generation of Th2 subpopulation.

Programmed death-1 molecule (PD-1) belongs to CD28/CTLA-4 family of molecules expressed on T cells, B cells, and macrophages. It is a co-inhibitory molecule in the interactions between T cells and APCs. Compared to CTLA-4 it inhibits more broadly the T cell responses. It seems that co-inhibitory action would stop or prevent T-cell activation started by TCR-peptide/MHC ligand (signal 1) interaction. This is done probably by recruiting SHP1 and SHP2 phosphatases to the cytosolic tails of PD-1 molecules. PD-1 has two ligands PD-1L and PD-L2. Both are expressed by DCs (and induced), whereas PD-L1 can be upregulated also on macrophages upon treatment with LPS and GM-CSF. PD-L1 is also upregulated on T and B cells after activation (via BCR/TCR). Cancer cells also express ligand for PD-1. Mice with ablated gene encoding PD-1 develop some form of autoimmune disease like *lupus-like glomerulonephritis* or *dilated cardiomyopathy*. Furthermore, it seems that PD-1 interaction with PD-1 ligands negatively regulates activation of CD8 T cells more than CD4 T cells.

SIGNAL TRANSDUCTION IN THE B CELL

Unlike T, B-lymphocyte activation (in germinal centers) starts with the first signal via BCR (antigen binding), the second signal being the help of CD4 T lymphocytes. The T–B interactions include a number of molecular bonds of which the most important are: (1) TCR–peptide/MHC ligand; (2) CD4–MHC; (3) CD28–CD80/86; (4) CD40L (CD154)–CD40; and (5) Secretion of cytokines in the immune synapse between T and B cells.

Molecular factors in B cells during BCR signal transduction are products of the genes similar or identical to those during the T-cell activation (compare Figure 3-9 with Figure 3-11). These include molecular adapters and enzymes that make cascades of phospho-kinases. Although different in the primary structure, many adapters are very similar to each other such as Syk and Zap70. Figure 3-11 emphasizes the interaction with T cells that contributes to the signal via MHC class II molecules, CD40, as well as possibly through cytokine receptors for cytokines secreted by CD4 T cells in the immunologic synapse.

Many pharmacological studies have been directed towards the modulation of expression of the above-mentioned signaling molecules. Namely, the

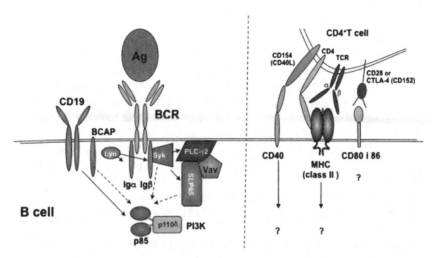

Figure 3-11 Signal transduction during activation of B lymphocytes. Dotted line separates additional signals in interaction with a helper T cell. BCR (B-cell receptor) is the antibody "anchored" in cell membrane with help of Igα i Igβ chains; Ag (antigen); Lyn: tyrosine kinase of Src family; Syk (spleen tyrosine kinase); PLC-γ2 (phospholipase C-γ2); SLP-65 (*SH2 domain containing leukocyte specific phosphoprotein of 65 kDa*); Vav (exchange factors for Rho-family of GTP-ases); PI3K (*phosphatidylinositol-6-kinase*); p110δ: catalytic subunit PI3K; p85: regulatory subunit PI3K; BCAP (*B cell adapter for PI3K*).

goals would be to disrupt T-B connection and produce specific inhibition of B-cell responses. This is justified as a therapeutic option in the treatment of autoimmune disorders where abnormal antibodies are present in the patient.

SIGNAL TRANSDUCTION IN MAST CELLS

Mast cells can become specific immune cells provided they bind by their Fc receptors the antibodies of the IgE class (see *Mast cells*, Chapter 2, p. 36). Thereby mast cells acquire weapons for a very quick response and attack on intruders who carry a specific antigen that can be recognized by IgE. This mechanism results in degranulation and the release of mediators including histamine. Factors in signal transduction are analogous or similar to those in T and B cells (Figure 3-12).

Summary

A. Lymphocyte activation is a process that usually starts with specific recognition of antigen or peptide/MHC ligand by B or T cells, respectively. We call it the "first" activation signal. This signal is sufficient to trigger (release) the effector T and B cells' function. However, for the activation of quiescent cells (naïve and resting memory cells) it is necessary, but not sufficient. To complete the activation process, additional signals are required.

B. Antigen receptors of B lymphocytes can recognize different conformations on the surface of macromolecules (antigens; i.e., proteins and polysaccharides).

C. T cells recognize particular conformation of macromolecules comprising antigenic peptide residing in the cleft of MHC molecule(s) by binding to this shape with $\alpha\beta$TCR.

D. CD4 T cells recognize by $\alpha\beta$TCR the complex of MHC class II molecules with peptide of about 6–8 amino acids in length.

E. CD8 T cells recognize the complex of MHC class I molecules with a peptide of 13–18 amino acids in length via their $\alpha\beta$TCR.

F. CD4 is a coreceptor, because it participates in recognizing antigen by binding to a conserved domain of the class II MHC; CD8 is coreceptor, because it joins in recognition of antigen by binding conserved moiety of the class I MHC. Coreceptor attaching sites on the MHC molecules differ from those to which TCR binds, but are located on the same molecule of MHC that is in contact with it.

G. Binding sites for TCR to MHC molecules have a similar general conformation, which differ in fine structure, because there are several hundreds of alleles of MHC class I and class II genes in almost all species that possess them.

H. MHC (HLA) molecules are polygenic and polymorphic (they have large numbers of alleles in a species). Hence they are highly confident genetic markers of individuality, but on the other hand they are a problem for organ and tissue transplantation (because they need to be matched in order to avoid rejection).

I. The "second" signals for activation of naïve lymphocytes are thought to be costimulatory molecules for T lymphocytes (including CD80/86), and for B cells –help by helper CD4 T lymphocytes. Other molecules including various cytokines are considered to have a modulating function and some call them a "third" signal.

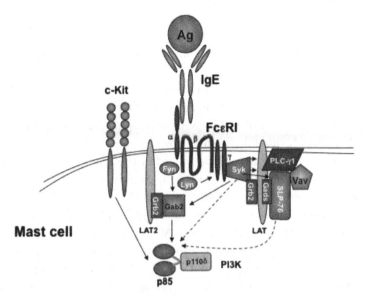

Figure 3-12 Signal transduction during activation of mast cells. Ag (antigen); IgE (immunoglobulin, epsilon isotype); FcεRI: receptor-1 for Fc part of IgE molecule (α, β, γ); c-Kit: receptor-tyrosine kinase for stem cell factor SCF. Fyn and Lyn: tyrosine kinase of Src family; Syk (spleen tyrosine kinase); LAT (*linker for activation of T cells*); LAT2 (*LAT, member 2*); PLC-γ1 (phospholipase C-γ1); Grb2 (*growth factor receptor-bound protein 2*); Gab2 (*Grb2-associated binding protein2*); Gads (*Grb2-related adapter downstream of Shc [SH2 domain-containing transforming protein]*); PLC-γ1 (phospholipase C-γ1); SLP-76 (*SH2 domain containing leukocyte specific phosphoprotein of 76 kDa*); Vav (exchange factor for Rho-family of GTP-ases); PI3K (*phosphatidylinositol-6-kinase); p110δ*: catalytic subunit of PI3K; p85: regulatory subunit of PI3K.

FURTHER DEVELOPMENT OF IMMUNE CELLS UPON ACTIVATION

Descendants of a clone that has been activated have two choices. Either continue to develop and express new morphological and functional differences with regard to the mother cell, or homeostatically divide under a slow pace (without acquiring new markers or functions). Those that developed further, according to the strict definition, the appearance of new markers means that they would no longer be of the same clone. However, we still use the term "clone" since all the descendants still carry the same receptor specificity, which is the most important feature of the immune cells. Peripheral development of specific clones can move through several stages. The last step of the development of specific clones of B or T lineage cells have either effector or memory functions, and most of the effector cells undergo apoptosis over time, after an initial burst of proliferation, which is a usual consequence of the immune response following infection (Figure 3-13).

We can distinguish three main phases of CD4$^+$T, CD8$^+$T, and B cells: (1) precursors or naïve (virgin) cells; (2) activated stage; and (3) effector cells. Activated cells are a transitional stage of development that lasts a few days. The cells appear larger (blasts) than unstimulated cells, because of rapid growth and cycling (persistent division). After the activation stage, effector B and effector CD8 T cells become again smaller in size being similar to naïve ones, but only in size, as they express different markers. All stages secrete cellular mediators and factors, and helper T cells (activated and effector CD4 T) up to 20 different cytokines. After proliferation, the CD4 T cells differentiate into different types of effectors, by which we define types of immune response. This happens under the influence of cytokines, signals from APCs and the microenvironment. Effector cells have a distinct range of cytokine production and secretion. So far, for peripheral CD4 T lymphocytes, this is the safest and sometimes the only way by which we can distinguish their developmental stages. Thus, helper CD4 T cells can be grouped into several groups as a result of activation, which are considered to be the final stages of their differentiation. Initially, there were just a few groups that

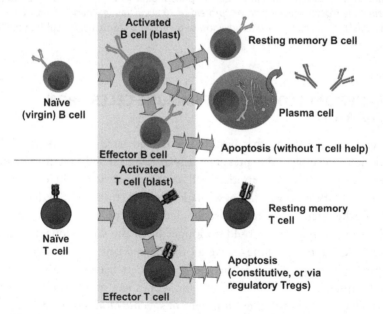

Figure 3-13 Peripheral development of lymphocytes after their activation.

were named in sequential order, like Th1, Th2, Th3. However, recently, the groups tend to bear a name that relates to their function or after the major cytokine product, such as Th9, Th17, and Th22.

Types of Effector Cells

The following types of effector cells have been described so far:

1. The effector helper CD4$^+$ T cells (T helper) type 1, 2, 3, 9, 17, and type 22 (Th1, Th2, Th3, Th9, Th17, and Th22), the follicular helper Tfh cells (in germinal centers), the regulatory type 1 (Tr1), natural T regulatory (nTreg), induced T regulatory (iTreg) as well as CD4$^+$CD25$^+$Foxp3$^+$ (*Forkhead/winged helix transcription factor, Foxp3*) type (Treg) of regulatory cells.
2. Effector cytotoxic CD8$^+$ T cells type 1 and type 2 (Tc1 and Tc2).
3. Germinal center B cells.
4. Plasma cells (antibody-secreting B lymphocyte lineage).

Ad 1

In lymph nodes (Figure 3-14) or spleen white pulp (Figure 3-15), effector CD4$^+$T cells (of type 1) help the development of effector cytotoxic CD8 T cells. Namely, activated naïve CD8 T cells (via TCR and costimulatory signals) need additionally a CD4 signal to proliferate. Hence this kind of "help" is called *licensing* to distinguish it from the B-cell help function of CD4 T cells. Licensing is mainly provided by Th1 type of helper T cells when they

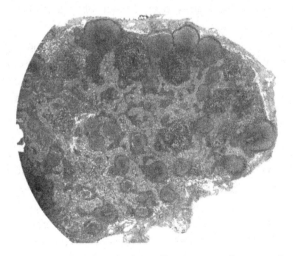

Figure 3-14 Human lymph node (magnification × 1.6; hematoxylin–eosin).

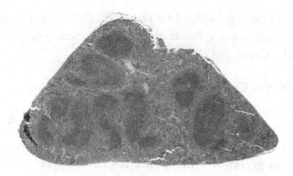

Figure 3-15 Mouse spleen (magnification × 2; hematoxylin–eosin).

interact with CD8 T precursors usually sharing the same APC (DC) in the paracortex of lymph nodes, for example, in the course of viral infection.

In lymphatic tissues, CD4$^+$T effector cells (T helper cells of various types) help B cells to develop into plasma cells. The help is mainly based on direct contact between B-T cells accompanied by the secretion of many cytokines (including IL-2 and IL-4). It is thought that Th2 type is involved by default in this process. Other helper types usually help B cells to develop different classes of antibodies. This is induced by cytokines during somatic hypermutation of BCRs in B cells in germinal centers. An organism uses the switch to another class of Ig to better fit the defense against microbes (see below, *Ad 3*, p. 87).

In somatic tissues (outside lymphatic germinal centers), Th1 effector cells have two main jobs: (a) activation of macrophages (by IFN-γ); and (or) (b) killing neighboring cells by Fas-Ligand (FasL, CD95L). Through these actions Th1 promote inflammation and rejection of dangerous intruders. The activation of macrophages involves secreting IFN-γ, usually triggered by molecular interaction involving TCR binding to its ligand (antigenic peptide in clefts of MHC class II molecules). Therefore, the effector CD4 T cells in their contact with macrophages do not need any more a costimula-tory (second) signal (by binding of CD28 to either CD80 or CD86) to execute their functions. We will refer to this kind of stimulation as "trigger-ing" (in other words, activation without a need for the second signal).

Furthermore, in order to kill target cells (the other effector function), CD4 T cells require expression of Fas molecule (CD95) on targets. The target cells also have to be in the neighborhood of the triggering interaction (effector CD4 T–macrophage). Since there can be many effector cells of the same clone surrounding such interaction, the CD4 T cells can cause killing of their own clone. This is so, because the activation of naïve CD4 T cells usually induces the appearance of Fas molecules on the cell surface (but, later than FasL expression). The killing of the same clone is called fratricide or suicide.

Effector Th17 cells recruit granulocytes by secreting IL-17 in tissues. There seems to be a balance between Th17 and regulatory T cells in tissues, but the controlling factors remain unknown. There are other kinds of effector helper cells, and their role will be described in Chapter 4 (Th9 and Th22 cells).

Tregs inhibit the activation of the previously mentioned CD4 T cells (specific for peptide/MHC ligand), through direct contact and/or by secretion of inhibitory cytokines such as IL-10 and NF-κβ. Tregs can do this by cross-inhibition (of neighboring clones) during the activation phases (in lymph nodes) or triggering phases (in tissues). For example, the antigenic peptide (p/MHC ligand) that "activates" Tregs need not necessarily be the same as the one that can activate (or trigger) previously mentioned CD4 Th1 or Th2 cells. For further discussion on the identity and role of Tregs, see: *T-cell development*, Chapter 2, p. 44, and *Theories about the function of the immune system*, Chapter 9, pp. 283–300).

Ad 2

The effector function of cytotoxic CD8 lymphocytes is recognizing targets in tissues (e.g., virus-infected cells) and killing them by direct contact provided targets were recognized. They utilize a special mechanism that induces apoptosis in target cells. It involves the secretion of perforin (which makes holes in the membrane of target cells) and insertion of serine proteases enzymes (so-called granzyme). The process is triggered by the recognition of the complex of antigenic peptide in clefts of the MHC class I molecules via TCR. Since MHC class I molecules are expressed by all somatic cells in a body with a nucleus, this is an efficient way of identifying those infected by microorganisms like viruses and intracellular bacteria. It is important to mention that for triggering these functions, costimulatory (second) signal is also not required (as for the effector CD4 T cells).

Ad 3

Germinal center B cells are known as centroblasts when they proliferate, and centrocytes when they stop. Germinal centers have a dark and light zone surrounded by the mantle zone (see germinal center in the tonsil, Figure 3-16). They can form in the lymph node follicles and they are a site

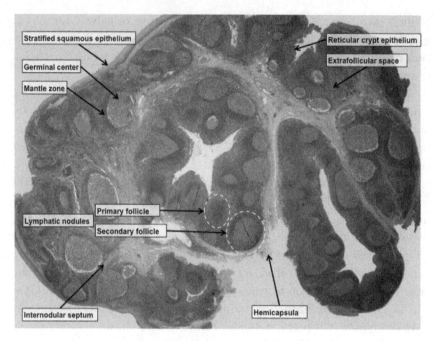

Figure 3-16 Human tonsil with germinal centers (hematoxylin–eosin).

where B cells become activated, proliferate, switch Ig class, and increase affinity for the antigen by somatic hypermutation. They constitute the primary T-B collaboration event. They proliferate as a result of their activation, which needs at least two events: recognition of antigen and help by T helper cells while recognizing the antigen. The first signal for the activation of B cells in germinal centers is the BCR–antigen interaction. Here the antigen is held by the antibody that is attached by its Fc portion to FDC in the light zone of the germinal center. In the dark zone, B cells (centroblasts) proliferate and undergo somatic hypermutation. Then they compete for the antigen binding on FDCs in the light zone, and only those that can attach themselves to the Ag-Ab-FDC complex, and in a due time window receive T-cell help will be rescued from death (apoptosis). It is clear here, that the tolerance to self-antigens works at the level of T-cell help. If there is no T-cell specific for the self-antigen, the self-specific (autoreactive, and potentially pathogenic autoimmune) B cells would not receive help and normally should be eliminated. Thus, only foreign (nonself) antigens should give successful T-B collaboration, in that B cells would differentiate into plasma cells to produce antibodies against the foreign antigen. In the course of this process, cytokines play an important role in promoting this development, and in addition control class switching of Ig isotypes.

Ad 4

Plasma cells secrete immunoglobulins and are terminally differentiated B lymphocytes. Immunoglobulins can destroy microbes (bacterial cells, viruses) directly by utilizing complement, or indirectly by guiding macrophages (and phagocytes) to express cytotoxic activity on cells marked by antibodies. Cells recognize Ig-labeled bacteria or viruses by binding to the Fc part of antibodies with Fc receptors.

Effector cells undergo blast phase (growth and proliferation) over the first several days after activation and are relatively large in size (cells are bigger than naïve immunocytes, but smaller than phagocytes). They are difficult to distinguish from other lymphocytes in tissues. There are markers, however (i.e., CD27), through which detection by immunohistochemistry or flow cytometry may suggest their belonging to a particular type of effector cells. Effector cells are usually difficult to distinguish from the next group of cells, which are called memory cells.

Memory Cells

They are divided into:
1. memory CD4 T cells;
2. memory CD8 T cells; and
3. memory B cells.

B- and T-cell memory cells are small and resting (with respect to cycling) but not stationary (they can re-circulate, i.e., from lymphatic to other tissues). The main task (with the exception of Tregs) for them is to be activated again upon encounter with the same antigen, and create an immune defense as soon as possible. This is called the secondary immune response (see *The course of the immune response*, Chapter 4, p. 105). The secondary activation is fast and it takes less than half of the time needed for the primary response. Such a rapid response is caused by already existing conditions: (a) recirculating memory cells in the body; (b) increased clonal number; and (c) in some cases a shortened activation pathway, like, for example, when memory B cells use a short-cut signaling to become plasma cells and secrete antibodies. The secondary immune response, in general, is characterized by the appearance of protective (neutralizing) antibodies in the blood or body fluids after 7 days, which means that the helper (CD4 T) response is also present a few days earlier than in the primary immune response. For viral diseases, in principle, secondary-response CD8 T cells can already be present in sufficient quantities after 6–8 days to destroy all virus-infected cells in an organism.

Not all infectious diseases have similar courses of the primary or secondary immune responses, as some microorganisms can modulate them. Furthermore, some hereditary immunodeficiencies can allow a number of microorganisms to cause diseases, because the immune defense is insufficient. In a dominant kind of immunodeficiency, the lack of a single gene can cause such symptoms. There is also a multifactorial genetic predisposition to immunodeficiency (e.g., only 10% of people can get sick from tuberculosis, but under severe decrease of immunocompetence, in acquired immunodeficiency caused by HIV virus, their percentage increases). There are many that are known; however, there should be still a number of yet unidentified immunocompetence genes.

Predilection for many (if not all) diseases can be modified by complex genetic inheritance of predisposing alleles. The genetic makeup can probably also modify severity of a disease, the latter's course as well as gender differences in predisposition to it.

The research on complex genetic susceptibility for diseases is in its infancy, and apart from the occasional known genetic factors (alleles) for several diseases, not much is known, although the last decade has shown increased progress. Of course, the phenotypic expression of each genotype is dependent on numerous environmental factors including nourishment, microorganisms, and the rest of the physical world, but the questions for research remain *how*, *why* and *to what extent*. For example, if just 60% of identical twins develop a disease (which has a predisposition involving many genes), then it is clear that the environment plays an important role in this disease development. We will probably witness a great increase in knowledge about susceptibility factors in the coming years due to *Next Gen* typing and sequencing techniques that will individualize medical research and open up novel therapies and health care opportunities.

Differences between Naïve, Effector, and Memory Immunocytes

For the development of T lymphocytes following activation, it is important to note that there is a difference between effector and memory cells in the accessory interactions with APCs during antigen (p/MHC ligand) recognition. The process of specific antigen (p/MHC ligand) recognition is in the central position for effector cells. This is identical to the activation of naïve (precursor) T lymphocytes. Differences between the activation of precursors on the one hand and eliciting the functions (triggering) of effector cells is that the latter does not need costimulatory molecules (CD28-CD80/86), nor additional factors from the microenvironment such as cytokines. Thus, the main difference between the activation of naïve T cells and the triggering of effector T cells is in the "second" signal. The role of cytokines in the triggering of effector-cell functions in tissues is still incompletely understood. Probably, cytokines can further regulate the type of the immune response in finer details (e.g., activation of innate immunity or other cells in vicinity), or they can silence the effectors. However, an additional type of signal was discovered (via membrane molecules) that many researchers also call costimulatory (and sometimes co-inhibitory). In order to avoid confusion, here we would use the term costimulation as a description of the activating "second" signal, because these other kinds of signal usually have an inhibitory influence on both cell function and "cross-talk" between T effector and the APCs. Although the role of such signals is not completely understood, they may stop immune responses, generate regulatory T cells or modulate B-cell responses. It has been suggested that they represent a kind of a negative feedback during the immune response, perhaps hindering potential autoreactivity, and thus contributing to maintaining individually suitable balance among clones of the immune repertoire.

Regarding the function of (resting) memory cells of both T and B cells, their activation requires (again) the two signals that are, in principle, equal to those during the activation of naïve cells. However, there seems to be a short cut for some resting memory B cells. Namely, the second signal (T-cell help) can be imitated by interactions with several different soluble mediators, making unnecessary help from CD4 T lymphocytes.

The latter might be similar to so-called T-independent antigens, which are usually multivalent and can induce cross-linking of BCR on naïve B lymphocytes. These antigens do not require the help of T lymphocytes (and hence the name) in order to elicit an immune response (that results with antibody production). Similarly, resting B-cell memory cells specific for the T-independent antigens do not need the second signal (T-cell help) for activation.

Research on regulation of the immune response is ongoing, as our knowledge about the immune system is still incomplete. Understanding these processes should come from discovering cytosolic mediators and defining all intracellular signal transduction pathways during the immune response. Likewise, the future therapeutic interventions aiming to control the immune system depend on this research.

During laboratory analysis of activated T cells it is important to distinguish effector cells from naïve and resting memory cells, as well as from B lymphocytes. As a marker of activated T cells the following molecules were used for flow cytometry: CD25, CD27, CD69, CD44, and CD45RA (RO, RA, RB, and RC).

Naïve T (CD45RA$^+$CD27$^+$) and memory T cells (CD45RA$^-$CD27$^+$) have homing receptors for colonizing the lymph nodes. Both have high frequency and number, but do not possess effector functions. Furthermore, cells rare in lymph nodes are the effector T cells (CD45RA$^-$CD27$^-$) and terminally differentiated effector T cells (CD45RA$^+$CD27$^-$) that express receptors for migration to inflamed tissues. They are mainly found in inflammatory areas of somatic tissues (outside lymphatic areas). Some researchers call the latter two groups *effector memory* T cells, and the memory T cells frequently found in lymph nodes (CD45RA$^-$CD27$^+$)—*central memory* T cells.

Summary

A. B lymphocytes after activation multiply and become effector B cells in germinal centers. During this process B cells have at least three fates: (1) they develop further into plasma cells, if successful in binding antigen (held by follicular dendritic cells in complex with antibodies); (2) they develop in memory cells, if they can bind antigen; and (3) undergo apoptosis, if they cannot bind to antigen.

B   T lymphocytes after activation multiply and become various types of effector cells that undergo apoptosis after a certain time or become memory cells.

C. The accessory costimulatory molecules are necessary for the activation of naïve and resting memory T cells, but not for triggering the function of effector T cells.

D. Tregs are thought to contribute in downregulating the clonal size of effector T cells after the infection has been dealt with (negative feedback).

T LYMPHOCYTE HOMEOSTASIS

Homeostatic or basic proliferation of T cells is required to keep normal concentrations of T lymphocytes in the blood ($1.5–3.5 \times 10^9$/L), tissues and body fluids, as well as to maintain a constant ratio between T-cell subgroups (i.e., CD4:CD8 = 2:1) found in humans and in other species. It is also called lymphopenic proliferation; because lymphopenia is a state with lower than normal blood concentration of lymphocytes.

Different types of T cells require various signals for homeostatic expansion. It is important to mention that it is not necessary to specifically recognize the whole part of the peptide/MHC ligand. Namely, specificity for antigenic peptides "does not matter" in TCR binding to peptide/MHC ligand. It is likely that any (usually self-derived) peptide that can fit and lie "flat" in the cleft of the MHC molecules would suffice for this interaction (such that perhaps it does not disturb TCR binding to alpha helices of the MHC molecules). (For details of the MHC–TCR interaction, see *Specific receptors for antigen (BCR and TCR), p. 59*).

Thus, naïve CD8$^+$T require binding to MHC class I molecules and cytokine IL-7. Similarly, naïve CD4$^+$T require MHC class II molecules together with IL-7, but they additionally need chemokine CCL21. Furthermore, CD4$^+$CD25$^+$FoxP3$^+$ Tregs can homeostatically divide by recognizing "flat" MHC II molecules under influence of cytokine IL-2.

Furthermore, in lymphopenia, CD4 and CD8 T memory cells can divide homeostatically without a need to interact with MHC molecules. This happens with the action of cytokines IL-7 and IL-15 on CD8 T memory cells, while CD4 T memory cells require only IL-15 (in humans). The homeostatic signals seem to differ between species. Although we have learned a lot from the mouse immune system, because it is very similar to human it differs in some details (up to 10%). For example, human CD4 T memory cells constitutively produce IL-15, while the mouse memory cells do not. Thus human memory CD4 T cells support their own homeostatic division by autocrine and paracrine modes (explaining their long survival in cell culture).

Summary
A. Homeostatic (lymphopenic) proliferation of T cells maintains constant concentration and subset ratio by the action of several key cytokines.
B. CD4 and CD8 T memory cells require IL-7 and IL-15 for homeostatic proliferation.
C. Naïve T cells require cytokine IL-7, and a nonspecific contact with the MHC molecules (naïve CD4 T cells require additionally chemokine CCL21).

REPERTOIRE AND TOLERANCE

Immunologic Repertoire of Recognition

The overall potential of an individual to develop an immune response to a variety of macromolecules derived from microorganisms and parasites is called a repertoire. It consists of the sum of all clones of B and T lymphocytes of an individual. The original repertoire is generated in the central part (thymus, bone marrow) of the immune apparatus. It depends on:

Genetic Organization of the Species

The most important genes are the immunoglobulin genes in B cells (BCR; Ig), receptor (TCR) genes in T lymphocytes (for antigenic peptide in the context of MHC; pMHC ligand), and major histocompatibility complex (MHC) genes (HLA in humans, H-2 in mice).

Negative and Positive Selection of T- and B-cell Clones on the Basis of Their Specificity for Self-Antigens

This in turn depends on the expression of specific receptors (BCR;TCR). Selection of specificity primarily takes place in the central lymphoid organs during development of lymphocytes. Negative selection eliminates those clones that can recognize self-antigens (B-cells in the bone marrow, and T-cells in the thymus). Furthermore, the T-lymphocyte clones that do not recognize "thymus–peptide/MHC ligand" in the epithelial cells of the thymus are also destroyed (as a result of neglect, or selection on the basis of the lack of such signals from the microenvironment). Only those clones that can recognize "thymus–peptide/MHC ligand" with low to moderate affinity can continue their development (positive selection). They will be able to recognize in the periphery (of the immune system) a different ligand (i.e., "virus–peptide/MHC ligand") most likely with greater affinity (then the positively selecting one) and thus initiate the specific immune response.

Exceptions are Tregs, which should regulate specific responses by negative feedback, or by additional ways that are still incompletely understood.

Affinity of Treg TCR towards self-peptide/MHC ligand is probably between moderate and strong in induced iTregs. The natural regulatory T cells (nTreg) have very high affinity for self-peptide/MHC. However, for the $CD4^+CD25^+Foxp3^+$ Tregs, the binding affinity for self-peptide/MHC ligand is unknown, and their mode of operating could be different from iTregs and nTregs.

Furthermore, it is not completely clear how Treg cells actually operate. For example, let us take the case with iTregs that have a repertoire nearly identical to T cells defined as those that upon encounter with antigen would become activated and then proliferate starting the immune response that ends with formation of effector cells. It is unknown *when and where* iTregs would respond to antigen challenge (i.e., when will they allow an immune response to be mounted as a defense and when or where would they inhibit the normally responding T cells). Moreover, their existence is not required to explain the immune response in the simplest model of immunity. The problem is that there exist more than one Treg subset of cells that can inhibit an immune response, and some of them may not necessarily be physiologic. It is also known that Tregs need not be specific for the same antigenic peptide/MHC ligand as the T cell that they inhibit. This Treg action is called bystander inhibition (suppression). It is possible that an antigen can have more than one peptide that can be presented to T cells, and that some would stimulate the immune response, and some could inhibit it. The question is whether this choice is a property inherent to the structure of antigenic peptide (i.e., conformation of p/MHC ligand; TCR orientation) or of microenvironment (i.e., other co-stimulatory or co-inhibitory signals; cytokines).

In a typical immune response, contact with foreign-antigen primed APCs stimulates naïve T cells to proliferate and differentiate into effector cells. Once the pathogen is destroyed, most of the effectors are destroyed too, which brings their concentration to undetectable levels. However, some effectors survive and become memory cells, maintaining their clonal concentration at a level that is a bit higher than the one they had in the primary repertoire of responses. With time and after a number of immune responses, increased concentration of memory cells eventually modify quantitatively the peripheral repertoire. If the frequency of a clone is reduced below a certain threshold (it is considered that there are about 10^6 different clones in 1 mL of blood) a homeostatic-like mechanism of division might maintain its frequency at constant levels.

The final immune repertoire is formed in the adult individual, and hypothetically it can change with each immune response that is a consequence of infectious diseases, cancer, organ transplantation or pharmacological therapy. However, no detailed information is available about how and when the repertoire changes. In AIDS, it is considered that the reduction of CD4 T lymphocyte repertoire is the cause of secondary infections, and eventually, death. Even nonpathogenic microorganisms and environmental factors (chemical, physical, and biological) can further modulate the immune repertoire in the periphery. The mechanisms of formation of the repertoire in the periphery are different. Some reduce activity of immunocytes like inhibition, anergy, nonspecific suppression of cell activation, or elimination (clonal deletion) of cells on the one hand, and on the other hand activation of immunocytes that increases frequency of memory cells after infection.

Immunologic Tolerance

Tolerance is defined as the lack of specific immune response to antigen. There is a **central** and **peripheral tolerance** of B or T cells.

Central tolerance of T cells, which makes the repertoire of T cells in the periphery non-responsive to self-antigens, is clonal deletion in the thymus (or negative selection).

In contrast, opinions about the peripheral T cell tolerance differ, and this area of immunology is not yet fully understood. There is clonal deletion (when T cells only receive the signal via TCRs without costimulation); and it is assumed that there is anergy (experimentally determined *in vitro,* but some researchers deny the existence of anergy *in vivo*). The existence of the third type of peripheral tolerance, which is called "regulation" or suppression (of activated T lymphocytes) by various Tregs is still controversial. Despite this, we will assume that various kinds of Tregs have a role in maintaining peripheral tolerance in the CD4 T cell compartment.

Central self-tolerance by clonal deletion in the thymus is not flawless. In fact, by chance some "forbidden" auto-reactive clones may escape negative selection and come out to the periphery. They can become accidentally activated by antigen (similar to self-antigen) during infection and thus damage the host organism. The symptoms and effects of such auto-reactive cells are classified as various autoimmune diseases or autoimmunity depending on which tissues they affect.

In B-cell repertoire, central tolerance (in the bone marrow) is made by clonal deletion of developing B cells that can recognize self-antigens associated with cell membranes or solid surfaces. When encountering the soluble antigen, developing B cells become anergic (and can be re-activated under certain conditions later in the periphery). Mature B cells will be clonally deleted in adult individuals provided they do not get help from T cells while receiving the "first" signal (i.e., by recognizing antigen in germinal centers). Exceptions are B cells that are specific for T-independent antigens. Namely, antigens that can aggregate or cross-link BCR by their multimeric structure (polysaccharides, etc.) can activate B cells without T-cell help.

In B-lymphocyte repertoire, "forbidden" clones can also by mistake escape clonal deletion and appear in the periphery. Such clones are generally not activated because there is no help from the T cells specific for the same antigen. This is called split tolerance. In other words, the establishment of helper (CD4) T-cell tolerance to (self)-antigens by clonal deletion is of paramount importance to hold back the destructive autoimmune attack should autoreactive B-cell clones sneak through negative selection.

Split Tolerance

In the *split tolerance* setting of an adult individual one might find autoreactive B- and CD8 T-cell clones, but CD4 T cell repertoire would be (ideally) properly clonally deleted and have no reactivity against self-antigens. Unfortunately, any foreign antigen (or a hapten) that can bind to the self-protein carrier can short cut such CD4 T-cell tolerance. In detail, foreign-peptide/MHC specific CD4 T-cell clones would be activated (as they were not clonally deleted), and subsequently help two kinds of B cell clones: one specific for foreign- and another one for self-antigen. Because the foreign protein is bound to the self-protein carrier, B cells specific for self-antigen can pick up the combination of the two proteins into the cell, process them and present peptides to T cells. There are two kinds of p/MHC ligands: one would have nonself-peptide and the other one self-peptide in the cleft of MHC molecules. Thereby CD4 T cells—that can recognize nonself-peptide/MHC ligand—would provide help to "sneaked" autoreactive (self-specific) B-cell clones and activate them causing autoimmunity. Perhaps we can add here Tregs, as just another fail-safe mechanism to preserve the integrity of tissues in an organism. They might be the last guardians of self-tolerance by preventing such scenarios.

The similar rule would also keep re-energized anergic autoreactive B-cell clones in check, because they would still require help from CD4 T cells to become activated and to develop into cells producing abnormal (autoreactive) antibodies.

Lastly, administrations of antigens together with antibodies, which can bind them, strongly influence the antigen-specific humoral immune responses. This phenomenon is called the antibody feedback regulation. It can result in almost complete suppression or thousand-fold enhancement of the specific antibody response, depending on antibody isotype and antigen. If suppressed, then it could be equaled as tolerance to a specific antigen.

It is known that passively administered IgG can inhibit the specific antibody response against large antigens such as erythrocytes, widely known as Rh(D)—prophylaxis that is used to prevent hemolytic disease in newborns. However, the mechanism behind this IgG-mediated suppression is not clear at all. Experiments in mice with knockout genes encoding Ig Fc receptors, complement factors or their receptors show that this suppressive capacity of IgG is not affected by the absence of FcRγ, FcγRIIB, CR1/CR2, or C1q. It is because of such mysteries that the understanding of immune tolerance seems to be of paramount importance, and its regulation stands in the focus of immunological research.

Summary

A. The immune repertoire is the potential of an individual to generate an adaptive immune response.

B. The immune repertoire comprises the sum of specificities carried by all clones of B and T lymphocytes in an individual.

C. Each individual has its own initial (primary) repertoire made during development in the central immunologic organs (thymus and bone marrow in adults).

D. Final mature (individually acquired) repertoire is formed in the periphery of the immune system, which is subject to constant homeostatic and clonal-selective changes during life of an individual.

E. Immunologic tolerance means a lack of the specific immune response to an antigen. It is a result of at least one or a combination of the following processes: deletion, anergy and suppression of B- or T-cell clones.

F. Central self-tolerance is acquired by clonal deletion (negative selection) of immunocytes during their development in thymus or bone marrow. Peripheral self-tolerance is established through processes outside primary (central) immunologic organs.

G. Split (divided) tolerance is a term that describes a condition in which autoreactive (not self-tolerant) B and CD8 cytotoxic T cells exist in an organism, due to imperfect clonal deletion in establishing central self-tolerance. However, they cannot be activated, because the helper (CD4) T-cell compartment is tolerant to the same self-antigens.

CHAPTER 4

The Role and Regulation of the Immune Responses

If microorganisms breach the physical and chemical barriers of the body, upon entering the tissues they are faced with a biological barrier—the immune response, which is, as we have already learned, twofold (innate and adaptive). Innate response is usually heralded by nonspecific inflammation and precedes adaptive immune response. Combination of innate immunity and adaptive, which will be described in the following paragraphs is called (according to the functional division) central immunity. It consists of dendritic cells (DCs; innate immunity), αβT cells, and B cells (adaptive immunity).

THE COURSE OF THE IMMUNE RESPONSE

The immune response begins when microorganisms such as bacteria or viruses start destroying the integrity of tissue in which they enter (Figure 4-1). Dendritic cells (DCs) in tissues are equipped with so-called pattern recognition receptors (PRRs). Toll-like receptors (TLR) can recognize patterns of molecules typical for microorganisms including peptidoglycan, lipopolysaccharide (LPS), DNA (especially unmethylated islands of CpG), and double- or single-stranded RNAs. There are 11 types of TLR, each binding a different molecular pattern (Figure 4-2). TLR 1-2, 4-6, 8, and 10-11 are cell surface molecules. However, TLR 3, 7, and 9 are found in the endosomes of cells that express them, where phagocytosed RNA or DNA can bind to them. DCs of type 1 do not have endosomal TLRs, whereas DCs of type 2 do. Some TLRs can bind necrotic tissue products or those from stressed and shocked cells. Besides TLRs, there are cytosolic PRRs like NOD-like receptors (NLP), and another PRR on the cell surface such as the mannose receptor.

The NLRs represent cytosolic PRR that include over 20 family members, which recognize a wide range of pathogen-associated molecular patterns (PAMPs). The specificity of many NLRs is still unknown, thus not only pathogen-associated pattern might be recognized with PRRs, but perhaps also Danger- and Integrity-associated molecular patterns (DAMPs and IAMPs, see *Theories about the function of the immune system*, Chapter 9, pp. 283–301).

The Cytokines of the Immune System
http://dx.doi.org/10.1016/B978-0-12-419998-9.00004-3

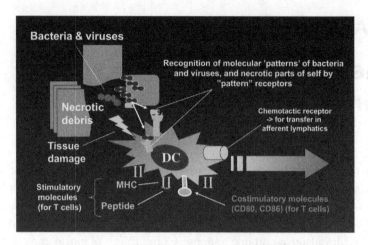

Figure 4-1 The beginning of the immune response in tissues.

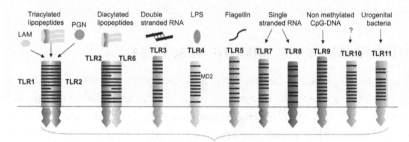

Toll / IL-1 Receptor (TIR) homologous domain
Signal transduction via specific adapters, NF-κB & MAP kinases

LAM = Lipoarabinomannan (*Mycobacteria*)   LPS = Lipopolisaccharide (gram-negative bacteria)
PGN = Peptidoglycan (gram-positive bacteria)

Figure 4-2 Human Toll-like receptors (TLR) and their ligands.

Three NLRs can form inflammasomes, which are protein complexes that can activate inflammatory and immune responses. Inflammasomes can activate pyroptosis, or caspase-1–dependent programmed cell death. Activation of any of four PRR family members (AIM2, NLRC4 or IPAF, NLRP1, and NLRP3) initiates the formation of an inflammasome. By activating caspase-1, they can upregulate the proinflammatory cytokines IL-1beta and IL-18. Other NLRs can signal through RIP2, a factor that by activating NF-κB signaling leads to proinflammatory cytokine release. Further analyses of inflammasomes should give new understanding about innate immunity and the link with specific adaptive response that might be essential in host–microbial response.

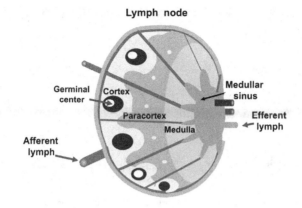

Figure 4-3 Schematic depiction of a lymph node.

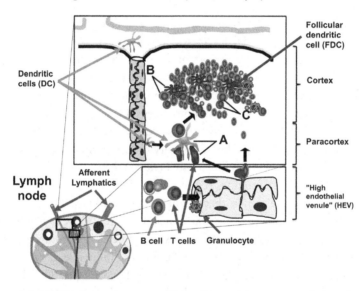

Figure 4-4 DC-T in the paracortex and T–B cell interactions cortex of a lymph node.

All these PRRs are involved in the activation, or rather, the maturation of DC. During maturation DCs phagocytose surrounding microorganisms as well as damaged tissue, then process the ingested and express peptides in clefts of the MHC molecules of both classes (the expression of peptides on MHC class I is called cross-presentation). At the same time, DCs upregulate costimulatory molecules and particular chemokine receptors (Figure 4-1) that allow them to migrate from tissues by afferent lymph vessels in lymph nodes (Figure 4-3), where they home in the paracortex (Figure 4-4). There they encounter resting (naïve and memory) T cells. DC–T cell interaction can activate T cells provided they specifically recognize the peptide/MHC ligand by TCR (interaction A in

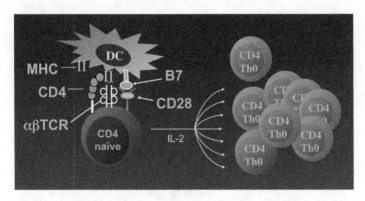

Figure 4-5 Activation of CD4 T cells in the paracortex of lymph nodes.

Figure 4-4). The T-cell activation also super-stimulates DCs in contact with them, which prolongs their life for a few days engaging in some sort of molecular crosstalk, which might be important for the type of the ensuing immune response. The naïve T helper cell has the following cell surface markers: $CD25^{lo}$, $CD44^{lo}$, CD62L (L-Selectin), $CD69^{lo}$; bears chemokine receptors CD184 (CXCR4) and CD197 (CCR7); and produces CD127 (IL-7).

Activated T cells proliferate in several stages. For CD4 T cells, the first stage is Th_0, which is characterized by the activity of Ki-67, the proliferation intracellular marker. Initially, it was previously believed that this stage also produces IL-2, IFN-γ, and IL-4 cytokines (Figure 4-5). However, this is only for those transitions towards the subsets that produce such cytokines. The activated Th stage bears the following cell-surface markers: $CD25^{hi}$, $CD44^{hi}$, $CD69^{hi}$, CD71, $CD98^{hi}$ and upregulates the expression of HLA-DR molecules. In the next phase, CD4 Th_0 becomes polarized under the influence of various cytokines, and develops into one of the following effector types: Th1, Th2, Th3, Th9, Th17, Th22, Tr1, or Tfh (follicular helper) cells, each of which secrete type-specific cytokines and perform typical "immune response" functions. This interaction can also generate $CD25^+Foxp3^+$ regulatory T cells. Although the conditions for the generation of all these cell types have been ascertained *in vitro*, the *in vivo* rules are still not yet fully elucidated. Effector CD4 T cells can migrate into the cortex of the lymph nodes where they can help resting B cells to get activated (interaction C in Figure 4-4). Various T helper types help development of different classes of B-cell responses. Follicular Tfh type help organizing germinal centers where B cells proliferate, affinity mature

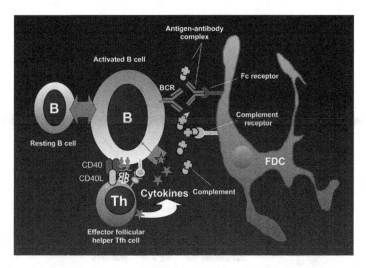

Figure 4-6 Activation of B cells. FDC–T–B interaction in lymph node cortex.

(by somatic hypermutation) their BCRs and switch their immunoglobulin isotype.

Activation of B lymphocytes occurs in parallel with CD4 T cells. In blood, antigens travel in complex with natural antibodies or complement and home in the cortex of lymph nodes where they adhere to the follicular dendritic cells (FDC; residual in the cortex) (Figure 4-6). The FDCs express Fc receptors on their surface by which they hold antibody–antigen complex. Resting B cells, they can bind such complexes with BCR (interaction B in Figure 4-4), are activated if they get the help of T cells (interaction C in Figure 4-4). B cells then proliferate making a germinal center. The B cells further develop into plasma cells that secrete Ig molecules. In the germinal centers B cells are selected for a higher affinity for an antigen. By somatic hypermutation of variable parts of immunoglobulin genes, B cells can generate BCRs with a higher affinity for the contacting sites (epitopes) on antigens. Furthermore, the activated B cells can switch the constant region of the BCR and generate another class of Ig molecules depending on the cytokines secreted in their microenvironment (see below in the section *Important control functions of cytokines: Effects on B lymphocytes*, p. 113). The development of B cells in the lymph nodes ends with the generation of effector B cells—plasma cells, which leave and populate somatic tissues, usually where the microorganisms made invasion and damage. Some home to the bone marrow where they can produce and secrete large amounts of antibodies. Figure 4-7 shows schematically

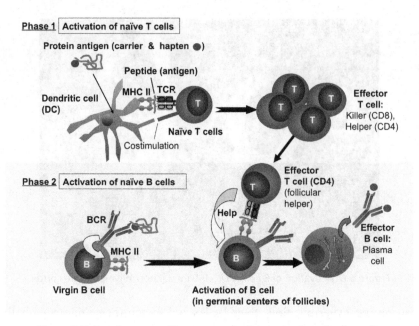

Figure 4-7 Development of immunocytes after activation of naïve cells.

activation of T and B cells and the development of effector cells that usually occurs in the lymph nodes.

Effector CD4 T cells that form in paracortex can also travel to the target somatic tissues where they can enhance the immune response, depending on the type. For example, they recruit monocytes, DCs, and activate macrophages by secreting cytokines like IFN-γ, recruit and activate neutrophils (IL-17) or other granulocytes like eosinophils (IL-5).

The cytotoxic CD8 T lymphocytes are generated in the course of viral infections or infections with bacteria that live inside cells. They are activated by DCs that present viral (or bacterial) antigens in the paracortex of lymph nodes. They need help (called licensing) by CD4 T lymphocytes stimulated with the same antigen (probably on the same DCs) to develop into effector cytotoxic T cells (CTL). The CTLs migrate to the target tissues where they can kill virus-infected cells.

Primary and secondary immune responses differ in the time it takes to mount them (Figure 4-8). If we measure the concentration of antibodies in the blood after immunization with an antigen (A), we will notice that it increases during the primary response with the growing tendency that

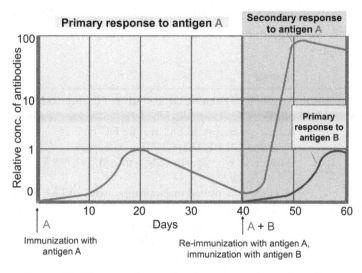

Figure 4-8 Primary and secondary immune responses to antigen.

reaches a peak after a couple of weeks. During re-immunization with the same antigen (A) after a month, serum antibody levels peak earlier than under the primary response. Because of clonal organization of the immune system, antibodies specific for another antigen (B) will follow the primary response, even if B was injected simultaneously with antigen A at the time of A's secondary challenge (Figure 4-8).

REGULATION OF IMMUNOCYTE DEVELOPMENT AFTER ACTIVATION

Numerous factors can modify the immune response, and not all are fully understood, such as in cases where the appearance of nonself antigen causes the opposite of that expected, namely—suppression, unresponsiveness, or even death of precursors of immune cells (clonal deletion) leading to tolerance. In addition to the B- or T-cell antigen receptors, CD4 and CD8 coreceptors, there are other molecules in the cell membranes of lymphocytes that play a role in the activation of B and T cells. These are known as costimulatory, coinhibitory, and crosstalk molecules. Interleukins and other cytokines play an important role in the activation of innate immunity and determining the class of response of cells of adaptive immunity. Their physiological roles are still being intensively investigated.

Here are some of the most important cytokines that can regulate development of innate immunity cells and adaptive immunocytes after activation in the periphery:

Name	Sources
IFN-γ	Activated CD4 and CD8 T (Th1, Tc1); activated NK and NKT
IFN-α/β	Mature plasmocytoid DC; mature DC type 2
IL-2	Activated CD4 T; Th1; CD4 T memory cells
IL-4	Innate cells type 2; mast cells; activated Th2, NKT
IL-5	Activated Th2
IL-6	Monocytes; activated macrophages; activated Th2; fibroblasts
IL-9	Activated Th9
IL-10	Immature DCs; quiescent Mø, activated Th2; Th3; Th9; Tregs
IL-12	DC type 1; activated macrophages; activated B cells
IL-13	Activated Th2, innate type 2 cells
IL-17	Activated Th17
IL-22	Activated Th22 (and Th17)
IL-23, IL-27	DC type 1; macrophages
IL-35	Regulatory T cells (IL-35 producing)
TNF	Activated macrophages (TNF-α), activated Th1 (TNF-β)
TGF-β	Quiescent macrophages; Tregs (CD4, CD25, Foxp3), Th3, Th9

IMPORTANT CONTROL FUNCTIONS OF CYTOKINES

Various cytokines modulate the fate of cells of the immune system.

The Generation of Th1-Type Effectors

Figure 4-9 shows development of CD4 T cells into Th1 type of response that is influenced by products of cells of the innate and adaptive immunity. The cytokines influencing Th1 development are IL-2, IL-12 (p70), IL-18, and IL-27.

The Th0 cells can develop into Th1-type effector cells under the influence of the master transcription factor T-bet, which is promoted by microbial agents and viruses. The cytokines involved include IFN-γ, but at the very beginning it seems that IL-27 (in the early response) and IL-12(p70) has the major influence, but IL-18 and also RANK ligand can promote their development. IL-12 increases the expression of receptor for IFN-γ, which in turn can act on the polarization of this subpopulation. Their differentiation is halted by IL-4, IL-10, and IL-21.

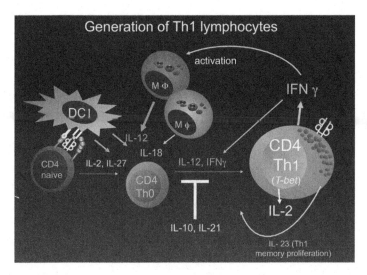

Figure 4-9 Role of cytokines in the generation of Th1 immune response.

The master regulator T-bet is the characteristic nuclear factor for Th1 pathway. It is stimulated by the Jak–Stat pathway and involves the following nuclear transcription factors: STAT1 and STAT4 and Runx3, that drive the expression of Th1-type genes. The hallmark of Th1 type is the secretion of IFN-γ, TNF-β, lymphotoxin α, cytokines, and furthermore cytotoxic proteins such as Perforin, Granzyme A and B (and in humans, Granulysin). The markers expressed by this subset include CD26, CD94, CD278 (ICOS), and Tim-3. Cytokine receptors expressed by this type of cell are: CD178 (FasL), CD212 (IL-12Rβ2), CD218a (IL-18Rα), IL-27Rα, NOTCH3, and RANKL, and these include the following chemokine receptors: CD183 (CXCR3) and CD195 (CCR5). Some cytokines are involved in the positive feedback loop in the generation of a single type of response like IFN-γ, and have at the same time a cross-inhibitory effect on other type(s) like Th2, Th17, and Tregs. IL-23 promotes the proliferation of Th1 CD4 memory cell population.

The Generation of Th2-Type Effectors

In Figure 4-10 the generation of the Th2 subset is shown. The master regulator transcription factor is GATA3, which can be upregulated via IL-4 action and STAT-6. IL-4 is sufficient, but is not the only necessary factor for Th2 development. Th2 can develop under the influence of cytokines such as TSLP, IL-25, and IL-33 (and IL-15 in humans, as well as IL-31). Indirectly,

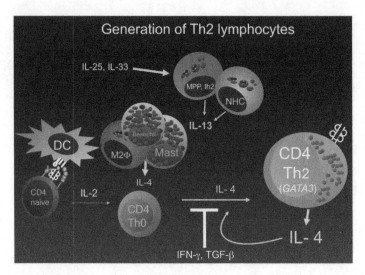

Figure 4-10 Role of cytokines in the generation of Th2 immune responses.

IL-13 is also involved. The cells of innate helper type 2 (Ih2) also called nuocytes, MPP, and NHC cells upon stimulus from IL-25 and IL-33 produce IL-13 that in turn promote mast cells, macrophages (type 2), and basophils to secrete IL-4, effectively steering the response towards the Th2 type.

GATA-3 is the characteristic transcription factor for the Th2 pathway. It also involves additional nuclear factors like IRF-4, GFI-1, MAF, STAT5, and STAT6. The hallmark of Th2 type is the secretion of IL-4 and IL-10, but it also secretes IL-3, IL-5, IL-6, IL-13, and IL-31 and GM-CSF. Markers on Th2 cells include Tim-1. Cytokine receptors expressed by the Th2 subset are: CD30, IFNγRβ, IL-17RB, IL-23Rα, NOTCH1 and NOTCH2, and with the following chemokine receptors: CD184 (CXCR4) and CD193 (CCR3), CD194 (CCR4), CD198 (CCR8), and CD294 (CRTH2). IL-4 is involved in the positive feedback loop that can generate more of the Th2 subset cells from the Th0 stage. This pathway can be inhibited by the action of IFN-γ or TGF-β. IL-13 can possibly act via a wider loop by generating more Th2 cells via mast cells, basophils, and type-2 macrophages.

The Generation of Th9-Type Effectors

In Figure 4-11 the generation of the Th9 subset is shown. The cytokines influencing Th9 development are IL-2 and IL-4 in initial phases and then TGF-β.

GATA-3 is the early master regulator that is followed by the PU.1 transcriptional activity, as a characteristic for the Th9 pathway. It also involves

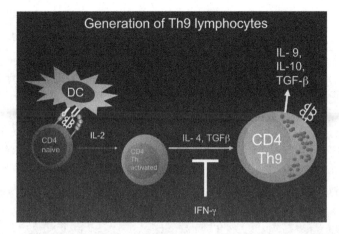

Figure 4-11 Role of cytokines in the generation of Th9 lymphocytes.

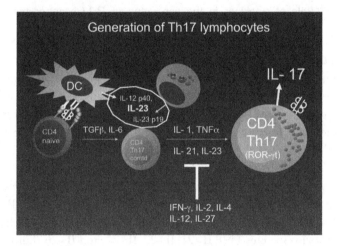

Figure 4-12 Role of cytokines in the generation of Th17 lymphocytes.

additional nuclear factors like IRF-4, STAT6, and SMADs (2, 3, 4, and 7). Th9 subpopulation secretes IL-9, which is a hallmark of this subpopulation (murine Th9 cells produce in addition IL-10), but they also produce TGF-β, and two chemokines: CCL17 (TARC) and CCL22 (MDC). Negative regulator of Th9 differentiation is IFN-γ.

The Generation of Th17-Type Effectors

Figure 4-12 shows development of the Th17 subset. The cytokines influencing Th17 development are TGF-β and IL-6 from the naïve T cells, and from

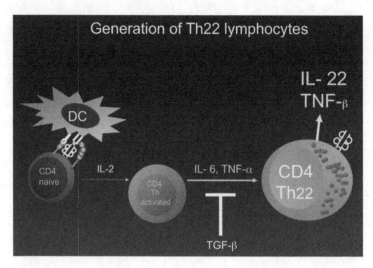

Figure 4-13 Role of cytokines in the generation of Th22 lymphocytes and their function.

the activated CD4 T cell stage IL-1, IL-21, and IL-23 are involved. There are some concerns as to whether this is a stable population, because two recipes *in vitro* for their generation can yield the same result. TGF-β plus IL-6 and IL-1 can generate Th17 cells, but also TGF-β plus IL-21 followed by IL-23 can do the same. Furthermore, some sources also mention TNF for the formation of an unusual sub-subset of Th17. Human Th17 cells are very hard to establish *in vitro*, unlike mouse Th17 subsets, which are easily polarized.

RORγt is the master regulator for the Th17 pathway. It also involves additional nuclear factors like IRF-4, Batf, Runx1, STAT3, and RORα4. The hallmark of Th17 type is the secretion of IL-17A, IL-17F, and IL-17A/F cytokines, but it also secretes TNF, IL-21, IL-22, IL-24, and IL-26 (human) and a chemokine CCL20 (MIP-3α). Markers on Th17 cells include CD161 (NK1) and CD278 (ICOS). Cytokine receptors expressed by Th17 subset are: CD126 (IL-6Rα), IL-13Rα1, IL-21R, and IL-23R that are followed by chemokine receptors CD194 (CCR4) and CD196 (CCR6). The generation of Th17 can be inhibited by IFN-γ, IL-2, IL-4, IL-12(p70), and IL-27.

The Generation of Th22-Type Effectors

Figure 4-13 shows the generation of the Th22 subset. The cytokines influencing Th22 development are IL-2 (from naïve to Th0 stage), and IL-6 and TNF (from the activated phase to the Th22 effector stage). The latter transition can be inhibited by TGF-β. The nuclear factor detected in the Th22 subset is the aryl hydrocarbon receptor. Th22 cells have CD140 (PDGFR)

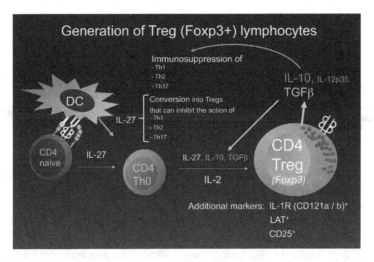

Figure 4-14 Role of cytokines in the generation of Treg lymphocytes. *Foxp3* is the master regulator (transcription factor) for the Treg response. TGF-β initiates Treg development.

cytokine receptor and the following chemokine receptors CD194 (CCR4), CD196 (CCR6) and CCR10 on their cell surface. The hallmark of Th22 type is the secretion of IL-22 and TNF cytokines.

The generation of Treg cells

Figure 4-14 shows development of the Treg subset. First, IL-27 promotes development to activated interphase during the T-cell activation from naïve T cells. And from the activated CD4 T cell stage the cytokines influencing inducible Treg (iTreg) development are TGF-β and IL-10. IL-2 is required for the survival of Treg population.

Foxp3 is the master regulator for the Treg pathway. The hallmark of Treg type is the secretion of IL-10, IL-12 (p35), and TGF-β. Markers on Tregs include LAT, CD25, and PGE2. Cytokine receptors expressed by the Treg subset are: CD121a/b (IL-1R). The generation of Tregs can be inhibited by IFN-γ, IL-4, and IL-12(p70). Their action can inhibit the Th1, Th2, and Th17 types of response.

The naturally occurring Tregs (nTregs) have been selected in the thymus (see Chapter 2, *T-cell development*, p. 44) having the highest TCR affinity for self-antigens (pMHC combinations on thymic epithelial cells) and are exported in the periphery of the immune system with a phenotype that includes expression of $CD4^+$, $CD25^{int}$, and $Foxp3^+$ markers as a hallmark for the nTregs lineage.

The generation of NKT cells

Another important subset should be mentioned here, namely the NKT cells, that have NK receptors such as CD314 (NKG2D) and TCRs.

They can be generated under the influence of the IL-15 (from thymic emigrants). Upon activation by cells that modulate their MHC antigens, or by directly recognizing some pMHC combinations, they secrete IL-4, IL-17A, and IFN-γ, influencing the generation of other subsets in the initial phase as well as in the regulation of the immune response.

Summarized below is the list of some important effects of cytokines involved in the immune responses:

IFN-α/β: have activating or inhibitory effect on Th1—they stimulate production of IFN-γ in effector T cells, and inhibit IL-12 in DC (under particular conditions, see "IFN-α/β", Chapter 5, p. 2).

IFN-γ: promotes development of Th0 into Th1 type; inhibits development of Th2, Th9, and Th17.

IL-2: promotes development of naïve T into Th0 stage; exerts a homeostatic effect on Tregs (regulatory CD4⁺CD25⁺FoxP3⁺ T cells); maintains survival of effector T lymphocytes.

IL-4: promotes Th2, and Th9 (with TGF-β) development, inhibits Th1 and Th17 development.

IL-6: promotes generation of Th17 (with IL-1, IL-21, IL-23, and TGF-β), Th22 (with TNF) and Tregs (with TGF-β).

IL-7: promotes growth of developing T and B cells in the thymus and bone marrow.

IL-10: inhibits the development of Th1.

IL-12: promotes development of Th1 helper CD4 T cells (from TH0).

IL-7 and IL-15: maintain the survival of naïve T lymphocytes (homeostatic proliferation).

IL-15: maintains homeostasis of CD8 memory cells; generates NKT cells.

IL-23: promotes the development of Th17 CD4 population that produces IL-17 (stimulates recruitment of neutrophils).

TGF-β: inhibits the proliferation of activated precursors of Th2 and Th22 immune cells, while together with IL-6 induces the generation of Tregs; and together with IL-1, IL-6, IL-21, and IL-23 generates the Th17 subset.

TSLP (thymic stromal lymphopoetin, similar to IL-7) has variety of important effects: it works on the DC cells that can polarize naïve CD4 T cells to develop into Th2-like (quasi-Th2) cell type (Th2'). These Th2' then secrete TNF-α (and IL-2, IL-4, and IL-13), but do not secrete IL-10. Important to note is that in the presence of IL-12, all of the effects of TSLP are lost. Furthermore, dendritic cells that are induced by the TSLP have a unique homeostatic effect on Th2 cells in the periphery, which consists of inducing proliferation of Th2 memory cells, and maintaining their pro-allergic phenotype. Lastly, TSLP triggers expression of FoxP3 factor in some thymocytes that will become precursors of natural Tregs (nTregs).

Effects on B lymphocytes

Antibodies secreted by plasma cells are immunoglobulin molecules that belong to five classes (and several subclasses). All antibodies are highly resistant to enzymatic degradation and have a very long half-life in the blood.

Class and specificity are clonally distributed. It means that any plasma-cell clone produces antibody of a single specificity that belongs to a unique class. Likewise, the pool of memory B cells with the single (or very similar) specificity can consist of various clones that can have all known isotypes (classes). The reason for specificity conservation is that the V region of the heavy chain (consisting of V-D-J rearrangement initially associated with the IgM or IgD constant part of the antigen receptor of B lymphocytes) will remain expressed after the switch of IgM (IgD) constant regions with IgG, IgA, or IgE regions. The switch occurs during the development of B lymphocytes after activation in germinal centers (Figure 4-15). B memory cells can have all possible classes of BCRs on the cell surface. In the dark areas of germinal centers, the replacement of the heavy chain constant regions of the Ig genes is influenced by the following factors:

IFN-γ: causes switch to IgG1 and IgG3 isotypes (in the mouse—IgG2a).

IL-4: causes development of plasma cells that secrete IgE and IgG4.

TGF-β: causes development of plasma cells that secrete IgA antibodies; reduces proliferation of activated B-lymphocytes.

Among other cytokines that act on B cells it is important to mention:

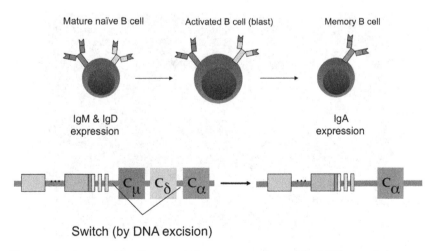

Figure 4-15 Activated B cells can switch constant regions of the BCR heavy chain genes (in germinal centers).

IL–2: enhances growth and multiplication of B lymphocytes.

IL–6: stimulates development of activated B cells into plasma cells.

IL–7: promotes development of precursors of B cells during development in the bone marrow.

THE ROLE OF Th1-TYPE OF IMMUNE RESPONSE

In the Th1-type of immune response, the effector T cells secrete Th1 cytokines and have a variety of functions (Figure 4-16). The first is the switch of B cell isotype to IgG1 and IgG3 in humans, which is influenced by IFN-γ. Depending on the affinity of these antibodies for the immunizing antigen, they will participate in the neutralization and opsonization of microorganisms that carry these antigens. Antibodies facilitate phagocytosis of microorganisms or their parts, as phagocytes can bind constant (Fc) parts of antibodies by Fc receptors. The second function of the Th1 response is exerted by cytokines IFN-γ and IL-2, which stimulate the amplification of the Th1 response. The third function is the amplification of the inflammation made by the intrusion of microorganisms by TNF-β. This way macrophages and other inflammatory cells are attracted to the site of inflammation. The fourth function of the Th1 response is that it activates macrophages (via IFN-γ). Macrophages can then kill intracellular bacteria (if they live in them) such as *Mycobacteria, Salmonella,* and *Leishmania.* Activated macrophages further enhance inflammation by secretion of

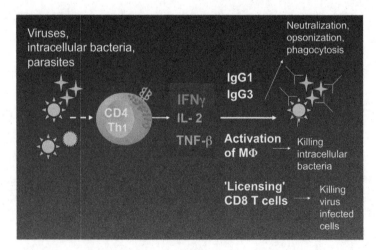

Figure 4-16 Role of Th1 effector lymphocytes in the immune response. Immunity to viruses, intracellular bacteria, and parasites.

TNF-α and IL-1. These cytokines cause fever, as they can elevate the threshold of the body's thermostat in the brain and thus raise body temperature (some bacteria and viruses cannot tolerate temperatures higher than 38°C). Furthermore, activated macrophages secrete chemokines (IL-8 or CXCL8) that attract other leukocytes at the site of damaged integrity. By the generation of oxidative radicals and hydrogen peroxide, macrophages can destroy cells in the microenvironment, phagocytose (clear) cellular debris and thus heal wounds. The fifth function of the Th1 response is licensing CD8 cytotoxic T lymphocytes in lymph nodes. This role helps in generation of effector cytotoxic CD8 T cells that can recognize foreign antigenic peptides (in clefts of MHC class I molecules) and thus kill, for example, target cells infected with a virus. The mechanism of cytotoxicity is by creating pores in the membrane of target cells and inserting serine proteases (Granzyme B) that induce programmed cell death (apoptosis).

The Th1 subset, if self-tolerance becomes broken, is the major cell type to play a role in autoimmune diseases like *diabetes mellitus type-1, multiple sclerosis, and rheumatoid arthritis.*

THE ROLE OF Th2-TYPE OF IMMUNE RESPONSE

Effector cells of the Th2 response are CD4 T helper lymphocytes that produce IL-1, IL-3, IL-4, IL-5, IL-6, IL-10, IL-13, IL-25, IL-31 and GM-CSF cytokines.

Th2 cells stimulate specific humoral immunity mainly because they cause isotype switch in antibody response into IgG4 and IgE classes, in humans. Similarly, IgG1 subclass (which is similar to IgG4) has a function in tissues that is neutralization, opsonization and phagocytosis of microorganisms that carry immunizing antigen (Figure 4-17). Cytokines that cause Ig class switch are IL-4 and IL-10. In addition, IL-4 and IL-10 will cross-inhibit Th1 response and enhance Th2. Furthermore, IL-6 cytokine stimulates the maturation of plasma cells and has a proinflammatory effect which helps in the production of acute phase proteins in the liver. IL-13 is similar to IL-4 regarding the inhibition of the Th1 response (it inhibits secretion of Th1 cytokines by activated macrophages) and causes antibody isotype switch to IgE.

As a consequence of increased production of IgE antibodies, their concentration in the body also rises enhancing the pro-allergic phenotype. Namely, IgE antibodies bind with their constant parts to Fcε (epsilon) receptors on the cell surface of mast cells. These cells, coated with IgE, can then settle in various

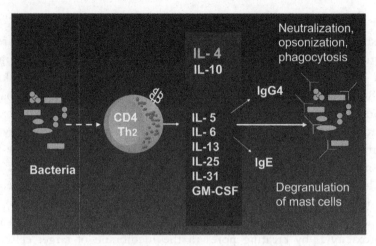

Figure 4-17 Role of Th2 lymphocytes in the immune response.

bodily tissues where they border the environment (i.e., skin, mucosa). Upon repeated encounter with antigen, IgE-coated mast cells can be triggered in a very short time, thus representing the first defense against possibly harmful microorganisms. Triggering causes degranulation with secretion of histamine and other mediators. If such a condition is not satisfactorily controlled (and its regulation is not yet fully clear) it may lead to anaphylaxis, atopy, and allergies. IgE antibodies also have a role in fighting parasites and parasitic worms.

Finally, IL-5 cytokine stimulates eosinophils, and the latter are involved in defense against parasites and helminths (Figure 4-18).

THE ROLE OF Th9 SUBSET

Th9 subset is involved in gut responses to parasitic helminths and worms (Figure 4-19), producing inflammation in the mucosa. Secretion of IL-9 by Th9 cells influences the induction of proliferation of mast cells in bone marrow and their differentiation (via IL-6). In addition, in animal models of diseases, Th9 play a role in allergic asthma, and experimental autoimmune encephalomyelitis as they produce slightly different set of cytokines (Figure 4-11).

THE ROLE OF Th17 SUBSET

The role of Th17 cells is in promoting defensive adaptive immunity to pathogens, while at the same time they support innate immunity such as inflammation and neutrophil recruitment and activation. It is possible that

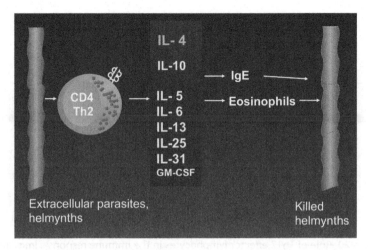

Figure 4-18 Role of Th2 lymphocytes in the anti-parasitic response.

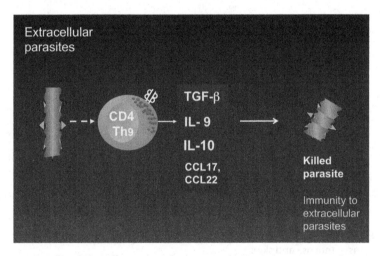

Figure 4-19 Role of Th9 effector lymphocytes in the immune response. Immunity to extracellular parasites.

Th17 cells are not terminally differentiated cells, because under the influence of other cytokines they can further either develop into Treg phenotype, or into a proinflammatory Th1-like subset.

Th17 have a key role in host defense against extracellular microbes such as bacteria and fungi and are instrumental in epithelial barrier immunity such as skin and mucosa (Figure 4-20). They have also a role in autoimmune diseases, primarily located in the areas where an organism borders with the environment.

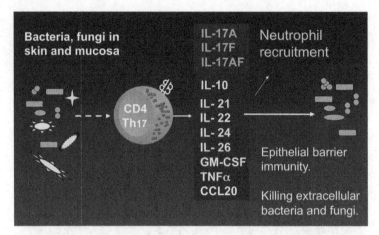

Figure 4-20 Role of Th17 effector lymphocytes in the immune response. Immunity to extracellular bacteria, and fungal infections.

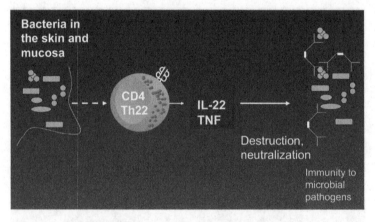

Figure 4-21 Role of Th22 lymphocytes in the immune response. Immunity to microbial pathogens in mucosa and skin.

THE ROLE OF Th22 SUBSET

This subpopulation produces IL-22 but not IL-17 (as Th17 also shows the ability to secrete IL-22), and neither IFN-γ nor IL-4. Apart from Th22, this subset produces TNF, and also IL-13 and fibroblast growth factor (FGF). It expresses chemokine receptors CCR4, CCR6 and CCR10 that make them home to skin and mucosal surfaces (Figure 4-21). They act on keratinocytes, epithelial cells, and myofibroblasts helping them in wound repair and healing of the skin. In general, they have a protective role in the skin, gut, and lungs.

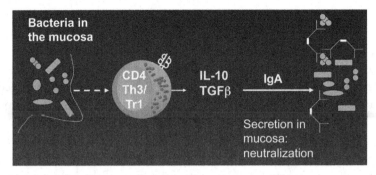

Figure 4-22 Role of T lymphocytes with TGF-β secretion in the immune response: Th3 and Tr1 subsets produce TGF-β (and IL-10) cytokines.

THE ROLE OF Th3, AND Tr1 CELLS

The existence of Th3 and Tr1 cells was proven *in vitro* by generating long-term cell cultures or T-cell cloning, respectively, using differentiation factors such as TGF-β, IL-10, IL-4, with anti-IL-12 mAb for Th3 cell culture, and IL-10 and IFN-α cytokines for Tr1 cloned lineage. The role for Tr1 effector cells is based on the secreting cytokine profile (IL-10, TGF-β) that has an inhibiting effect on proinflammatory Th1 response. As Tr1 effector cells are not toxic *in vivo*, they show potential for therapeutic use in *chronic inflammatory diseases*. Interestingly, dexamethasone or vitamin D3 addition to cell cultures stimulates Tr1 clones to secrete high amounts of IL-10. The profile of *in vitro* generated Tr1 cells is similar to Tregs (Foxp3, GITR, and CTLA-4)⁺.

Similarly, it can be supposed that the secretion of TGF-β (by both Tr1 and Th3) should calm down inflammation in general, as well as downregulate the Th1 type of the immune response. Regarding defense, Th3 cells are the highest producers of TGF-β that causes IgA isotype switch in B cells (Figure 4-22). IgA antibodies are extremely important, because they are secreted in the mucosa. Their presence outside bodily tissues shows that they have a role in preventing intrusion of microorganisms through the mucosa. IgA is found in breast milk and is very important for the defense of infants (intestinal epithelium possesses specialized receptors that can transfer undigested IgA antibodies in the circulation of children).

THE ROLE OF REGULATORY CD4 T LYMPHOCYTES—Tregs

If the activation of B or T cells fails or stops (due to various factors in the microenvironment), they may enter a state of inactivity called anergy, which is the inability to be successfully activated for a prolonged period of time. Sometimes peripheral lymphocytes that were unsuccessfully activated can undergo apoptosis (programmed cell death), and thus be clonally deleted. These mechanisms are collectively called peripheral tolerance.

Another type of tolerance is silencing the immune response by specific suppression. Many believe that the suppression is a multifaceted phenomenon, and the result of a complex regulation of the immune response. An explanation could involve anergy, or the cytotoxic effect of CD8 T cells. An alternative, which dates back to the beginning of the 1970s immediately after the discovery of helper T cells, involves inhibition of the immune response by supposedly "antigen-specific suppressor T cells." Unfortunately, many such clones were thrown into oblivion after discovery of the TCR genes, because it was found that they lack a part of TCR. The absence of fully functional TCR made suppressor T cells perform poorly (i.e., they were inactive) and suppressed other cells in standard laboratory assays. Thus today many researchers are cautious when they write about suppression, as it invokes such connotations. The solution was the introduction of the concept of regulatory T cells (Tregs), which can suppress (inhibit) the immune responses, but differ from previously described suppressor T lymphocytes by having expression of TCR. So, several decades later, when T cell clones were discovered that have inhibitory (suppressive) effects, they were named regulatory T cells. These include natural (nTregs), induced (iTregs), (CD4+CD25+FoxP3+) Tregs, IL-35 producing Tregs, Th17-derived regulatory T cells, and Tr1 cells.

Recent studies have shown that Treg cells (CD4+CD25+Foxp3+) can silence the immune response to particular antigens (for Treg development, see the *T-cell development,* Chapter 2, p. 44).

The transcription factor FoxP3 is a hallmark of one lineage of Tregs and has an essential role in maintaining their inhibitory activity. There are three splice forms of FOXP3 mRNA in humans, which give rise to protein isoforms with different functional properties. Two isoforms including full length and a smaller one (d2) confer suppressive phenotypes to Tregs, whereas (d7) isoform inhibits the function of the other two isoforms in a dominant negative fashion.

Activated Tregs become immunosuppressive to other T cells (CD4 and CD8) by direct contact, and by secreting TGF-β, IL-10, and IL-35 cytokines. Tregs function reduces inflammation. While Tregs are activated by specific recognition of particular antigenic (peptide/MHC) ligand using their TCRs, they can inhibit other clones having different specificities—thus exhibiting a nonspecific or cross-specific suppression. Probably such suppressed clones reside in the vicinity of Tregs. The inhibition is manifested as the absence of activation of resting immunocytes, and perhaps also as the absence of triggering their effector functions. Therefore, suppression (by Tregs) leads to the lack of defensive type of the immune response. Cytokines can have important roles in the generation of Tregs. For example, IL-28 and IL-29 secreted by plasmocytoid DC (in tissues) are involved in development of Tregs.

Tregs are believed to be important from negative feedback of the immune response to fail-safe mechanism for autoimmunity. In tolerance to self-antigens, evidence shows that autoimmunity occurs in the absence of Tregs. However, it remains unclear when, how, and why an antigen (or part thereof) would generate the defensive immune response (like in vaccination), and when, how, and why the same antigen would generate the opposite, namely, suppression (via Tregs) for itself (for further discussion, see *Theories about the function of the immune system,* Chapter 9, pp. 283–301).

Signal transduction in Treg cells is similar to other T cells after activation and recognition of antigenic peptide/MHC ligand on the presenting cells. The PI3K p110δ is important but not specific as a marker of Tregs. The FoxP3 is in combination with CD4 and CD25 a marker for one type of Tregs, as it is not present in some other regulatory T cells (like Tregs that secrete IL-35). The only detected difference is perhaps that Tregs preferentially use NFκB2 (p52p65), while other types of T cells use NFκB1 (p50p65) transcription factor. Probably soon the other differences will be detected, and thus offer better explanation of the origin, development, and the role of Treg cells.

THE ROLE OF THE Tfh SUBSET

T follicular helper (Tfh) subpopulation can be distinguished by the cytokine profile and cell markers from other Th subsets. The master regulator of differentiation is the Bcl6 transcription factor. They have a high expression of chemokine receptors CXCR5 (a receptor for CXCL13—a chemokine secreted by follicular stromal cells) and low CCR7 that keep them migrating towards the edges of the B-cell zones of germinal centers, where they help developing B cells to mount specific antigen responses and develop into plasma cells or memory B cells. Tfh form stable contacts with follicular B cells and produce IL-4, IL-10, IFN-γ, and IL-21 cytokines, which promote formation of germinal centers, development of B cells, and their class-switch.

Summary

A. Effector function of plasma cells (the last stage of development of a clone of B lymphocytes) is the production of antibodies. Effector function of CD4+ T cells is helping B-cells or helping (licensing) precursors of cytotoxic CD8+ T lymphocytes. The effector function of CD8+ T cells is the killing of virus-infected cells. Memory T and B lymphocytes are important for the secondary immune response (which is faster than the primary).

B. Effector T cells have identical specific recognition as the resting (or naïve) cells from which they have developed. Effector B cells are subject to mutation of their antigen receptors in germinal centers, by which they can increase the affinity of BCR for antigen (somatic hypermutation).

C. Effector CD4 T and memory CD4 T cells secrete many different cytokines, which characterize various types of the immune response.

D. The Th1 and Th17-type responses stimulate mainly cellular adaptive immunity of the proinflammatory kind.

E. The Th2, Th9, and Th22 type of responses stimulate proinflammatory humoral adaptive immunity, and are likely involved in the development of allergies.

F. The regulatory type of Th response (nTreg, iTregs, Th3, and Tr1) is involved in the inhibition of Th1-type immune response and the modulation of specific Th2 type response. It also includes help in B-cell isotype switch (to IgA, due to TGF-β), and the inhibition of licensing cytotoxic CD8 T lymphocytes.

CHAPTER 5

Cytokines of the Immune System: Interferons

Cytokines stimulate, influence and control growth, development, survival, and effector functions of cells of hematopoietic tissues. They are divided into families of regulatory molecules such as interferons, interleukins, chemokines, growth factors, and colony stimulating factors according to historical view of their function.

Interferons are proteins (divided in three types) that act on neighboring cells stimulating intracellular defense against viruses. Interferon-α, -β, -γ, and -λ (IFN-α, IFN-β, IFN-γ, and IFN-λ) are produced in response to viral infections, and directly affect the uninfected neighboring cells preventing replication of some viruses. However, apart from that role, interferons have a function in the regulation of immune responses. Most prominent is IFN-γ, as it activates phagocytic cells like macrophages in somatic tissues. Activated macrophages can destroy all the bacteria around them as well as those who live in them (*Leishmania, Salmonella, Mycobacteria*). They can also attract leukocytes promoting inflammation by secreting proinflammatory factors and cytokines (including IL-1, TNF-α). However, recently, many interleukins and other cytokines showed effects that overlap with the functions of interferons (with the exception of antiviral roles). We see it ever more often that the difference between the individual groups of cytokines is blurred. Cytokines apparently possess many more redundant functions than previously imagined.

In this chapter, I give a short description of cytokines important for the immune system which focus on interferons. The subsequent chapters will describe interleukins IL-1 to 38 (with the exception of IL-14 and IL-30, because they do not exist in the databases). In Chapters 7 and 8, I will describe chemokines, *tumor necrosis factor* (TNF-α/β), *transforming growth factor* (TGF-β), and many other factors important for growth and development of cells of the immune system, as well as for other somatic tissues.

The Cytokines of the Immune System
http://dx.doi.org/10.1016/B978-0-12-419998-9.00005-5

INTERFERON-α/β

Structure

Interferon-α (alpha) is a group of about 20 highly related proteins. This group includes IFN-β (beta), IFN-ω (omega), IFN-δ (delta), and IFN-τ (tau), and they are also called type I interferons. All members can bind to the single heterodimeric receptor to exert their action.

Source

All somatic nucleated cells can produce type I interferons. The initiator is the presence of the double-stranded viral RNA or induction through other cell-membrane receptors. Specialized types of hematopoietic cells can also secrete them. These are generated by monocytes and lymphoid precursors, called plasmacytoid dendritic cells (pDC) that have a characteristic marker on the surface—CD123 in blood and somatic tissues. (Immature pDC wander through the tissues, like other types of DCs, and possess the ability of antigen presentation to T lymphocytes after homing in paracortex of the lymph nodes.) Somatic cells that express the pattern recognition receptors like TLR3 and TLR4 can produce IFN-β after their activation. It seems that signal transduction that engages nuclear factors IRF3 and IRF7 can promote synthesis of type I interferons.

Function

Type I interferons act in a paracrine manner and have numerous effects on the surrounding cells, preparing them to ward off possible infection. The primary function is to induce protection against viruses in neighboring, non-infected cells. In the target cells they cause digestion of viral DNA and viral proteins. Interferon-α/β that are secreted from mature pDC may regulate the immune response under certain conditions. It has been shown that they can induce, but also inhibit the secretion of IFN-γ of monocyte-derived DCs (moDC), and thus stimulate or inhibit the development of Th1-type cells (which secrete IFN-γ). Generally, they show anti-proliferative effect on most somatic tissues.

Receptor

Receptor for IFN-α/β group of interferons is the IFNα/βR, and consists of two polypeptide chains (R1 and R2) in the cell membrane (Figure 5-1). Signal transduction goes through tyrosine kinases Jak1 (Janus kinase) and Tyk2.

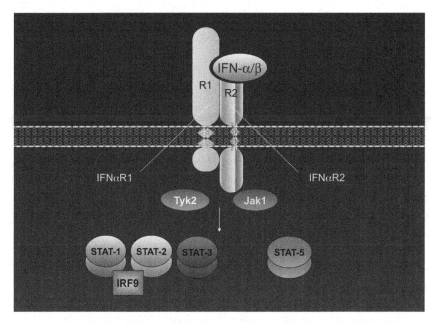

Figure 5-1 The IFN-α/β receptor and signal transduction factors.

The name for *Janus* kinase comes from the Roman god of doors—lat. *ianua*—with two faces turned in opposite directions, indicating a dual function of Jak molecules—the tyrosine phosphorylation in the receptor and phosphorylation of other molecules bound to these phosphorylated sites. Tyk2 was discovered by another group of researchers, and although it has a similar function as Jak, it has been named differently by simply abbreviating its (tyrosine kinase) function. By phosphorylation, the kinases change conformation of the receptor such that other molecules can now bind. The signal is then transferred further in the cell via such an interaction. Particularly, it was shown that *signal transducer and activator of transcription 1* (STAT-1) and STAT-2 can bind and be activated (by phosphorylation via Jak/Tyk complex). Activated STAT-1 and STAT-2 form homodimers and heterodimers, and associate with *interferon response factor 9* (IRF9; a protein of 48 kDa; the older name is p48) in cytosol (Figure 5-1). This complex can then enter the nucleus, and bind to the specific *interferon-specific response elements* (ISRE) in DNA, as for example in the promoter of the gene for *interferon stimulated gene factor 3* (ISGF3). In addition, STAT-3 and STAT-5 are involved in signal transduction, whose effects on cellular responses and genes are still being investigated. Also, in some tissues, PI3 kinase participates in the signal transduction like for example in neutrophils. The IFN regulatory factor 5 (IRF5) is a regulator of type I IFN expression.

Other Features

Genes coding for IFN-α/β members are located on human chromosome 9p22. In genetics (and it is especially important to bear in mind when searching databases), the use of *Latin* letters represent genes, whereas symbol fonts symbolize proteins, and thus each gene member of this group is designated with the name abbreviated as IFNA (IFND, IFNT) or *Ifna* (species annotation is: capital letters for human; lowercase italics for mouse) followed by the number in sequence. However, there is only a single gene for IFN-β, called IFNB1 and it is close to IFNA cluster on chromosome 9p21 (other names for IFNB1 are IFB, IFF, IFNB, MGC 96 956).

The action of type I interferons includes phosphorylation and thereby induction of oligoadenylate synthase (OAS-1), an enzyme with whose activity the cell can prevent viral replication.

Interferons can inhibit the effect of HIV Tat protein. However, interferons can suppress synthesis of mRNA in HIV provirus with defective Tat gene, suggesting that the effect of Tat and the replication of the virus is still stronger in the HIV infection. Furthermore, interferons inhibit the assembly and release of HIV from cells.

Hepatitis C virus (HCV) does not cause activation of IFNA genes in hepatocytes (which opens the possibility for therapy).

Anti-tumor effects of IFN-α/β can be divided into two modes of action: (1) direct anti-proliferative effect on some tumors; and (2) increased antigenicity (rejection potential) of tumors due to the increased expression of MHC molecules, increased expression of TNF receptors, and stimulation of NK activity.

Type I interferons (IFN-α/β) are the early molecular effectors of the innate immune response against microbes. Their action can further regulate the adaptive immune response by promoting Th1 response. It seems paradoxical that IFN-β can be useful in the treatment of *multiple sclerosis*, because it is thought to enhance and not inhibit Th1 autoimmune processes. Important roles perhaps have other functions of IFN-β or the conditions under which the IFN-β acts on dendritic cells during differentiation of Th1 cells. In particular for the latter explanation, if IFN-β is present during TNF-induced maturation of DCs, then it greatly increases the capacity of DCs to generate Th1 population (and inhibits the formation of the pDC) *in vitro*. But if the IFN-β is present (in the cell culture) when mature DCs (not treated with TNF) stimulate naïve CD4 T cells, then one gets the opposite effect, namely, reduced generation of Th1 population and promotion of the generation of IL-10 secreting T lymphocytes. The latter result might explain the beneficent *in vivo* effect observed in clinical trials as therapy against autoimmune disease like *multiple sclerosis*. Studies with blocking antibodies suggest that these effects of IFN-β are caused (at least partially) by suppression of secretion of IL-12-related cytokines (IL-12p70, IL-23, and IL-27) and IL-18 by DCs. Furthermore, *in vivo* neutralization of endogenous IFN-α (with anti-TNF antibodies) can sustain secretion of IFN-α by immature pDC. All these treatments seem to counteract generation of auto-reactive Th1 that are believed to be involved in etiology of *multiple sclerosis*.

In experiments using human skin (from body mass reduction surgery) cell-surface marker analyses of migratory (crawling-out) dermal dendritic cells (CD14$^+$, CD1a$^+$, not Langerhans cells) were studied after intradermal, intramuscular (i.m.), or subcutaneous (s.c.) injections of IFNβ—1a and 1b. Intradermal injection with IFNβ-1a and IFNβ-1b greatly enhanced the maturation status of such dermal dendritic cells (DC) migratory cells (marked by upregulation of activation markers such as CD86 and HLA-DR). In addition, there was a difference between migratory dermal DCs from IFNβ-1a (i.m. and s.c.) injected skin and those injected by IFNβ-1b. Namely, in the mixed lymphocyte reaction (which measures T-cell proliferation) in the former case (IFNβ-1a) migratory dermal DCs induced Th1-type cytokine IFN-γ, whereas in the latter case (IFNβ-1b) DCs stimulated the production of Th2-type cytokine IL-4 in primed T-cells.

Associations with Human Diseases

IFN-α overproduction by pDC seems to have a pathogenic role in *systemic lupus erythematosus* (SLE), an autoimmune disease that can affect nearly every organ or tissue in the body. It is characterized by immune attack on the parts of the cell nucleus (or lack of tolerance to them), such as the generation of antibodies against double helical DNA (anti-dsDNA), also called anti-nuclear antibodies (ANA). However, while most people with lupus have a positive ANA test, most people with a positive ANA test do not have *lupus*. *The American College of Rheumatology* has set forth 11 diagnostic criteria for SLE, including positivity to ANA as the 11th, and the patient must present with at least four of them.

Predisposition to some diseases might be hereditary and complex, implying more than a single gene or genomic factor to be involved including interferon type I genes. For example, genetic risk for sarcoidosis might be influenced by the IFNA17 gene single nucleotide polymorphism (SNP) at +551, T/G. The G allele with higher production of IFN-α was significantly associated with the disease. Furthermore, the genes associated with the regulation of action of type I interferons like TYK2 and IRF5 genes have SNPs that displayed strong association ($p < 10^{-7}$) with SLE in Nordic Caucasian populations.[1]

Infectious diseases can also have a genetic susceptibility component. For example, respiratory syncytial virus (RSV) is a common cause of severe lower respiratory tract infection in infants. A genetic association study involving 470 children hospitalized for RSV *bronchiolitis*, their parents, and 1008 random, population controls was performed recently in European Caucasians. The authors analyzed 384 SNPs in 220 candidate genes involved in airway mucosal responses, innate immunity, chemotaxis, adaptive immunity, and *allergic asthma*. Results showed associations with *bronchiolitis* of SNPs in the IFNA5 gene (rs10757212; $p < 0.01$) among other innate immune genes (including vitamin D receptor, VDR; rs10735810; JUN, rs11688; and NOS2, rs1060826).[2]

Additional conditions might occur more often in humans with a particular genetic constellation or profile. In Koreans, an SNP was identified that seems to be associated with increased risk for intracranial hemorrhage. Namely, T allele of nonsense polymorphism (rs2039381, Gln71Stop) of IFN-ε gene is a risk factor for the development of intracerebral *hemorrhage*.[3]

The receptor IFNAR1 has been investigated for genetic polymorphisms regarding susceptibility to various complex hereditary diseases. Although an SNP in the IFNAR1 gene (rs17875871) was found to be linked with predisposition to *hepatocellular carcinoma* in Chinese, the authors suggest that in fact a miR-1231 binding site polymorphism in the 3'UTR of IFNAR1 gene is the risk factor for *hepatocellular carcinoma* in relationship to HBV infection, because the association was more pronounced in HBsAg positive subgroup.[4]

Therapeutic Options

The therapeutic use of IFN-α cytokines applies to *hairy-cell leukemia*, *cutaneous T-cell lymphoma*, and *metastatic renal cell carcinoma*. It also has a therapeutic role in the forms of malignancies that respond poorly to conservative treatment (chemotherapy or radiotherapy) or as adjuvant therapy in a variety of tumor immunotherapy. Furthermore, it is used as a local therapeutic agent for warts (*genital warts*, however, this option has been rarely in use, lately), *Herpes keratoconjunctivitis, basalioma (basal cell carcinoma)* and *Laringeal papillomatosis.*

IFN-α has anti-tumor activity in advanced melanoma, and high-dose IFN-α reduces relapse and mortality by up to 33%. However, a large majority of patients experience side effects and toxicity that outweigh the benefits.

Systemic administration is used for *hepatitis B* and *C* infections, *Kaposi* sarcoma in AIDS, *Cytomegalovirus* and *Herpes zoster* infections as well as in immunocompromised patients. However, there is little effect in AIDS.

Until 2012 the standard for treatment of adult *chronic hepatitis C* consisted of pegylated interferon alpha (peg-IFNα) and ribavirin. The development of first-generation direct antiviral agents such as protease inhibitors *boceprevir* and *telaprevir* has changed this concept (in patients infected with genotype 1). It seems that a cocktail of drugs using additional protease inhibitors to hepatitis C virus would be capable of curing almost 100% of chronic patients, albeit at a high treatment cost.

IFN-β is used in the treatment of *multiple sclerosis.*

INTERFERON-γ (IFN-γ)

Structure

IFN-γ is a homodimer composed of two anti-parallel chains with a molecular weight of 20–25 kDa (monomer has 123 amino acids in mouse, 147 in humans). It belongs to the type II interferons.

Source

It is secreted by Th1-type cells, cytotoxic Tc1 cells, and activated NK cells. Human DC type I cells secrete it under certain conditions, such as stimulation through TLR2.

Function

IFN-γ has antiviral activity, which is less compared to IFN-α/β, in terms of the strength of intracellular response and viral range. More pronounced are its immunomodulatory effects. IFN-γ promotes Th1 development, inhibits Th2 development (see next paragraph for more details), stimulates development of B lymphocytes after activation, and causes BCR isotype switch in IgG2 and IgG3. It is the major activation factor of macrophages (see *Other features of IFN-γ* below). Furthermore, it has anti-proliferative effects on many tissues and tumors (with the exception of Th1, Tc1, B, and NK cells whose development it promotes; see *Cellular adaptive (specific) immune system,* Chapter 2, p. 42). Its action is specific to the species (the human does not work in the mouse).

On T helper (CD4) cells, IFN-γ stimulates development of the Th1 subset from the Th0 stage. On the other hand, it can inhibit development of three other Th subsets: it blocks Th2 subset development (TGF-β inhibits their development too; Th2 subset arises *in vitro* when T cells are activated in medium supplemented with IL-2, IL-4, IL-25, IL-31, IL-33, and TSLP). Then, IFN-γ suppresses the formation of Th9 subset (whereas a combination of IL-4 and TGF-β promotes it). And, IFN-γ suppresses development of Th17 cells (together with IL-2, IL-4, IL-12, and IL-27) from the Th0 activated stage. (Th17 can be developed using IL-1, IL-6, IL-21, IL-23, and TGF-β).

Receptor

IFN-γ acts through a cell-surface receptor that is a heterotetramer. The receptor has two chains encoded by two unique genes on different chromosomes (R1 and R2; Figure 5-2). IFN-γ binds to preformed combination of two heterodimers; each made of IFN-γR1 and IFN-γR2 chains. In the cell membrane they are associated with Jak1 and Jak2 kinases with their cytosolic parts, respectively (Figure 5-3). Binding of the ligand causes a conformational change in intracellular parts of both chains due to tyrosine phosphorylation by Jaks. It is likely that Jak can cross-phosphorylate when the ligand aggregates them in the heterotetrameric conformation. The sites on the receptor chain R1 with phosphorylated tyrosines have higher affinity to bind STAT1 monomers. The receptor–ligand complex opens up intracellularly, and allows binding of two STAT1 molecules. Upon binding, the Jaks immediately phosphorylate STAT1 molecules. This creates a shift in the structure of STAT1, which then homodimerizes. As a homodimer, STAT1 has an increased affinity to enter the nucleus, and after entering it acts as a transcription factor. However, it was then discovered that in addition to homodimeric STAT1, intracellular components of IFN-γR1 and IFN-γ itself also participate in the process of signal transduction into the nucleus (Figure 5-4). Complex STAT1/IFN-γR1/IFN-γ (probably as hetero-hexamers) enters the nucleus where it affects the transcription of genes that can be induced by IFN-γ. This is the first description of an extracellular ligand to be involved as a nuclear (co)-factor in gene transcription, which has a cell-surface transmembrane receptor with otherwise viable signal transduction

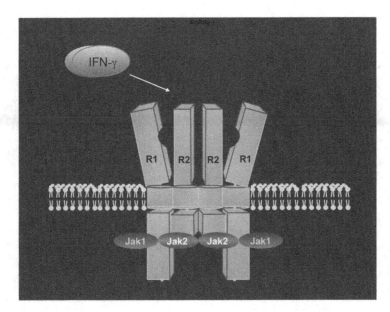

Figure 5-2 The IFN-γ receptor R1 and R2 chains in cell membrane before ligand binding: a suggested mode of action.

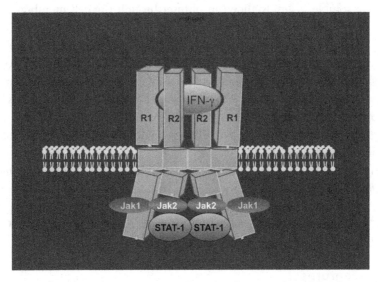

Figure 5-3 The IFN-γ receptor: suggested mode of action. Ligand binding to IFN-γ receptor causes a change in conformation of the complex.

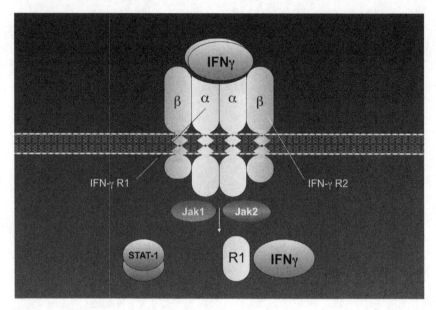

Figure 5-4 The IFN-γ receptor and its signal transduction factors. R1 = intracellular portion of the first (α) receptor chain.

mechanism. (Corticosteroids have a similar mechanism of action, but since they are soluble in lipids, they can diffuse through the cell membrane and bind to cytoplasmic receptor, with which they then enter the nucleus in form of the receptor-ligand complex and bind to DNA.) Apart from the above, probably other factors, such as STAT2 and STAT3, might be involved in the transfer of IFN-γ signal in some cells. Recently it has been found that an intracellular factor called *mammalian target of rapamycin* (mTOR) is also important for the action of IFN-γ. This factor may be defining a new path of signal transduction not only for IFN-γ, but also IL-12, as mTOR acts on the phosphorylation of STAT-3.

Signaling by IFN-γ into the cell can be inhibited the *suppressor of cytokine signaling* (SOCS) factor-1, whose gene is induced by the action of IFN-γ. SOCS-1 can inhibit the activity of Jak kinase by negative feedback (see *IL-6 receptor, regulatory feedback loops in signal transduction,* Chapter 6, p. 170 for details on the members of SOCS factors as inhibitors).

Other Features

The gene coding for IFN-γ, designated IFNG, is located on human chromosome 12q14 (other names: IFG, IFI). The receptor has another name in use besides IFN-γR1, as CD119; its gene (IFNGR1) is located on human chromosome 6q23-q24. The receptor's second-chain gene, IFNGR2, is located on chromosome 21q22.11 (other names for the IFNGR2 gene that are usually not found in latest literature are the AF-1, IFGR2, and IFNGT1).

IFN-γ is induced by the activity of IL-12 in activated T cells (Th1). This action can be inhibited by *rapamycin*, but not with *cyclosporine* (CsA). IL-18 participates in this interaction by inducing the expression of IL-12 receptor on the cell surface in Th1 lines. IL-23 can also stimulate secretion of IFN-γ in T cells.

IFN-γ induces cell-surface expression of MHC class II molecules and enhances the expression of (already existing) MHC class I glycoproteins on antigen presenting cells (B cells, macrophages, and dendritic cells; APCs). Some cells, such as DC, have a constitutive expression of MHC class II molecules.

Monocytes, under the influence of IFN-γ, probably through autocrine influence of M-CSF and IL-6 cytokines, can develop into macrophages (but not in the DCs). Macrophages are activated by IFN-γ, causing a multitude of changes. Among them, the following important functions should be mentioned (Figure 5-5): (1) MØ can destroy intracellular bacteria that normally live in their vesicles; (2) they produce nitric oxide, oxidative radicals, and hydrogen peroxide, which they secrete into their microenvironment and thereby destroy microorganisms as well as normal or damaged cells of the surrounding tissue, all of which they then phagocytose; (3) they express the receptor for the constant region of antibody (Fc); (4) they induce cell-surface expression of the TNF receptor; (5) they produce proinflammatory cytokines such as TNF-α, IL-1, and IL-12; and (6) macrophages produce chemokines such as IL-8, which attract other leukocytes and lymphocytes (Figure 5-5).

The effect of IFN-γ on DCs is somewhat more complicated. If monocytes were incubated with GM-CSF and IL-4 *in vitro*, the procedure can generate immature monocyte-derived DC. Maturation of DCs can be then further induced with TNF-α. Then, if naïve T cells were added to the culture, the interaction between DCs with naïve T cells can cause an interesting phenomenon. Namely, the interaction between cell-surface anchored molecules, CD40 and its ligand (CD40L) on DCs and T cells, respectively, can cause DCs to produce small amounts of IL-12p70, IL-18, IL-27, and possibly IL-23. These cytokines then act in synergy on DCs that produced them (autocrine signaling) and induce IFN-γ. The further (autocrine) effect of IFN-γ on mature CD40-activated DCs extensively increases the secretion

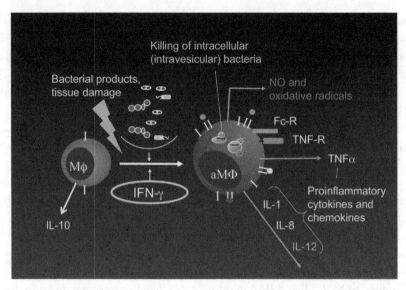

Figure 5-5 Consequences of macrophage activation by IFN-γ. Mφ—not activated macrophage. aMφ—activated macrophage. I and II—MHC molecules (class I and class II).

of IL-12 (p70) cytokine, thereby supporting the development of naïve CD4 T cells into Th1 type effector lymphocytes. It is interesting that such induction of Th1-type responses can be inhibited by the IFN-β, but only if immature DC were pretreated with it (before incubation with TNF). However, if immature DCs were pre-incubated with both TNF and IFN-β, a reverse effect will ensue, for example, increased secretion of IL-12 (p70), and hence skewing towards the Th1-type immune response. Probably because of the former effect of IFN-β (inhibition of Th1 response) one expects some beneficent effects in treatment of patients with *multiple sclerosis* (in whose pathophysiological basis is an autoimmune Th1 type attack on myelinized sheath of neurons).

IFN-γ downregulates the action of IL-13 by expression of its decoy receptor (IL-13R2). Namely, although it has a high affinity for the ligand, IL-13R2 does not transduce the signal when expressed on the cell membrane (and, it is usually withheld inside the cell). IFN-γ causes the appearance of the IL-13R2 decoy receptor on the cell surface, thereby diluting the action of IL-13.

IFN-γ provokes migration of lymphocytes into the lungs via the chemokine CXCL10 causing inflammation of the alveolar wall (*alveolitis*) and granuloma formation.

IFN-γ has an important anti-angiogenesis effect. In neural tissue, it is possible that it participates in the development of neurites (neurogenic effect); the latter are projections of the cell body of a neuron (either as dendrites or axons). Furthermore, IFN-γ inhibits collagen synthesis in connective tissue and skin (thus opening a possibility in therapy for *scleroderma*).

Cells of human metastatic prostate cancer (M12) can be killed (by apoptosis) if treated with IFN-γ *in vitro*.

To illustrate further the multifaceted action of IFN-γ, it activates 66 genes in human bronchial epithelial cells after incubation *in vitro* for 8 hours, as determined by the oligonucleotide *microarray* hybridization with their mRNA (with 5% errors). After 24 hours, the number of induced genes increased by 287 to a total of 353 genes while 376 of them were inhibited by 50%. Most of these genes encode cytokines and secreted products of epithelial cells. Dexamethasone inhibits two (after 8 hours) and 45 genes (after 24 hours) induced by IFN-γ. Also, dexamethasone increased the expression of 65 of the 376 inhibited with IFN-γ. Most of the latter genes encode proteins of the nucleus and the cell cycle. (Dexamethasone alone increased expression of only 22, and inhibited seven genes after 24 hours.)

Association with Human Diseases

IFN-γ causes disruption of tight junctions between intestinal epithelial cells (with the help of TNF), and thereby allows the entry of bacteria into the tissues, which opens the possibility of contributing to development of *inflammatory bowel disease* (IBD).[5]

In a mouse model of restenosis after coronary lesions, it seems that IFN-γ plays a role in the etiology of coronary disease (atherosclerosis). In the mouse, IFN-γ is a central factor in vascular endothelial dysfunction, manifested by inhibition of *endothelial nitric oxidase synthase* (eNOS), and stimulation of inducible NOS (iNOS) (in infiltrating T lymphocytes). The lack of sensitivity of vessels to (relaxing effect of) NO is probably the main reason for late complications of *atherosclerosis*.

SNPs are common in studies of susceptibility to various diseases with complex inheritance. Allelic frequencies for SNPs differ significantly by race and Asian, African-American, and Caucasian frequencies of each SNP are listed in the NCBI SNP database at www.ncbi.nlm.nih.gov/snp/. Furthermore, racial groups do not have simple proinflammatory or anti-inflammatory genetic profiles implying complex inheritance of predisposition for most (if not all) inflammatory diseases.

Some of SNPs are used as markers, and some affect the stronger or weaker expression (transcription) of the respective alleles. The most frequently used for IFNG are SNPs at +874 T>A (rs2430561), +2109 A>G (rs1861494), and for the receptor, the polymorphisms at IFNGR1 C-56T and IFNGR2 A+839G.

IFNG +874 T>A (rs2430561) SNP is associated with *leprosy* among Brazilians.[6]

In addition, the SNP -764 G>C in the IFNG gene promoter is functionally important during IFN-α-induced spontaneous recovery in HCV-infected patients. The authors suggest that in determining treatment response it could be used as a genetic marker to predict anti-viral response in HCV-infected patients.[7]

Significant correlation was observed of one SNP in IFNG with oral *lichen planus*.

T allele of the SNP in the promoter of the IFNG gene at position -179 G>T (rs2069709) increases the influence of TNF on IFNG allowing for higher production of IFN-γ. This allele was significantly correlated with faster development of AIDS (measured by reduction of CD4 T lymphocytes in the blood), which can be used for prognostic purposes. Probably TNF decreases the threshold for activation of T cells, and thus accelerate their destruction (T-tropic HIV retrovirus is silent in resting infected CD4 T cells, but it kills them upon activation. The spreading mechanism includes coating viral particles with the patches of cell membrane as they burst out of the cells).

It seems that functional polymorphisms of IFNG gene, especially −1616T/C (rs2069705), and +874A/T (rs2430561), are strongly associated with *pneumonia*-induced sepsis in the Chinese population.[8]

IFN-γ gene polymorphisms (SNP: rs1861493, and microsatellite CA together with others unrelated to IFNG) showed significant allelic associations with the *idiopathic inflammatory myopathies* in a UK Caucasian population.[9]

In *atopic asthma* the association of the IFNG-gene +2109 A>G (rs1861494) SNP polymorphism (A/G) was observed in a case–control cohort study, which was replicated in a family study.[10] There is another study implicating IFNG genotype in sex differences in the risk of childhood (allergic) *asthma*. Two IFNG SNPs (rs2069727 and rs2430561) showed significant associations with disease. Namely, genotype–sex interaction on *asthma* was characterized by nonadditivity; that is, heterozygous boys had the highest risk for *asthma*, and heterozygous girls had the lowest risk.[11]

Polymorphisms in the genetic area close to the IFNG gene on chromosome 12 (which includes a larger region including genes encoding IL-22 and IL-26 cytokines) is associated with gender differences in the predisposition to *rheumatoid arthritis* (women have higher incidence), as well as to *multiple sclerosis*. Recent results point to a conclusion that IFNG allelic variants are associated with susceptibility to *multiple sclerosis* in men but not in women. Carriers of rs2069727*G polymorphism had higher expression of IFN-γ than non-carriers, and the polymorphism was linked to disease susceptibility.[12] Therefore, there is a link between the (IFNG-associated) sex bias (in susceptibility to disease) and the expression of IFN-γ in *multiple sclerosis*.

In the Korean population, several SNPs in the IFNG gene are associated with the risk for developing *systemic lupus erythematosus*. The predisposing allele of the linked SNP (rs2430561) has an NF-kB binding site. This could imply that augmented IFNG expression might increase disease susceptibility.[13]

Variants in some cytokines' genes are linked to modification of the risk in development of *non-Hodgkin lymphoma (NHL)*, such as the influence of environmental factors like organochlorine exposure. Associations between studied exposures and NHL risk were limited to genotype including that of the **IFNG** gene (C-1615T) TT and **IL4** (5′-UTR, Ex1-168C>T) CC. Associations with *NHL* risk were also found to be limited to particular genotypes for **IL16** (3′-UTR, Ex22+871A>G) AA, **IL8** (T-251A) TT, and **IL10** (A-1082G) AG/GG genes. This study was one of the first examples of a potential gene–environment interaction in forming the risk for *NHL* in the USA population.[14]

Epidemiologic studies showed four times increased risk of *acute lymphoblastic leukemia* in children of women with *multiple sclerosis*. Furthermore, *multiple sclerosis* shows a risk association with HLA-DRA SNP rs3135388, (a proxy marker for DRB1*1501; see Chapter 3; *MHC associations with disease*, p. 68). There seems to be a male-specific protective association of IFNG SNP rs2069727 in both *multiple sclerosis* and *childhood acute lymphoblastic leukemia* (in combination with other factors like HLA-DRB1*1501, -Cw*05, and tenascin XB genes) in South Wales (UK) and Mexican populations. In other words, only girls born to mothers with *multiple sclerosis* may have an increased susceptibility to *childhood acute lymphoblastic leukemia*.[15]

It is thought that EBV infection might contribute to development of *breast cancer*. Serum levels of EBV viral capsid antigen IgA and nuclear antigen-1 (EBNA-1) IgA are associated with the polymorphisms of IFNG (rs2069705) and IL10 (rs1800871) genes with *breast cancer* susceptibility in the Asian population. This result suggests that EBV may be a risk factor and its contribution is further modulated by genetic variations in the IFNG and IL10 genes.[16]

Recent profiling of the IFNG genotypes showed correlation with *imatinib* therapy in *chronic myeloid leukemia* (*CML*) and predicts cytogenetic and molecular response to the disease. This suggests a probable contribution of the IFN-γ signaling pathway in the mechanism of action of *imatinib* in *CML*.[17]

Genetic deficiency of the IFNGR gene on both chromosomes causes *Mendeleev type* of hereditary predisposition to disease caused by infection with *atypical mycobacteria* including *Bacille Calmette–Guerin* (BCG), which can lead to a fatal outcome in these children.

Seven SNPs located in the IFNG and IFNGR1 genes were genotyped in the Chinese Han population, and a significant association between rs7749390 and *tuberculosis* was observed.[18] Similar studies in other human populations gave controversial results, and some showed that associations were only with IFNG polymorphisms and severity of the disease in Caucasians. In African-Americans, however, nitric oxide synthase (NOS2A) variants may contribute to *tuberculosis* susceptibility that may act synergistically with SNPs in TLR4 and IFNGR1 genes.

Patients with *atopic dermatitis eczema herpeticum* have reduced IFN-γ production, and IFNG and IFNGR1 SNPs are significantly associated with *atopic dermatitis eczema herpeticum* disease that may contribute to an impaired immune response to *herpes simplex* virus.[19]

Genome-wide linkage analysis identifies polymorphism in the human interferon-gamma receptor that affects *Helicobacter pylori* infection.[20]

There is an important influence on *cancer* risk, especially colon and rectal cancer, of the interferon-signaling pathway that was performed in two population-based studies of *colon cancer* (1555 cases and 1956 controls) and *rectal cancer* (754 cases and 959 controls) in USA (Northern California and Utah). For *rectal cancer*, IFNGR1 rs3799488 polymorphism was directly associated with risk. Five other SNPs in IFNG, IRF2, and IRF3 genes were associated with *colon cancer* and eight SNPs in IFNGR1, IFNGR2, IRF2, IRF4, IRF6, and IRF8 were associated with *rectal cancer*. IRF3 rs2304204 was associated with the strongest direct association and IRF2 rs3775554 with the strongest (protective) inverse association for *colon cancer*.[21]

The IFNGR1 -56C/T gene polymorphism (rs17175350) is associated with increased risk of early *gastric carcinoma*.[22] Polymorphisms in IFNGR2 (Ex7-128 C>T) (and also TNFA -308 A>G) may increase the risk of *gastric cancer*.[23]

IFNGR2 and other cytokine and cytokine receptor genes of the adaptive immune response are differentially associated with *breast cancer* risk in American women of African and European ancestry. Multivariate logistic regression found SNPs in genes important for T helper type 1 (Th1) immunity (IFNGR2 rs1059293, IL15RA rs2296135, LTA rs1041981), Th2 immunity (IL4R rs1801275), and T regulatory cell-mediated immunosuppression (TGFB1 rs1800469) associated with *breast cancer* risk, mainly among AAs. The combined effect of these five SNPs was highly significant among AAs. (When stratified by estrogen receptor [ER] status, LTA rs1041981 was associated with ER-positive *breast cancers* among EAs and marginally among AAs. Only among AA women, were IL15 rs10833 and IL15RA rs2296135 associated with ER-positive tumors, and IL12RB1 rs375947, IL15 rs10833, and TGFB1 rs1800469 were associated with ER-negative tumors.) The study has identified genetic variants in the adaptive immune response pathway associated with *breast cancer* risk, which differs by ancestry populations, menopausal, and ER status.[24]

Therapeutic Options

Inhibition of IFN-γ and its action is considered in the treatment of various diseases, including autoimmune diseases. Furthermore, small molecules that can inhibit Jak kinases and thus the signal transduction through the JAK-STAT pathway were recently discovered. This opens the possibility to test strong inhibitors for the therapeutic effects in the future.

IFN-γ showed a modest success in anti-tumor therapy alone, and it is currently being used in a number of anti-cancer clinical trials. It can be used as adjuvant in immunotherapy, or in therapeutic immunizations, like for example those with killed autologous tumor cells. Therapy with IFN-γ has many adverse effects (shivering, anemia, fatigue, nausea or vomiting, and orthostatic hypotension), but most of them are transient. Lower or higher doses of IFN-γ are usually either ineffective or show unwanted immuno-modulatory properties. Targeted delivery to the vascular endothelium using CD13 molecules (a hallmark of angiogenesis) might be able to improve the performance of anti-tumor therapy. In therapy of *melanoma* and *renal cell carcinoma*, in order to maintain the induction of IFN-γ in the body, clinical trials with i.v. recombinant human IL-12 (rhIL-12) with the addition of sc IL-2 are being conducted.

Experiments in mice transgenic with constructs of IFNG gene driven by tissue-specific promoters have shown that IFN-γ expressed by such methods could help anti-tumor therapy, particularly in cancers in which DNA viruses were an etiologic factor.

Similarly, injections of IFN-γ into the skin with a fine needle may help the treatment of *scleroderma* according to preclinical results.

Analysis of epidemiological, preclinical and clinical studies (1966–2005) of IFN-γ1b in *idiopathic pulmonary fibrosis* has been recently published and conclusions state that the benefit of treatment is controversial. Although little advantage was shown in the largest clinical study, further clinical trials and analyses are needed to better evaluate treatment with IFN-γ. IFN-γ is one of two drugs of choice for this disease (with perphenidon), because it has a potential to modulate the balance of various T helper subsets (enhancing Th1 while diminishing Th2) and inhibit fibroblast activation.

With disseminated BCG infection in children with *Mendeleev type* predisposition to *mycobacteria* like in hemizygotic absence of genes encoding either receptor for interferon-γ (IFNGR1) or IL-12 (IL12RB1) due to natural defects, therapy with IFN-γ showed modest results, but such cases are too infrequent for clear evaluation.

More successful results were achieved with IFN-γ as anti-fungal (adjuvant) therapy of *chronic pulmonary aspergillosis*.

INTERFERON-λ (IFN-λ)

Synonyms

Interleukin 28A, 28B, and IL-29 (see under *Interleukins 28 and 29*, Chapter 6, p. 224).

The group designated as IFN-λ belongs to type III interferons that have both anti-viral and immunomodulatory actions.

REFERENCES

1. Sigurdsson S, et al. Polymorphisms in the tyrosine kinase 2 and interferon regulatory factor 5 genes are associated with systemic lupus erythematosus. *Am J Hum Genet* Mar, 2005;**76**:528.
2. Janssen R, et al. Genetic susceptibility to respiratory syncytial virus bronchiolitis is predominantly associated with innate immune genes. *J Infect Dis* Sep 15, 2007;**196**:826.

3. Kim SK, et al. T Allele of nonsense polymorphism (rs2039381, Gln71Stop) of interferon-epsilon is a risk factor for the development of intracerebral hemorrhage. *Hum Immunol* Jan, 2014;**75**:88.

4. Zhou C, et al. A miR-1231 binding site polymorphism in the 3'UTR of IFNAR1 is associated with hepatocellular carcinoma susceptibility. *Gene* Oct 1, 2012;**507**:95.

5. Chiba H, Kojima T, Osanai M, Sawada N. The significance of interferon-gamma-triggered internalization of tight-junction proteins in inflammatory bowel disease. *Sci STKE* Jan 3, 2006;**2006**:pe1.

6. Cardoso CC, et al. IFNG +874 T>A single nucleotide polymorphism is associated with leprosy among Brazilians. *Hum Genet* Nov, 2010;**128**:481.

7. Huang Y, et al. A functional SNP of interferon-gamma gene is important for interferon-alpha-induced and spontaneous recovery from hepatitis C virus infection. *Proc Natl Acad Sci USA* Jan 16, 2007;**104**:985.

8. Wang D, et al. Functional polymorphisms of interferon-gamma affect pneumonia-induced sepsis. *PloS one* 2014;**9**:e87049.

9. Chinoy H, et al. Interferon-gamma and interleukin-4 gene polymorphisms in Caucasian idiopathic inflammatory myopathy patients in UK. *Ann Rheum Dis* Jul, 2007;**66**:970.

10. Kumar A, Ghosh B. A single nucleotide polymorphism (A → G) in intron 3 of IFN-gamma gene is associated with asthma. *Genes Immun* Jun, 2008;**9**:294.

11. Loisel DA, et al. IFNG genotype and sex interact to influence the risk of childhood asthma. *J Allergy Clin Immunol* Sep, 2011;**128**:524.

12. Kantarci OH, et al. Interferon gamma allelic variants: sex-biased multiple sclerosis susceptibility and gene expression. *Arch Neurol* Mar, 2008;**65**:349.

13. Kim K, et al. Interferon-gamma gene polymorphisms associated with susceptibility to systemic lupus erythematosus. *Ann Rheum Dis* Jun, 2010;**69**:1247.

14. Colt JS, et al. Organochlorine exposure, immune gene variation, and risk of non-Hodgkin lymphoma. *Blood* Feb 26, 2009;**113**:1899.

15. Morrison BA, et al. Multiple sclerosis risk markers in HLA-DRA, HLA-C, and IFNG genes are associated with sex-specific childhood leukemia risk. *Autoimmunity* Dec, 2010;**43**:690.

16. He JR, et al. Joint effects of Epstein–Barr virus and polymorphisms in interleukin-10 and interferon-gamma on breast cancer risk. *J Infect Dis* Jan 1, 2012;**205**:64.

17. Kim DH, et al. The IFNG (IFN-gamma) genotype predicts cytogenetic and molecular response to imatinib therapy in chronic myeloid leukemia. *Clin Cancer Res* Nov 1, 2010;**16**:5339.

18. He J, Wang J, Lei D, Ding S. Analysis of functional SNP in ifng/ifngr1 in Chinese Han population with tuberculosis. *Scand J Immunol* Jun, 2010;**71**:452.

19. Leung DY, et al. Human atopic dermatitis complicated by eczema herpeticum is associated with abnormalities in IFN-gamma response. *J Allergy Clin Immunol* Apr, 2011;**127**:965.

20. Thye T, Burchard GD, Nilius M, Muller-Myhsok B, Horstmann RD. Genomewide linkage analysis identifies polymorphism in the human interferon-gamma receptor affecting *Helicobacter pylori* infection. *Am J Hum Genet* Feb, 2003;**72**:448.

21. Slattery ML, Lundgreen A, Bondurant KL, Wolff RK. Interferon-signaling pathway: associations with colon and rectal cancer risk and subsequent survival. *Carcinogenesis* Nov, 2011;**32**:1660.

22. Canedo P, et al. The interferon gamma receptor 1 (IFNGR1) -56C/T gene polymorphism is associated with increased risk of early gastric carcinoma. *Gut* Nov, 2008;**57**:1504.

23. Hou L, et al. Polymorphisms in Th1-type cell-mediated response genes and risk of gastric cancer. *Carcinogenesis* Jan, 2007;**28**:118.

24. Quan L, et al. Cytokine and cytokine receptor genes of the adaptive immune response are differentially associated with breast cancer risk in American women of African and European ancestry. *Int J Cancer* Mar 15, 2014;**134**:1408.

FURTHER READING

Bekisz J, Schmeisser H, Hernandez J, Goldman ND, Zoon KC. Human interferons alpha, beta and omega. *Growth Factors* Dec, 2004;**22**:243.

Chiba H, Kojima T, Osanai M, Sawada N. The significance of interferon-gamma-triggered internalization of tight-junction proteins in inflammatory bowel disease. *Sci STKE* Jan 3, 2006;**2006**:pe1.

CHAPTER 6

Cytokines of the Immune System: Interleukins

IL-1

Structure

Interleukin-1 (IL-1) represents a group of 17–20 kDa cytokines with a broad range of biological functions centered on the generation and maintenance of inflammatory processes. The best-known members are IL-1α, IL-1β, and IL-1Ra (receptor antagonist). Similarity between IL-1 family members is relatively small. According to primary protein structure, IL-1α and IL-1β are about 30% different from each other. Prior to secretion, the active forms are made from precursors by caspase complex 1/5.

Source

The main physiological source of IL-1 is activated macrophage (Figure 5-5), and it is created as a precursor called pro-IL-1. Its secretion can be triggered by varying proinflammatory stimuli, including cell injury, products of the bacterial cell membranes, zymosan, leukotrienes, activated complement components, TNF, immune complexes (Ig-antigen), granulocyte-macrophage colony stimulating factor (GM-CSF), and IL-1 itself (autocrine). On the contrary, its production can be reduced with corticosteroids (e.g., dexamethasone), TGF-β, and retinoic acid. IL-1β, can be detected in the serum unlike IL-1α, which is secreted from the dendritic cells (DCs) only on the activation stimulus.

Function

IL-1 represents a group of pleiotropic cytokines with proinflammatory, immunoregulatory, and hematopoietic effects. It can cause an increase in body temperature, bone resorption, muscle proteolysis, cachexia (indirectly via tumor necrosis factor (TNF)), an increase in the amount of circulating acute-phase proteins such as C-reactive protein (CRP), and a decrease of iron and zinc plasma concentrations. The central function of IL-1 in the connective tissue is wound healing probably due to the angiogenic effect. Active forms of IL-1 cytokine (that can be secreted) are formed by

The Cytokines of the Immune System
http://dx.doi.org/10.1016/B978-0-12-419998-9.00006-7

conversion of the inactive cytosolic protein pro–IL-1 with caspase 1 enzyme (CASP1/ICE).

During T cell activation, IL-1 promotes development of the Th17 phenotype of helper T cells (from Th0 stage) together with IL-6, IL-21, IL-23, and TGF-β (whereas IFNγ, IL-2, IL-4, IL-12, and IL-27 block their development).

Receptor

On the surface of target cells (Figure 6-1), IL-1 and the antagonistic molecule called IL-1Ra can bind to the IL-1 receptor (IL-1R, type-1; two chains IL-1RI and IL-1RacP) or to the decoy-IL-1 receptor (type-2; IL-1RII). Also, there is a second receptor for IL-1 (type 3; two chains of IL-36 and IL-1RacP), which binds other agonistic molecules of IL-1, namely IL-36A (IL-1F6) and IL-36G (IL-1F9). The latter two cytokines are specifically inhibited by the action of the IL-36Ra (IL-1F5), which is similar in activity to IL-1Ra (as well as IL-38, which is another IL-36 receptor antagonist). The soluble form of IL-1RacP, which can bind IL-1 and further inhibit its action, joins the antagonism of IL-1.

Importantly, granulocytes predominantly have type-2 IL-1 receptor (decoy) (90%). Upon binding to the ligand, type-2 receptor is rapidly internalized,

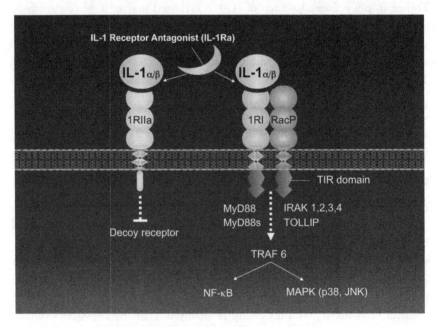

Figure 6-1 IL-1 homologs, IL-1R antagonist, and IL-1 receptors.

releases the ligand and recycles back to the cell surface. This probably contributes to the rapid disappearance of IL-1 from the circulation.

Signal transduction into the cell is similar to the signal transduction of the Toll-like receptor (TLR, see the section on dendritic cells and innate immunity; they are important for recognition of molecular *patterns* of microorganisms). IL-1 signal transduction into the cell is controlled via TIR (*"Toll/interleukin-1 region"*) domain in the intracellular part of IL-1 receptors. It can bind various mediators (adapters) which help in protein kinase activation, resulting in ubiquitination (and activation) of TRAF6, and there are adapters–inhibitors of these bonds (TOLLIP, IRAK3, and MyD88s). This ultimately results in the activation of nuclear factor *kappa* B (NF-κB) and MAP kinase dependent nuclear factors (c-Jun, ATF-2, and CREB), which further participate in the transcription of IL-1 stimulated genes in the target cell.

Other Features

IL-1α has previously been named: hematopoietin-1; preinterleukin-1-alpha; pro-interleukin-1-alpha. Previous names for IL-1β were catabolin; preinterleukin-1-beta; pro–interleukin-1-beta. The gene coding for IL-1α is called **IL1A** (alias: IL-1A, IL1, IL1-ALPHA, IL1F1), and the one encoding IL-1β —**IL1B** (alias: IL-1, IL1-BETA, IL1F2). They are on chromosome 2q12-21. Other members of this group are also encoded in this segment of the chromosome and form a gene *cluster*. The IL-1 receptor antagonist (IL-1Ra) is encoded by a gene in the same *cluster*, called **IL1RN** (alias: IRAP; IL1F3; IL1RA; IL-1ra3; ICILA-1RA; MGC10430).

The IL1 gene cluster includes nine genes encoding IL-1-alike cytokines on human chromosome 2. Six of these genes are located in-between IL1A/IL1B on the one side and IL1RN gene on the other in the following order (in direction from centromere to telomere): **IL37** (alias: IL1F7), **IL36G** (alias: IL1F9), **IL36A** (alias: IL1F6), **IL36B** (alias: IL1F8), **IL36RN** (alias: IL1F5), and **IL38** (alias: IL1F10).

Interleukin-1 receptor I chain (IL-1RI) is also called "*antigen* CD121a" (and frequent aliases are "interleukin 1 receptor alpha, type I"; or just interleukin 1 receptor). Its gene is named **IL1R1** (aliases: CD121A, IL-1R-alpha, IL1R, IL1RA, p80, D2S1473). It is located on chromosome 2q12, 10 Mb centromeric to genes of the IL-1 gene *cluster*, close to the receptor of the IL18R gene.

Interleukin-1 decoy receptor chain (IL-1R, type II; IL-1R2) is also called "*antigen* CD121b" (aliases: IL1RB; IL1R2c; CDw121b; IL-1R-2; IL-1RT2; or IL-1RT-2).

IL-1β together with TNF and IFN-γ stimulate gamma-secretase-associated cleavage of *amyloid precursor protein* (APP) via JNK-dependent MAPK, which may be the reason for increased production and accumulation of amyloid in *Alzheimer's disease.*

Gamma rays stimulate the body to secrete IL-1 and IL-6, probably because of radioprotective impact. The level of secretion of these cytokines may be taken as a measure of received radiation doses.

Interleukin-4 (IL-4) antagonizes the activity of IL-1 by inducing the decoy receptor (IL-1R2) expression and activity as well as release in its soluble form.

Association with Diseases

IL-1 and its receptor are involved in the pathogenesis of various acute and chronic inflammatory diseases including *septic shock, rheumatoid arthritis, atherosclerosis, Alzheimer's disease, kidney diseases, migraine, endometriosis* (RA), and in the tumors like *liver, bladder,* and *gastric* cancer. Apart from diseases, it seems that variations in vaccine-induced cytokine responses are modulated by genetic polymorphisms in many cytokine and cytokine receptor genes.

Inflammatory diseases, which show complex genetic predisposition in inheritance, are suggested to be associated with alleles of IL-1 group of cytokines or their receptors. Such alleles should theoretically change the physiological function of IL-1. Studies which investigated genetic predisposition for developing certain diseases through association with single nucleotide polymorphisms (SNPs) of the IL-1/R group alleles are numerous and often contradictory. Thus, there have been suggestions about association of the IL1A with predisposition for developing certain diseases, but only in certain ethnic groups (probably due to genetic drift) with diseases such as *ankylosing spondylitis, systemic sclerosis, Alzheimer's disease, severe periodontitis* (similar to the IL1B) and the development of nephropathy (last stage renal disease, *"end-stage renal disease"*; ESRD), and back pain syndrome (*"low back pain"*), as well as adverse conditions such as miscarriage. Furthermore, one IL1A allele is associated with a negative outcome of allergy skin-prick test (in non-asthmatics).

Associations of the IL1-gene-cluster-loci genetic polymorphisms with diseases are as follows:

Asthma, Osteoarthritis, Autoimmune Diseases

Increased risk for childhood asthma (in the first decade of life) was suggested after analysis of the gene–environment interaction of the IL-1 receptor antagonist gene (IL1RN) polymorphism rs2234678 regarding maternal smoking during pregnancy.[1]

In addition to the SNP, variable tandem repeats of nucleotides in DNA sequence (*"variable nucleotide tandem repeats"*; VNTR) are also used as markers for the alleles of certain genes or alleles in the gene cluster. By testing VNTRs, association of IL1 gene cluster with *knee osteoarthritis* (OA) was found, but, interestingly, not with *hip* OA in the UK. Recent meta-analyses gathered data from various human subpopulations of Caucasians and showed that the influence of IL-1 gene cluster on the risk of acquiring *large joint OA* is still controversial, and likely to be differently spread among various (sub)populations. In detail, one meta-analysis does not confirm but only suggests that some *hand* and *hip OA* risk could be associated with the IL-1 region, particularly centered in IL1B and possibly also IL1RN.[2] On the other hand, another meta-analysis showed that common genetic variation in the IL-1 region is not associated with prevalence of *hip or knee* OA, but that IL1RN might have a role in severity of *knee* OA.[3] Along with this, a greater likelihood of radiographic progression of *knee OA* was shown to be associated with a commonly occurring IL1RN haplotype marked by three IL1RN SNPs (rs419598, rs9005, rs315943). Thus, IL1RN gene markers could be useful in monitoring patients for medical management and possibly drug development.[4]

Analysis of SNPs in the IL1R1 gene revealed an association with severe *hand OA* in family-based and case–control studies, with the strongest candidate for predisposition to disease being the SNP rs2287047.[5]

Some IL1 gene cluster polymorphisms seem to affect risk of *small joint OA* as well. A case–control study in bilateral *distal interphalangeal joint osteoarthritis* (DIP OA) in dentists and teachers were investigated, as they professionally use such joints in their everyday work. Results showed that two IL1B SNPs (rs1143634 and rs1143633) are associated with DIP OA, implying that the IL-1-gene-cluster variants may predispose DIP joints to the effects of mechanical overload.[6]

Meta-analysis of the risk for *systemic juvenile idiopathic arthritis* showed that three IL-1 gene cluster SNPs (rs6712572, rs2071374, and rs1688075) and one IL-1 receptor cluster SNP (rs12712122) are associated with disease.[7]

The genetic susceptibility for *ankylosing spondylitis* may be associated with the IL1A gene polymorphisms.[8] According to meta-analysis the following polymorphisms in the IL-1 gene cluster contribute to increased risk: IL-1RN (VNTR), IL-1A (rs1800587), and IL36B (rs1900287), with a distinct discrepancy for these associations among races.[9] Additional meta-analysis suggested three IL-1 gene cluster polymorphisms (rs2856836, rs17561, and rs1894399), as well as the IL-38 (rs3811581) and IL1A (rs1800587) polymorphisms to be associated with the development of *ankylosing spondy-litis* in Europeans but not in Asians.[10] The association between several poly-morphisms located in the IL-1 gene cluster and *spondyloarthritis* as a whole was also found. The IL1A locus was strongly associated with *ankylosing spon-dylitis* phenotype, whereas IL38 gene was associated with non-*ankylosing spondylitis* phenotype of *spondyloarthritis*.[11]

There is also an association between the interleukin-1 family gene clus-ter and *psoriatic arthritis*.[12]

RA susceptibility seems to be revealed in meta-analysis. Namely, the IL-1 promoter region polymorphism IL-1B −511A/G (rs16944) variant seems to be associated with *rheumatoid arthritis*.[13]

In *morbus Behcet*, the homozygous genotype IL1B (+3954 T, rs1143634) SNP allele has been suggested to be associated with risk for the disease.

IL-1 genetic polymorphisms (and those of TNF-α) contribute to the development of *juvenile dermatomyositis* as risk and severity factors.[14]

The risks for *Graves' disease* and *Graves' ophthalmopathy* might be associ-ated with the rs1800587 (IL1A) and rs16944 (IL1B) polymorphisms in the Asian population.[15]

The interleukin-1 cluster gene region seems to be associated with *multiple sclerosis* in an Italian Caucasian population.[16]

A Chinese study suggests that variations in the IL1B and IL1RN genes are associated with increased susceptibility to *IgA nephropathy* in children. The results also suggest that the development of proteinuria is related to IL1A and that podocyte foot process effacement is associated with IL1B.[17]

The susceptibility to *alopecia areata* seems to be associated with the IL1A gene polymorphism rs3783553 in two independent Chinese populations.[18] This is an insertion/deletion polymorphism (ttca/−) at miRNA-122 bind-ing site in the 3′ untranslated region that was shown to be functional. In addition, it seemed to reduce the risk of *gastric cancer* in Chinese.[19]

IL-1Ra measurements in sera can predict the progression of *metabolic syndrome* to clinically incident *diabetes type 2* independently of CRP and other risk factors, according to two large Finnish cohort observational stud-ies (with over 12 thousands persons) carried over 7–10 years. Furthermore, genetic variation in the IL-1 locus may have gender-specific associations with the risk of *type 2 diabetes mellitus*.[20]

Infections, Chronic Inflammations

Two polymorphisms, one in the IL1B gene (rs1143634) and the other in the inflammasome's NLRP3 gene (rs10754558), were significantly associated with the HIV-1 infection in Brazilians.[21] High risk-human papilloma virus (HR-HPV) clearance rates were significantly (p < 0.001) associated with five SNPs (rs228942, rs419598, rs315950, rs7737000, and rs9292618) mapped to coding and regulatory regions in three genes (IL2RB, IL1RN, and IL7R). These data suggest that the analyzed genetic variants in interleukin family of cytokines modulate HR-HPV clearance in HIV-1 seropositive African-Americans.[22]

The IL1RN gene promoter SNP (C/T) rs4251961 plays a key role in the pathophysiology of *invasive pneumococcal disease*. Namely, plasma IL-1Ra concentrations were significantly higher in nonsurvivors compared with survivors, and the major (C) allele of rs4251961 was associated with a significant increase in plasma IL-1Ra.[23] The minor allele has been previously shown to be associated with decreased IL-1Ra production in healthy adults.

Recurrent aphthous stomatitis is strongly associated with one IL1B (−511) allele, but less with the VNTR marker of IL-1 receptor antagonist gene.

IL-1 genetic factors are associated with the severity of *chronic periodontitis* in four different ethnic groups (Caucasians, African-Americans, Hispanics, and Asians) as reported by large case–control study from patients recruited in USA, Chile, and China.[24]

Associations between *chronic rhinosinusitis* with *nasal polyposis* and SNPs in the IL1A (rs17561 and Ser114Ala) and IL1B (rs16944) genes were suggested as risk factors in Canadian and Turkish populations (the study also pointed to correlation with the TNF rs361525 and rs1800629 SNPs).[25]

IL1B SNPs rs1143634 and rs1143639 showed a consistent association with lung disease severity in *cystic fibrosis*, suggesting that IL-1β is a clinically relevant modulator of the lung disease.[26]

Myocardial Infarction, Stroke

The risk of *myocardial infarction* and *stroke* in young people has been significantly decreased in carriers of the genotype T/T (weak producer of IL-1β) in IL1B (T-511C, rs16944) SNP, and the T allele plays a co-dominant role. The SNP rs380092 in IL1RN showed an association with overall *ischemic stroke*.[27]

Genetic variation in IL1B and IL10 genes may also influence the risk of *idiopathic venous thromboembolism*.[28]

Cancer

Polymorphism in IL1RN is associated with *osteoporotic fractures*, as well as with the development of *gastric* cancer.

Increased risk of developing *non-small-cell lung cancer* was found in carriers of two markers: VNTR of the IL-1 receptor antagonist (IL1RN*1) gene and allele of the SNP in the IL-1B gene (IL1B-31T, rs1143627). IL1B allele that has a phenotype of strong producer (IL1BT-511C, rs16944) is associated with the development of *liver cancer* as a result of *chronic hepatitis B* infection.

One IL1B genotype is also associated with the risk of *gastric atrophy* and *cancer*. Some alleles and polymorphisms of the IL1B are associated with the success of therapy for *Helicobacter pylori*, as well as with predisposition for the development of the disease from the same microorganism.

A large study on predisposition to *ovarian cancer* found association with SNPs rs17561 and rs4848300 in the IL1A gene, which varied by histologic subtype,[29] that was corroborated with even larger recent one, which found additional risk factors in the NF-κB pathway and TNFSF10 genes.[30]

IL1B SNP at the +3954 C>T (rs1143634) site is associated with increased *breast cancer* risk, while IL-6 SNP at −174 G>C (rs1800795) seems to be protective in the Indian population.[31]

Carriers of IL1B rs1143634 polymorphism with T allele show association with the higher risk of developing *lung cancer* especially among smokers in the Japanese population.[32]

The genetic variation in the IL1RN gene (rs2637988 and, additionally, FCGR2A) may play a role in lymphomagenesis of *non-Hodgkin lymphoma (NHL)*, according to pooled analysis of three studies evaluating genetic variation in innate immunity genes with the risk of *NHL*.[33]

However, recent large-scale case–control study and meta-analysis excluded the IL1B SNP rs16944 as a major *multiple myeloma* risk factor.[34]

Other Conditions and Diseases

IL1B and IL1RN alleles are associated with the outcome of kidney transplantation.

Idiopathic pulmonary fibrosis (IPF) has been associated with genetic variations in the IL1RN gene. Recent meta-analysis of polymorphisms in IL1RN corroborated these findings. Furthermore, polymorphisms influencing low IL-1Ra mRNA expression and thus lower levels of IL-1Ra predispose to developing IPF. This suggests that the cytokine IL-1Ra plays a role in IPF pathogenesis.[35]

IL-1R2 (decoy receptor for the IL-1) gene variants along with other cytokine gene polymorphisms are associated with poor sleep maintenance in adults living with human *immunodeficiency* virus/ *acquired immunodeficiency syndrome* in USA. The study controlled for demographic variables such as race and sex, and clinical variables such as CD4+ count and medications. Results showed that higher percentage of wake-after-sleep-onset was associated with IL1R2-gene rs11674595 and tumor necrosis factor A (TNFA)–gene rs1041981 SNPs. In addition, these two SNPs were also correlated with short sleep duration.[36]

IL1B (G–511A; rs16944) genetic polymorphism is associated with cognitive performance in elderly males without *dementia*.[37] The authors suggest that since cognitive decline in the elderly is associated with local inflammation processes, genetic variants of cytokines and their receptors could be tested to improve gene-based prediction of general cognitive function in the elderly.

Therapeutic Options

Because IL-1 is a key mediator of inflammation, for clinical purposes there are attempts to inhibit the action of IL-1, particularly in *autoimmunity*, *osteoarthritis*, and other inflammation-related diseases, some using the addition of anti-TNF treatment. Also, targeted gene therapy with soluble natural inhibitors of the IL-1 system is being investigated in many preclinical studies.

IL-2

Interleukin-2 was detected as a growth factor for T cells, but has subsequently been shown to help the growth of many hematopoietic lines including regulatory T cells (Tregs).

Structure

Human IL-2 has 133 amino acids and in mature form it is a glycosylated globular protein of 15.5 kDa. In other species its peptide chain ranges from 133 to 149 aa. An *"improved sequence"* (IL-2IS) variant of human IL-2 (with a serine to cysteine substitution; alias: aldesleukin) has been constructed by recombinant genetic technology. Besides showing the same biological properties as natural IL-2, it additionally has increased stability and activity in cell culture.

Source

IL-2 is secreted primarily from activated T lymphocytes (CD4 Th0 cells; helper CD4 Th1 cells; and cytotoxic CD8 Tc1 cells). DCs of myeloid and lymphoid lineages can also produce IL-2, but only in the presence of IL-15 cytokine.

Function

IL-2 has an immunoregulatory role; it promotes the growth and development of peripheral immune cells in the initiation of the (defensive) immune response, and keeps them alive as effector cells. However, later in the response it has a pro-apoptotic effect. Although there is no effect on the generation of CD25$^+$FoxP3$^+$ regulatory T cells, IL-2 has a homeostatic effect by promoting survival and division of Treg clones when their numbers become critical. Thus, IL-2 has a role in tolerance to antigens.

Receptor

IL-2 receptor (IL-2R) has three subunits (Figure 6-2): α (CD25), β (CD122), and γ$_c$ (CD132, c = *"common"*; a shared chain with five other cytokine receptors: IL-4R, IL-7R, IL-9R, IL-15R, and IL-21R). Alpha chain (alias: Tac antigen or p55) of human receptor is encoded on chromosome 10p14-15 by the gene IL2RA. The gene for the human β chain (IL2RB, CD122) of the receptor is located on chromosome 22q11.2-12, while the gene for the common IL-2Rγ$_C$ chain (IL2RG) is on chromosome Xq13. Assembly of all three subunits of the receptor is important for the signal transduction into the B and T cells. IL-2R was found on the cell surface (either temporary or permanent) in almost all hematopoietic cells including lymphoid linages T, B, and NK cells, as well as myeloid ones like macrophages, monocytes, and neutrophils. The signal is transferred into the cell via the Janus kinases—Jak1 and Jak3. The phosphorylation of the intracytosolic part of

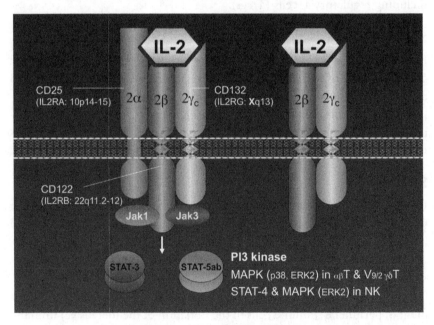

Figure 6-2 The IL-2 receptor with high (left) and medium affinities (right).

the receptor's β chain enables homodimer formation of STAT-3 and STAT-5 factors. Homodimers of STAT-3 and STAT-5 show increased affinity for the nucleus, where they bind to specific DNA elements enhancing the transcription of IL-2-dependent genes.

Jak3–Lck Activation at Different Stages in Life of T Cells

In resting and anergic T cells, signal via IL-2 receptor does not activate Jak3, but *lymphocyte-specific tyrosine kinase (LCK)*, and the latter has an anti-apoptotic effect. In activated T cells, the signal then includes the Jak3 kinase.

Other Features

After translation, the primary precursor of IL-2 is processed into the final secretory form by cutting off the signal peptide, glycosylation of threonine at position 3, and connecting two cysteines with disulfide bridge. According to the crystallographic data with X-rays, IL-2 is a globular protein with α-helical conformation in about 67% of the entire molecule. Disulfide bridge between Cys 58 and Cys 105 is critical for bioactivity.

Human IL-2 gene (IL2; alias: TCGF) is located on chromosome 4q (p26-28) near the gene encoding another cytokine—IL-21. The IL2 expression is inducible *in vivo* and it is primarily regulated at the transcriptional level via the 5′ enhancer. Regulatory elements that are cis-active include binding sites for transcription factors such as *nuclear factor and activator of transcription*-1 (NFAT-1), NF-κB, Jun (AP-1), and octamer. These factors are activated by signals from the TCR–CD3 complex. The expression of the IL2 gene is also regulated post-transcriptionally through a mechanism that involves the stabilization of its transcripts, and the latter depends on the AU-rich sequence at the 3′-end of the mRNA.

The biological function of IL-2 depends on its binding to specific receptors on the cell surface. IL-2 is synthesized *de novo* in mature T cells and is the result of their activation usually by antigen (peptide/MHC ligand) recognition (with TCR plus co-activation via CD28) or activation by mitogens like concavalin A (ConA). Activated T cells secrete transiently for a short period of time IL-2. IL-2 acts by autocrine and paracrine modes on cells in the microenvironment. Autocrine, because T cells after activation also express IL-2 receptor, and thereby enhance the growth of their own clone; paracrine, because, IL-2 is essential for development of adjacent:

1. Th0 cells from naïve CD4 T cells.
2. CD8 killer T cells from precursor CD8 T cells (precursor of CD8 T cells).

3. Development of Th1 and Th2 cells from the Th0 activated stage, and inhibition of Th17. For development of Th1 cells, IL-2 requires also IL-12 (p70), IL-18, and IL-27 cytokines (whereas IL-4, IL-10, and IL-21 can block their progress). Interestingly, *in vitro*, either IFN-γ or IL-12 (p70) is necessary and sufficient for Th1 development; however, *in vivo*, additional levels of complexity are encountered. Similarly, for development of Th2 cells, IL-2 has to be supplemented by IL-4, or either IL-25, IL-31, IL-33, or TSLP (and this development can be inhibited by IFN-γ or TGF-β, *in vitro*). Furthermore, IL-2 contributes together with other cytokines that promote Th1 development in blocking the development of the Th17 subset, which is characterized by secretion of IL-17A, IL-17F, and IL-22 (Th17 development is usually supported by IL-1, IL-6, IL-21, IL-23, and TGF-β cytokines from the Th0 stage).
   IL-2 further promotes:
4. the survival of Treg (CD4, CD25, FoxP3)+ cells[38];
5. the growth of B cells, production of Ig, and production of Ig joining (J) chains in developing plasma cells;
6. the growth and cytotoxic activity of NK-cells, with production of IFNγ
7. the growth and differentiation of monocyte precursors of macrophages, and it stimulates the increase of the tumoricidal effect of macrophages by *antibody-dependent cellular cytotoxicity* (ADCC); and
8. the growth of oligodendrocytes (in neural tissue).

The IL2 gene expression in thymocytes is mono-allelic; a feature that shows the unique regulation of the IL2 gene expression during thymocyte development, as a single allele can take precedence over the other (by yet unclear reasons).

Expression of human IL-2 and its receptor chains on the cell membranes of T lymphocytes are significantly reduced, upon inhibition of endogenously produced melanin. Exogenous addition of melanin increases their expression.

IL-2 increases the expression of human TLR4 on monocytes (but not on B lymphocytes, where this role is taken by IL-4).

Pro-apoptotic effect of IL-2 on effector T lymphocytes is reflected in the transition of sensitivity from mitochondrial-dependent apoptosis to the independent one in the effectors. The latter occurs in the interaction of Fas (CD95) and FasL. Since the T lymphocytes upon activation transiently express FasL, they can kill themselves as they already have Fas expressed on the cell surface. This is called *fratricide* or *suicide*. Killing own clonal "siblings" can lead to a reduction in clonal proliferation, but it does not happen immediately. Namely, although FasL begins to be expressed a day after T-cell activation, this reduction occurs only later, because internal factors (like Bcl-xL) inhibit mitochondrial-dependent death program, and the T cells are insensitive to apoptosis through Fas at that stage. However, after a while they stop being insensitive (by unknown factors induced by IL-2) and die. It is important to note that in the first phase of the activation of T lymphocytes, the lack of IL-2 will also result in apoptosis (mitochondrial dependent), because it is a factor of their growth. Furthermore, in combination with IL-7, which has an effect on the homeostatic proliferation of naïve T cells, IL-2 *in vitro* can also sensitize cells to undergo the Fas-dependent apoptosis, thus regulating their clonal number (but is still unknown why, and which factors participate in it). It is important to note that memory T cells are not sensitive to Fas-dependent apoptosis (or just minimally).

Other Features of the Receptor

In humans, IL-2 receptor has 251 amino acids in the α-chain (CD25), 525 in β-chain (CD122), and 347 in γ-chain (CD132). A protease (sheddase) can cleave off (from the cell membrane) these chains and make a soluble receptor, which can be detected in the serum.

Affinity for the ligand of the IL-2R depends on the composition of the subunits. A single chain such as the α-chain has a very low affinity for IL-2 ($K_d = 10^{-8}$ M), as well as the β-chain. However, the β/γ complex (CD122/CD132) has an intermediate affinity ($K_d = 10^{-9}$ M) and it can also signal, if expressed on the cell surface (Figure 6-2). High affinity for the ligand has heterotrimeric complex $\alpha/\beta/\gamma$ ($K_d = 10^{-11}$ M). In resting T-lymphocytes (small non-dividing and non-activated cells) the α chain (CD25) is inducible, while the β (CD122) and γ (CD132) chains are constitutively expressed. Upon activation of T cells, the CD25 gene begins to be transcribed under the influence of NF-κB. In infection with HTLV-I virus, virally encoded *Tax* product can disturb regulation of production and expression of the α subunit of the receptor for IL-2, increasing the amount of NF-κB and similar factors. This may be one of the changes during infection with HTLV-I virus that eventually leads to occurrence of *leukemia* or *lymphoma*.

For resting NK cells, it is sufficient to receive a signal through the IL-2R with intermediate affinity (β/γ) in order to proliferate and gain cytolytic (killer) function. Perhaps that is why there is a difference in the signal transduction between T and NK cells. Namely, in T lymphocytes (of both $\alpha\beta$ and Vγ9/δ2 lineages) signal transduction through IL-2 receptor uses additionally phosphoinositol-3 (PI3) kinase, p38 MAP kinase, and JNK.

However, in NK cells, IL-2 signal triggers STAT-4, MAPK p38, and ERK2 in contrast to the ones mentioned above for T cells (Figure 6-2).

Monocytes and neutrophils can also functionally respond to stimuli through IL-2R with intermediate affinity. But, B cells require the expression of IL-2R with high affinity, and the regulation of the response is done under the influence of IL-4 and membrane-bound IgM (BCR).

CD25 is also a characteristic molecule expressed on regulatory CD4$^+$Foxp3$^+$T cells (Treg). Foxp3 molecule is thought to be a key regulator of Treg development (Treg have other markers, such as CTLA-4, GIFR, and membrane-bound TGF-β). In experiments with mice, the generation of regulatory CD4 T cells (with one specific peptide/MHC ligand) makes them anergic and immunosuppressive to other T cells in the antigen non-specific manner (e.g., they can suppress activated T cells specific for a different peptide/MHC ligand). It is believed that Tregs are the last stage of development of CD4 T lymphocytes (i.e., they are terminally differentiated), like the memory cells. It is also thought that they were responsible for the emergence of mucosal tolerance to antigens.

Therapy with IL-2 in people with AIDS resulted in an increased number of naïve and memory CD4 T cells without being infected with HIV. It is also observed that during such treatment another naïve T cell subpopulation evolves having CD4$^+$CD25$^+$ markers on more than half of the total number of naïve T cells, which is usually significantly lower in (not IL-2 treated) healthy subjects where this discrete subpopulation makes only about 10% in the peripheral blood. These naïve CD4 T cells were detected by flow cytometry, as they expressed a combination of other typical markers such as CD45RO$^-$/CD27$^+$, used for cell sorting, and CD45RA$^+$CD62L$^+$. However, they were not regulatory T cells, as all tests prepared to detect inhibitory activity of CD4$^+$CD25$^+$ populations did not show any suppression or anergy. In fact, these cells could be activated, because they proliferated all kinds of activation stimuli (either by mitogens, or by antibodies to CD3 and CD28). It is believed that they originated by expansion of T cells as a result of stimulation with IL-2 treatment, but without antigenic stimuli.

In older people, naïve T cells cannot be found after the involution of the thymus. However, CD8 memory T cells have a subpopulation carrying CD25 antigen on the cell surface, which is sensitive to IL-2, but is not of the regulatory kind (i.e., it produces IL-2 and IL-4 upon activation). They are often double positive for coreceptors (CD4$^+$ CD8$^+$). Chromosomal telomeres of this population are longer than in other memory CD8

T cells (that do not express CD25), suggesting that they divided fewer times than the latter, although they may be of the same clone (sharing the same TCR). Probably, this subpopulation is a substitute for the lack of naïve T cells.

Phenotype with the Absence of Genes Encoding Either IL-2 or IL-2 Receptor

In mice with targeted disruption of the IL-2 gene, no major disruptions in the development and function of T lymphocytes were found. However, these mice developed later *ulcerative colitis*, suggesting an important role of IL-2 in immunoregulation. Many believe that the reason for colon pathology is the lack of Treg populations that maintain tolerance to self-antigens in the colon. More severe immunodeficiency of joint cellular and humoral type manifests itself in disruption of the gene encoding IL-2Rγc common chain (CD132), which leads to disorders in the actions of six cytokines (IL-2, IL-4, IL-7, IL-9, IL-15, and IL-21) called *severe combined immune deficiency* (SCID).

Association with Diseases

In humans, a condition known as *X-linked combined immunodeficiency*, or *X-linked SCID*, is congenital lack of the gene encoding the gamma chain of the IL-2 receptor (IL2RG or CD132) on chromosome X. By the beginning of symptoms, the disease was at first confused with congenital HIV infection. Mutations in the JAK3 gene that make it inoperative also manifest themselves with the SCID phenotype.

SNP at T-330G in the IL2 gene has a strong expression phenotype with the G allele, and genotype G/G has a higher frequency of *graft versus host reaction* in allogeneic bone marrow transplantation. On the other hand, genotype of the weaker IL-2 producer (T/T) is associated with a higher incidence of graft rejection in people with a kidney transplant, but, interestingly, not heart transplants.

Two SNP near the IL2/IL21 genes (rs6822844 and rs2069778) were found associated with *psoriasis*, which suggested that this genetic region might play a key role in the pathogenesis of *psoriasis*.

IL2 contributes to gene–gene interaction in assessing the diagnosis *of type 1 diabetes mellitus.*[39] It is known that the common genetic loci that independently influence the risk of *type 1 diabetes* have mostly been determined. However their interactions with the major susceptibility locus, HLA class II, remain mostly unfamiliar and these can affect age-at-diagnosis or gender skewing in various subpopulations. In a British study, more than 14,000 type 1 diabetes samples (6750 British diabetic individuals and over 8000 affected family samples of European descent) were genotyped at 38 confirmed type 1 diabetes-associated non-HLA regions. The alleles that confer susceptibility to *type 1 diabetes* at interleukin-2 (IL-2), IL2/4q27 (rs2069763) and renalase, FAD-dependent amine oxidase (RNLS)/10q23.31 (rs10509540), were associated with a lower age-at-diagnosis.

SNP rs6822844 in the IL2 region is associated with *type 1 diabetes* in the Polish population, and may affect serum levels of interleukin-2.[40]

Although the polymorphisms from the TENR-IL2-IL21 region in the 4q27 chromosome were found associated with *type 1 diabetes, celiac disease, RA*, and *psoriasis*, a study (with *Spanish* Caucasian subpopulation) did not find a correlation between IL2 (rs3136534, rs6822844, and rs2069762) SNPs, and another autoimmune disease – *multiple sclerosis* (using case–control study with 805 patients and 952 healthy controls).[41]

An over 10,000 large case–control study that included *systemic sclerosis* patients and healthy controls of various Caucasian origins (Spain, Germany, The Netherlands, USA, Italy, Sweden, UK, and Norway) tested several SNPs in the IL2–IL21 region (rs2069762, rs6822844, rs6835457, and rs907715). The results showed that allelic combination (haplotype) consisting of rs2069762A–rs6822844T–rs6835457G–rs907715T was associated with *systemic sclerosis* and limited *cutaneous systemic sclerosis* subtype.[42]

An association between IL2 and IgE-mediated *allergy, asthma*, and *atopic eczema*, has been mapped to the IL2 gene (but not IL15). Using 235 families to study the genetic predisposition to these diseases, two SNPs in the IL2 gene were found significantly linked, and one of them (rs2069762), located in the IL2 promoter, influences the level of IL-2 expression. The authors suggest that susceptibility to allergic disease might be due to skewing the Th1/Th2 response balance towards Th2 type.[43]

The IL2 G-330T (rs2069762) polymorphism (and IL4 SNP at T-168C; rs2070874) were analyzed in a case–control study of over 1000 patients with *gastric cancer* and compared to 1100 cancer-free controls in Han Chinese population.[44] Individuals carrying GT/TT genotypes of IL2 rs2069762 SNP had a reduced risk of developing *gastric cancer* (in stomach cardia), similarly to those carrying the IL4 (rs2070874) SNP.

IL2RB (–627C/C) homozygous genotype correlates with an increased predisposition to *endometriosis*. On the other hand, it is associated with lower susceptibility to *gastric atrophy* and low risk for *cancer* (outside *cardia*) during infection with *Helicobacter pylori*.

Therapeutic Options

IL-2 was used in cancer therapy in order to stimulate the maintenance of T lymphocytes. Its use was approved for *metastatic renal cell carcinoma* and *melanoma*.[45] However, since the finding of effects on survival of Tregs its therapeutic use is controversial, and could be counterproductive. Namely, it could lead to worsening of the disease by making tolerance to tumor antigens via Tregs rather than leading to killing of tumor cells via T killers.

Clinical trials have shown that, in the treatment of AIDS with HAART (*highly active antiretroviral therapy*), it is possible to use IL-2 intermittently, to increase the number of $CD4^+$ T cells.

It was found that HIV infection of Tregs decreases the expression of the alpha chain of the IL-2 receptor (IL-2Rα or CD25) and phosphorylated STAT5, suggesting an impaired capacity of Treg to control the expansion of activated CD4 T cells.[46]

Blocking antibodies against IL-2R is in use in organ transplantation follow-up treatment to control the numbers of activated anti-transplant T or B cells.

Cytokine receptors can be used as targets for targeted therapy with various drugs if they are attached to their ligands. Proteins such as *diphtheria* toxin can kill a cell if they bind and consume it. A molecular fusion between the toxic portion of such a molecule and a carrier such as cytokine can be made by genetic engineering. Such a fusion protein was made with IL-2 and *diphtheria* toxin. It is used in successful depletion of activated T cells in *cutaneous T cell lymphoma (cutaneous T cell leukemia)* and *chronic lymphocytic leukemia*. It is called Denileukin Diftitox or Ontake; (DAB389IL2). Furthermore, it was shown to be useful in the treatment of *psoriasis*. A full range of *immunotoxins* was made in a similar fashion; they await for approval for the treatment of various *chronic hematological neoplasms*. Perhaps, in the future, other cytokine receptors could be used as targets of similarly directed therapies in malignant and inflammatory diseases. In addition, inhibition of signal transduction through IL-2 receptor, with specific Jak3 inhibitors, could be used for therapeutic purposes in the future.

Considering congenital absence of a common gamma chain gene (IL2RG; CD132) in *SCID*, the therapy goal is to replace defective cells with ones that have a normal functioning IL2RG gene by transplanting allogeneic hematopoietic stem cells. Autologous stem cells can perhaps also be used. In such a case, they should be repaired by gene therapy using a transgenic procedure by which a healthy functional IL2RG gene would be introduced in the genome.

IL-3

Structure

IL-3 (alias: MCGF; the multi-CSF) is a glycoprotein of 20–32 kDa molecular mass. Human IL-3 is encoded by the gene on chromosome 5q21-32, near the genes for IL-4, IL-5, IL-13, and *granulocyte-macrophage colony-stimulating factor* (GM-CSF, also called *colony-stimulating factor 2*; CSF2).

Source

IL-3 is produced and secreted upon specific activation of T lymphocytes (Th1 and Th2), or mast cells that are activated by cross-linking of cytophilic antibodies binding to their cell membranes through specific antigen.

Function

IL-3 stimulates division, growth, development, and survival of several cell lineages: (A) pluripotent hematopoietic stem cells; (B) the progenitor cells of all the hematopoietic lineages with the exception of lymphocyte precursor; (C) neural tissue progenitor; and (D) many other mature cell lines. It is a cytokine with the widest range of action, and therefore had a large number of previous names such as *colony-stimulating factor of multiple lines, pan-specific hematopoetin, mast cell growth factor*, and *growth factor of hematopoetic cells*.

Receptor

IL-3R consists of two subunits (Figure 6-3): IL-3Rα and a common β_C chain (also part of the IL-5R and CSF2 [GM-CSF]) receptors. Molecular weight of IL-3Rα chain is 60–70 kDa, while the common β_C chain has 120–140 kDa. Human IL-3Rα gene (IL3RA, alias: CD123, IL3R, IL3RAY, IL3RX, IL3RY, hIL-3RA) is close to the CSF-2Rα gene (CSF2RA) in the pseudo-autosomal regions of chromosomes X or Y at Xp22.3 and Yp11.3, respectively (In mouse, *Il3ra* and *Il3rb* genes are separated on autosomal chromosomes; chr14 and chr19, respectively.) The gene for the common β_C chain is denoted CFR2RB (alias: CD131; IL3RB; IL5RB; CDw131) and located on chromosome 22q12-13.

IL-3R is expressed on numerous lines of hematopoietic cells, but not on CD3$^+$ T lymphocytes and the majority of B cells. The expression of IL-3R

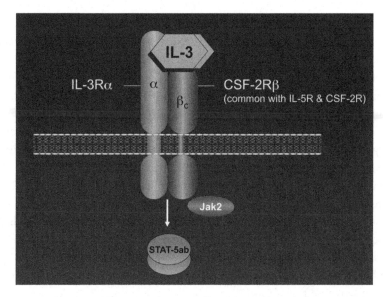

Figure 6-3 The IL-3 receptor and signal transduction factors.

is increased by addition of IL-1, TNF-α, or IFN-γ to cultures of CD34+ stem cells. Signal transduction inside the cells occurs via Jak2/STAT-5ab system (Figure 6-3), and other intracellular mediators such as tyrosine kinases *Lyn* and *Fyn*.

Other Features

IL-3 protein, as a monomer, has 133 amino acids (14 kDa), with two intra-molecular disulfide bridges. Crystallographic studies show that its structure is similar to that in CSF2. It is highly likely that the IL-3 and CSF2 genes evolved from a common ancestor and diversified after its duplication.

Eosinophils treated with IL-3 *in vitro* express MHC class II molecules and costimulatory molecule CD86, and can thus present peptide/MHCII ligands to CD4 T lymphocytes. However, eosinophils cannot process native antigens. It is thought that perhaps the presentation of this kind has a role in defense against parasites (helminths) or in allergies that are T cell mediated.

Of interest is the recent finding that IL-3, by regulating the division and survival of neural progenitors can influence the volume of the brain in humans. A polymorphic marker has been identified (rs31480) in the IL3 promoter that correlates with different expansion potential of neurons and their precursors.[47]

Associations with Human Diseases

IL-3 plays an important role in allergic diseases as the excess of IL-3 increases production, prolongs survival, and enhances the function of eosinophils and mast cells.

In young adult Japanese, the IL3 SNP rs40401 is significantly associated with the risk of *asthma*.[48]

Constitutive secretion of IL-3 was found to play a role in the generation of *myeloid leukemia* in mice, but there is no evidence that similar condition can cause *acute myeloid leukemia* (AML) in humans.

Abnormalities of the IL-3 receptor are frequently observed in AML. Expression of the IL-3RA chain on the surface of hematopoietic stem cells may be a marker for leukemic stem cells, because normal stem cells are negative. Defective gene CFR2RB coding for the common beta chain is associated with *pulmonary alveolar proteinosis*.

There is an association between IL3 gene SNP and risk for *rhinoconjunctivitis* in Japanese population.[49]

The IL3 SNP rs2073506 (G>A) is associated with risk for *esophageal cancer* in Chinese population.[50]

Since some IL3 genotypes of rs40401 SNP have a protective effect on recurrent *malaria* attacks, it is hypothesized that IL-3 might play a role in pathophysiology of (*falciparum*) *malaria*.[51] This is due to the complex inheritance of risk factors for *malaria*.

Therapeutic Options

Clinical IL-3 use is interesting because IL-3 enhances the restoration of hematopoiesis after cytotoxic cancer therapy or bone marrow transplantation. Also, antagonists of IL-3 are interesting as medicaments for the newer therapeutic approaches to allergy and *asthma*, in which the increased number of mast cells and basophils are found.

IL-4

IL-4 (alias: BSF-1, B-cell stimulatory factor-1).

Structure

IL-4 is a glycoprotein with 153 amino acids in humans (18–20 kDa). The gene is located on chromosome 5, near the gene encoding IL-3, IL-5, IL-13, and CSF2 (GM-CSF) cytokines.

Source

IL-4 is secreted mainly by activated T lymphocytes (CD4 helper Th2 type, and cytotoxic CD8 Tc2). B cells in germinal centers (tonsils and mucosa of the colon), mast cells, DCs type 2, and basophils also produce IL-4. Secretion requires cross-linking of TCR on T cells, and for the mast cells and basophils cross-linking of the IgE bound to Fcε receptor.

Function

IL-4 affects growth and development of B lymphocytes, and the switch of the Ig isotype from IgM/IgD to IgE or IgG_1 in germinal center B centroblasts. It also promotes the development of Th2 type of immune responses that in turn regulate humoral immunity, eosinophilia, mastocytosis, and deactivation of inflammation-activated macrophages (by secretion of Th2 cytokines such as IL-10 and TGF-β).

The action of IL-4 on mature activated T cells (from Th0 stage) is wide, as it promotes development of Th2 cells together with IL-2, IL-25, IL-31, IL-33 and TSLP (whereas IFN-γ and TGF-β inhibit their development). IL-4 also promotes formation of Th9 cells (and IFN-γ blocks this function) from Th0. On the other hand, IL-4 suppresses development of Th1 cells (together with IL-10 and IL-21) and Th17 cells (together with IFN-γ, IL-2, IL-12, and IL-27) from the Th0 activated stage.

IL-4 has a direct anti-inflammatory effect *in vitro* by suppression of the secretion of: (A) IL-1β, IL-12, IL-10, and TNF-α by monocytes and (B) IL-1β and IL-12 by macrophages.

In addition, IL-4 has a role in cartilage homeostasis.

Receptor

IL-4 binds to two receptors (Figure 6-4). The first is the proper receptor or IL-4R that is expressed by many human cells, such as T and B cells, myeloid lineage cells, fibroblasts, and endothelial cells. It consists of two chains: the IL-4Rα chain or CD124 (130–140 kDa) and the IL-2γ_C (CD132) common chain (shared with IL-2R, IL-7R, IL-9R, IL-15, and IL-21R; *see* IL-2R). Gene encoding the α-chain is called IL4R (alias: CD124, IL4RA), which is located on chromosome 16p11.2-12.1. The second receptor is composed of IL-4Rα subunit (CD124) and IL-13Rα1 subunit (CD213A1). The latter gene is located on chromosome X. The IL-13Rα1 is a subunit of the IL-13 receptor and can bind IL-13, thus endowing the second IL-4 receptor a possibility to bind and be activated by IL-13 binding.

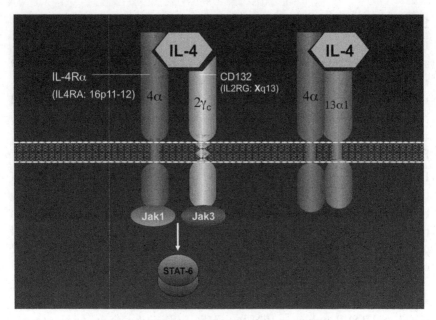

Figure 6-4 The IL-4 receptor and signal transduction factors.

Signal transduction through the IL-4R includes Jak1 and Jak3 kinases that phosphorylate the STAT-6 factor. The latter then forms homodimers, translocates into the nucleus where it induces transcription of IL-4 regulated genes. The signal through IL-4Rα/IL-13Rα1 receptor involves JAK1 and additionally TYK2 kinase resulting in activation of STAT3 and STAT6.

The IL-4R chain may have a soluble form that can inhibit the effect of IL-4. Soluble form (sIL-4R) is either made by alternatively splicing variant of IL-4R mRNA, or by shedding from the membrane via the action of proteases.

Other Features

Production of IL-4 in Th2 cells is inhibited by IL-12 (while IFN-γ has no effect).

In some animal models IL-4 has an anti-tumor effect.

IL-4 induces osteoprotegerin (OPG) and the transcription factor Cbfa1 in smooth muscle cells in the walls of coronary arteries, contributing to their calcification, and thus to development of *coronary heart disease*. OPG is an inhibitor of bone resorption; it is a decoy receptor for RANK ligand, RANKL. (RANKL is a primary factor for the development of osteoclasts.) OPG is also called *osteoclastogenesis inhibitory factor*, OCIF; or *tumor necrosis factor receptor superfamily member 11B*, TNFRSF11B). Reduction of the expression of OPG (induced by IL-4) can be caused by treatment with a drug D609, the inhibitor of phospholipase C (PLC), which can hinder the activation of STAT-6. The prolonged effect of IL-4 treatment for over 4 weeks (in a mouse model) changed smooth muscle cells in the walls of the coronary arteries' osteoblasts–like cells (via Cbfa1). Osteoblasts secrete bone matrix proteins that can be subsequently mineralized (calcified).

IL-4 has a role in the regeneration of muscle tissue. It induces migration of myoblasts to the site of the injury, and is important for the formation of myotubules (but not for the fusion of mononuclear myoblasts).

Associations with Human Diseases

Genetic analysis of the region encoding the IL-4R gene revealed several SNPs that were associated with a risk for hip osteoarthritis in British population.

Genetic analyses of polymorphisms in IL4R and IL13 genes reveal that carriers of particular SNP combinations of IL4R (S478P) and IL13 (–1111) alleles have about five times higher likelihood to develop *asthma* than others in the Dutch population.

SNPs in IL4 (C-590T) and TLR4 (A+896G) genes have an epistatic effect on the risk of developing *asthma* (in women), when both are present in the genome of the Finnish population. Namely, alleles analyzed alone are not associated with risk for *asthma*. However, women with a weak sensitivity to LPS (TLR4 G allele carriers) and strong producers of IgE isotype (IL4 T allele carriers) have a predisposition to *asthma*. This allelic combination is not associated with the risk for *atopy*.

Homozygous genotype (R/R) of the polymorphism detected in the receptor chain IL4RA (Q576R) is associated with susceptibility for *asthma* in the Chinese population, but not in the population from Hawaii.

Furthermore, the SNP IL4 (C-590T) is associated with *periodontitis* in the adult Korean population, but not in the Brazilian population of African descent.

Genetic polymorphisms in genes encoding IL-4RA and IL-13 are epistatically associated with the predisposition to developing *diabetes mellitus type I* in the Philippine population.

Some IL4 alleles are associated with *chronic disseminated candidiasis* in *acute leukemias*.

Some haplotypes of the genes encoding IL-4 and IL-10 are associated with *AIDS*. They can be used as prognostic factors for disease progression.

Therapeutic Options

Clinical trial (Phase II) treatment of *renal cell carcinoma* with IL-4 was proven minimally successful, and thus further clinical testing was abandoned.

Systemic administration of IL-4 may result (in over 10% of cases) with gastro-duodenal erosions and ulcerations, under anti-tumor therapy of malignant tumors at later stages.

IL-4 antagonists can be used in the treatment of persistent mildly severe *asthma*. Clinical trials (Phase II) with soluble sIL-4R show that it is well tolerated and has promising properties. As IL-4 induces IgE class switching, anti-IgE antibody called Omalizumab (a humanized IgG1κ) has been tried in clinical trials to combat allergies as well as being approved by FDA (in 2003) for treatment of moderate to severe allergic *asthma* (12 years and older).

Blocking IL-4 with Pascolizumab (a monoclonal antibody against IL-4) is planned for use in clinical trial with *tuberculosis*.

IL-5

Source

IL-5 is produced by activated T lymphocytes (mainly by a minor subpopulation of CD4 helper Th2 cells). Human Th2 cells have two major subpopulations: about 20% of them are capable of producing IL-5, having a phenotype (IL-5+, IL-4+, IL-13+). The rest do not secrete IL-5 despite being producers of IL-4 and IL-13.

Structure

IL-5 is a glycoprotein of 40–45 kDa (as monomer) that occurs in homodimeric conformation created by the inter-chain disulfide bond. The gene coding for IL-5 (IL5; alias: EDF, TRF, IL-5) is located on chromosome 5q13, together with the genes for IL-3, IL-4, IL-13, and CSF-2 (GM-CSF).

Function

IL-5 is the strongest cytokine that controls eosinophilia. It is a factor of development, growth, maturation, and activation of eosinophils.

Receptor

IL-5 receptor (IL-5R) is composed of two glycoprotein subunits: α chain (60 kDa), which is specific for the ligand, and β_C common chain (120–130

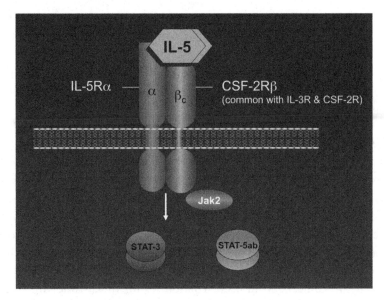

Figure 6-5 The IL-5 receptor and signal transduction factors.

kDa), which is also present in the receptors for IL-3 and GM-CSF (see *IL-3R*). The gene for IL-5Rα chain is located on chromosome 3p26. Transduction of signals inside the cells occurs via Jak2 kinase, STAT-3 and STAT-5ab factors, and some other tyrosine kinases (Figure 6-5).

Other Features

The majority of genes responsible for the Th2 type immune response are assembled together in the genome over a very large region of 120 kilobases. It has a number of gene regulatory elements.

Association with Human Diseases

Since eosinophils have a critical role in allergic diseases, IL-5 is one of the key cytokines responsible for the development of *asthma* and *allergies*.

There is a correlation between eosinophilia, IL-5 levels (which can be detected), and various diseases such as infections with various parasites, *idiopathic eosinophilia, eosinophilic myalgia, Hodgkin's lymphoma*, and *asthma*. Local eosinophilic infiltration was observed in some tumors and has a positive prognosis in *primary carcinoma* of the lung, stomach, and colon, as well as for *Hodgkin's disease*. In contrast, inflammatory infiltration of eosinophils after kidney transplantation has a poor prognosis for the maintenance of transplant, and in liver transplant patients eosinophils are specific indicator of acute rejection. Unfortunately, it is not established whether the eosinophils are only a marker (of infiltration by Th2 lymphocytes) or the cause of these pathological changes.

Genetic predisposition analysis showed that C allele of the IL5 gene SNP (C-703T) is associated with bronchial *asthma* in the Russian population.

Therapeutic Options

Reducing the production of IL-5 can be achieved with glucocorticoids that are its strong inhibitors, which is the standard therapy of *asthma* and some *allergies*. (Glucocorticoids additionally inhibit production of Th2 cytokines including IL-4, IL-13, and GM-CSF.) In cases when it is therapeutically desired to reduce the use of glucocorticoids, anti-IL-5 antibody (*mepolizumab*) is a safe and effective means of treatment of hyper-eosinophilic syndromes (like *atopic asthma*).

There are clinical and molecular rationales for therapeutic targeting of IL-5 and its receptor.[52]

IL-6

IL-6 was previously called interferon beta-2.

Structure

IL-6 is a member of a large group of cytokines that signal into the cell via receptor subunit gp130 (IL-6ST, interleukin-6 *signal transducer*), or via a protein very similar to gp130. The family includes 11 members: IL-11, IL-27, IL-31, CNTF (*ciliary neurotrophic factor*), CT-1 (*cardiotrophin-1*), CLC (*cardiotophin-like cytokine*), LIF (*leukemia inhibiting factor*), NPN (*neuropoetin*), OSM (*oncostatin M*), and viral vIL-6 of *Kaposi sarcoma* associated herpesvirus. IL-6 is glycoprotein of 21–26 kDa, which contains 184 amino acids. The IL6 gene (alias: BSF2, HGF, HSF, IFNB2) is located on human chromosome 7p21.

Source

IL-6 is a product of activated T and B lymphocytes, monocytes and fibroblasts, and activated macrophages.

Function

This is pleiotropic cytokine with a multitude of functions. The role of IL-6 is proinflammatory, with important effects in adaptive immunity especially after activation of T and B cells. It induces the final step of peripheral B lymphocyte development into plasma cells. IL-6 plays a role in the production of acute phase proteins in liver cells, developing neurons, the maturation of megakaryocytes, the activation of osteoclasts, the proliferation of keratinocytes, mesangial cells, and *myelomas/plasmacytomas*, as well as in wound healing. IL-6 is required for the development of Th22 helper cells, together with TNF (whereas TGF-β blocks their development). IL-6 is essential in the formation of the Th17 phenotype of helper T cells from the Th0 stage together with IL-1, IL-21, IL-23, and TGF-β (whereas IFN-γ, IL-2, IL-4, IL-12, and IL-27 can block their development). The hallmark of Th17 cells is the production of IL-17A, IL-17F, and IL-22 cytokines with neutrophil (granulocyte) mobilization.

Receptor

Functional IL-6 receptor is composed of two chains (Figure 6-6): IL-6R (alias: CD126, IL-6R-1, IL-6R-alpha, IL-6RA) in the strict sense (80 kDa, 468 amino acids; IL-6R gene is on chromosome 1q21) and the gp130 chain, which is the signal transducing chain, and also referred to as IL-6ST (alias: CD130, CDw130, G P130, gp130-RAPS, IL-6R-beta; IL6ST gene is chromosome 5q11).

IL-6ST is a common signal transducing chain for other cytokine receptors such as IL-11, LIF, CNTF, CT-1, CLC, NPN, OSM, and IL-27 (Figure 6-7).

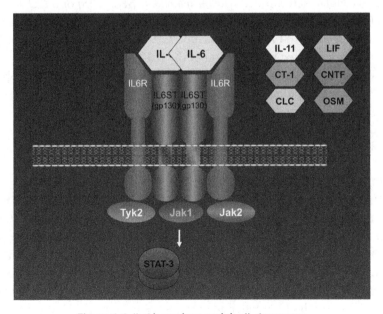

Figure 6-6 IL-6 homologs and the IL-6 receptor.

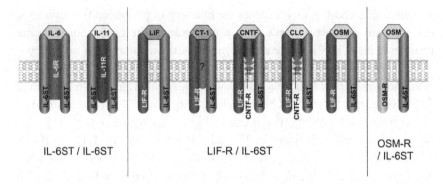

Figure 6-7 Receptors with IL-6ST (gp130) chain and ligands of the IL-6 cytokine family. (IL-27 receptor has also IL-6ST, and IL-31R has an IL-6ST homolog.)

Interestingly, the IL-31 receptor has a very similar relative of gp130 as a signaling chain (Figure 6-30). Binding of IL-6 to IL-6R/IL-6ST (Figure 6-6) causes homodimerization of IL-6ST, which in turn activates Jak1, Jak2 and Tyk2 kinases, and the transcription factor STAT-3.

Regulatory Feedback Loops in Signal Transduction

There is a negative feedback loop in the IL-6 signaling, which goes through the intracellular factors called *cytokine inhibitor of SH2* (CIS) or *STAT induced STAT inhibitors* (SSI). There are eight members of the group called *suppressor of cytokine signaling* (SOCS) that include CIS and SOCS1–SOCS7 factors, which are synthesized by the action of the JAK/STAT signal. SOCS inhibit the activity of Jak kinases and thus reduce signal transduction from respective cytokine receptors. The SOCS members that are involved in negative feedback mechanism during signal transduction are for:

IL–6: CIS, SOCS1, SOCS2, and SOCS3;

LIF: CIS, SOCS1, SOCS2, and SOCS3;

IL–11: SOCS3; and

OSM: CIS, SOCS1, and SOCS3.

Besides these, the signal can also be inhibited at the level of RNA/DNA by transcriptional repression of STAT molecules via *protein inhibitor of activated STAT* (PIAS) family of proteins (there are five members in the group).

On the other hand, there is a positive feedback loop that can amplify the signal via STATs. Here it seems to play an important role an oncogenic protein LMO4 that belongs to the *Lim only* (LMO) group of four nuclear factors carrying the Lim domain.

Soluble Receptor (IL-6R) is an Agonist Unlike Other Soluble Cytokine Receptors

IL-6R is expressed only in certain kinds of cells, including hepatocytes and some leukocytes, whereas IL-6ST is expressed in a wide variety of tissues. There are also soluble (s) forms of receptors: sIL-6R and sIL-6ST. Soluble IL-6R is synthesized and secreted by platelets upon their activation. Neutrophils (and probably monocytes too) have membrane receptors for IL-6, but they can release them as soluble. Releasing sIL-6R occurs via membrane sheddase (metalloproteinase) ADAM17.

Unlike other soluble cytokine receptors, sIL-6R is an agonist, which can signal through gp130. This means that a complex IL-6/sIL-6R can stimulate target cells that express only gp130 on the cell surface despite the lack of target cell's own IL-6R chain. This phenomenon is called trans-signaling. Along the same line of thought, the inhibitor of this process is called trans-signaling inhibitor, and in the IL-6 system of signaling it is a soluble form of gp130 (sIL-6ST). Soluble sIL-6ST has no effect on the activity of IL-6 via membrane bound IL-6R, which is important for therapeutic purposes.

Other Features

In experimental models of *arthritis* in mice, a series of experiments has proven a role of IL-6 in the destruction of joints, gathering of leukocytes, apoptosis, and activation of T cells. Knockout (KO) mice with targeted disruption of the IL6 gene (IL6$^{-/-}$) have very little or no pathological signs of *arthritis*, indicating that the lack of IL-6 generates a protective phenotype. Injection of IL-6 in the joints has no influence on the initiation of *arthritis*. In contrast, reconstitution of IL-6 trans-signaling results in increased migration of CCR2$^+$ mononuclear cells with the development of pathological changes in the joints.

Normal cells typically do not secrete IL-6. Secretion of IL-6 can be activated with the NF-κB, a factor that is activated in many signaling pathways, including those by TNF and TLRs. Stimulation by LPS (that binds to TLR4–MD2 complex on the cell membrane with a help of CD14 molecules) causes the secretion of IL-6 from monocytes and fibroblasts. Activated macrophages (with IFN-γ) also secrete IL-6. Neutrophils that have migrated to inflammatory sites release membrane form of the receptor chain (sIL-6R) after a few hours. Soluble sIL-6R can bind to IL-6, making a composite ligand that can act on other cells in the microenvironment provided they have IL-6ST (the remaining membrane-anchored part of the receptor for

IL-6). Consequently, all tissues that express gp130 become responsive to IL-6, and the process is named trans-signaling.

IL-6 can be secreted from some DCs; an action with which DCs can inhibit the activity of regulatory Treg cells (and thereby by suppression of suppression they might activate helper T cells and thus break tolerance).

IL-6 and IL-1 are secreted in response to radioactive gamma rays, and it is considered that they have a radio-protective effect. However, in testes, Sertoli cells secrete only IL-6 after radiation. It has been suggested that the level of secretion of these cytokines can be taken as a measure of received radiation dosage.

Colon cancer cells under the influence of IL-6 secrete IL-10 that has immunosuppressive effects.

Garlic increases the flow of blood through the solid tissue, and the effect may be regulated by secretion of IL-6.

IL-6 is produced in adipocytes and is regulated negatively with gluco-corticoids and stimulated with physiological concentrations of insulin and catecholamines. Short-term exercise induces the secretion of IL-6 from adi-pocytes, which immediately stops by ingestion of carbohydrates. At variance from the effect on fat tissue, 10-week training reduces the production of IL-6 in skeletal muscle. Acute muscular effort increases IL-6 in muscle cells, regardless of their fitness or glycogen levels.

High levels of IL-6 levels were correlated with poorer sleep quality in healthy people. Circadian rhythm of secretion of IL-6 has led some authors to speculate that the low levels of IL-6 are inducers of sleepiness, and that this contributes to homeostatic desire for sleep. Animal experiments indicate that IL-6 is somnogenic.

Associations with Human Diseases

In experimental models in animals, IL-6 is via trans-signaling critically involved in the pathogenesis of chronic inflammatory diseases such as *inflammatory bowel disease* (IBD), *peritonitis, RA, asthma*, and in *colon cancer* it is thought to have a role in maintaining the condition.[53] Specifically, the transition from acute to chronic phase of inflammation is thought to be generated under the influence of soluble sIL-6R.

Increased serum concentrations of IL-6 and sIL-6R were found in *RA* and *juvenile* forms of *RA*, which correlate with faster disease progression as well as the degree of joint destruction in *RA*. In *systemic juvenile RA (sJRA)*, sIL-6R was also significantly increased. Furthermore, osteoclasts produce large amounts of IL-6 in *Paget's disease*.

IL-6 is thought to play a role, along with other cytokines and factors, in the pathogenesis of *postmenopausal osteoporosis, Castleman's disease, multiple myeloma*, and *pituitary adenoma*.

Interestingly, the gene for IL-6 is constitutively active in a number of tumors such as *cardiac myxoma, cervical* and *kidney cancer, prostate cancer*, and *bladder cancer*. High serum concentrations of IL-6 correlate with the progression of these diseases. It remains to be seen whether these are causative associations or not. Although the expression of IL-6 is different among races and ethnic groups, it is considered to be a risk factor for *breast cancer*.

In patients with *prostate cancer* after radical prostatectomy, preoperative levels of TGF-β and soluble sIL-6R concentrations are associated with metastases to regional lymph nodes, occult metastases, and disease progression.

Serum levels of IL-6 and VEGF have been identified as independent prognostic factors in the treatment of *non-Hodgkin's lymphoma (NHL)*, and combined as prognostic factors in *aggressive lymphoma* or *T-cell leukemia/lymphoma*. The prognosis is worse in patients with higher concentrations of these cytokines.

Men who are predisposed to secrete higher levels of IL-6 (GG genotype of SNP: IL6 C-174G, rs1800795) have a reduced chance to achieve a long life. However, all carriers of C allele have a greater tendency to develop *atherosclerosis*. Severe *ischemic stroke* in young adults is associated with the GG genotype. Recently, a correlation was found between SNP (C-174G, rs1800795) and an increased predisposition to *cardiovascular* disease, *hypertension* and *left ventricular hypertrophy* in patients on dialysis in the US American population. The IL-6 (-572 G>C, rs1800796) polymorphism is associated with the risk of developing *acute coronary syndrome* in the Mexican population.[54]

In similar studies in the Netherlands and Germany, no relationship was found between this SNP and *cardiovascular* disease (in patients without other diseases). In patients with *diabetes mellitus* type 2 (with the GG genotype), there is a susceptibility to develop *peripheral vascular disease* of the arteries, which is accompanied with higher fibrinogen and CRP serum levels. Furthermore, the C allele carriers have a 3.7 times higher risk of rejection of the transplanted kidney. Therefore, it has been proposed to use this parameter (together with the level of IL-6 in serum) for prognostic purposes in transplantation.

Significant correlation was found between G (C-174G) and G (A-598G) alleles of SNPs in the IL6 gene and *diabetes mellitus* type 2 in the German population. The authors suggested that these are independent risk factors for the disease, and probably indirectly through the effects of IL-6 on MCP-1 (CCL2) chemokine and perhaps other factors. Studies in other populations (native Americans and Caucasians) confirm this association with the SNP in the promoter of IL6 (C-174G).

There was no association of this polymorphism with *migraine, endometriosis* (except *chocolate cysts*), *Graves' ophthalmopathy*, and *multiple sclerosis*. CC genotype (C-174G, rs1800795) polymorphism is represented more frequently in women with *Alzheimer's disease* (than in healthy subjects) in the Italian population. The similar and more extensive study in the UK, however, found no association with *Alzheimer's disease*.

Patients with *periodontitis* had significantly less frequent genotype with heterozygous IL6 (G-572C) polymorphism, suggesting a protective effect in the Czech population.

In tumors, SNP in the promoter of the IL6 gene (C-174G, rs1800795) is associated with *colorectal* and *breast cancers*. Carriers of C allele have increased risk for the development of these diseases. Increased IL-6 levels correlate with high serum carcinoembryonic antigen (CEA) in preoperative stage of patients with *colorectal cancer*. For *ovarian cancer*, carriers of C allele have a greater chance of disease-free survival (and survival in general) after treatment, and typing this SNP has proved to be the best parameter for prognostic purposes.

Similarly, for prognosis of *neuroblastoma*, the IL6 SNP rs1800795 (−174 G>C) correlates with lower survival of high-risk tumors.[55]

Therapeutic Options

Atlizumab (a neutralizing anti–IL-6R antibody) proved to be very effective in clinical trials (Phase I and II) in *rheumatoid arthritis* (*RA and JRA*), *Crohn's* and *Castleman's disease*. It is very well tolerated, and has few side effects or additional complications. It seems no better than the *Infliximab* therapy of *RA* (that uses anti–TNF antibody, *Infliximab*), but it may be beneficent in the treatment of *TNF-resistant RA*, or as a complement to *Infliximab* therapy.

In experimental animal models of diseases such as *chronic inflammation* and *colon cancer*, treatment with soluble sIL-6ST inhibits their progress by inhibiting trans-signaling. Soluble gp130 is thus a candidate for the treatment of people with similar diseases. The advantage of the use of sIL-6ST compared to *Atlizumab* is that it does not inhibit signal transduction through the cell surface IL-6 receptor (IL-6R). This is important, as sIL-6ST usage leaves the possibility of the IL-6 action on the liver (stimulating the synthesis of acute phase proteins) and B lineage cells (the maturation of plasma cells). Therefore, this treatment would prevent the side effects and possible complications of therapy with IL-6 neutralizing antibodies.

IL-7

Structure

Interleukin-7 is a glycoprotein of about 25 kDa (152 amino acids in humans). The gene is located on chromosome 8q12-13. It can make heterodimers with *hepatocyte growth factor* (HGF).

Source

IL-7 is constitutively secreted from adherent stromal cells of many tissues, including bone marrow, spleen, thymus, kidney, and epithelial and epithelial goblet cells lining the intestinal mucosa. It is also produced by keratinocytes, DCs, hepatocytes, and neurons. Its secretion is stringently controlled and is independent of mitogen or other growth factors.

Function

It has a role in development and survival of lymphocytes. IL-7 strongly stimulates proliferation of both lymphoid progenitor lines: pre-pro B cells (together with HGF, in bone marrow) and precursors of T cells (in the thymus). In T lymphocyte development, IL-7 is a co-factor in the rearrangement of TCR β chains during the early DN (CD4$^-$CD8$^-$) stage (see *T-Cell Development*, Chapter 2, p. 44, and *B-Cell Development*, Chapter 2, p. 51). Furthermore, it is a factor of homeostatic growth and division of mature resting functional T cells (naïve and memory cells). IL-7 can help the generation of active lytic CD8 killer T lymphocytes as well as the activation of NK cells to become *lymphokine activated killer* (LAK) cells. In monocytes, it also stimulates lytic activities and induces the secretion of cytokines such as IL-1α, IL-1β, IL-6, and TNF-α; IL-7 is an important factor for lymphangiogenesis, and is considered to play a role in the metastatic spread of cancer to the lymph nodes.

Receptor

IL-7 can bind to a cell surface receptor composed of two chains (Figure 6-8). The first is IL-7R, a receptor in proper sense (*in strictu senso*) (alias: CD127; the IL-7R gene is located on chromosome 5p12-14) with molecular weight of 75 kDa (comprising 459 amino acids), and the second

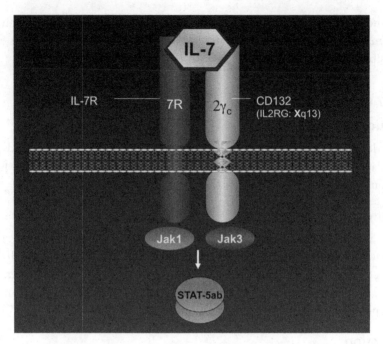

Figure 6-8 The IL-7 receptor and signal transduction factors.

chain is the common IL-2Rγc chain (CD132), found building five additional cytokine receptors (IL-2R, IL-4R, IL-9R, IL-15R, and IL-21R) (see the description of IL-2R on p. 9). The IL-7R is a member of a family of receptors that even includes hormone receptors like the ones for growth hormone and prolactin. There is a soluble form of the receptor's first chain, without transmembrane and cytoplasmic parts of the molecule, which is enzymatically cleaved by the action of shedding proteases.

However, IL-7R can bind another cytokine: thymic stromal lymphopoetin (TSLP). Namely, TSLP acts via a specific receptor, which has a similar chain composition as the IL-7 receptor, in which the common IL-2Rγc (CD132) is exchanged with structurally related TSLP-R chain thus making IL-7R/TSLP-R heterodimers (see *TSLP*, Chapter 8, p. 269).

IL-7R is expressed by progenitors of B and T cells, thymocytes, mature T lymphocytes, and monocytes. Signal transduction involves tyrosine phosphorylation via Jak1 and Jak3 kinases, STAT-5ab factor activity and metabolites of inositol phospholipids (Figure 6-8).

IL-7R is expressed on endothelial cells, and has influence in the formation of new lymphatic vessels.

Other Features

During development of T cells in the thymus, IL-7 is required at the double-negative CD4$^-$CD8$^-$ (DN) stage. It is secreted in response to pre-TCR signaling, but its actions must stop at the next one, the immature single positive stage, so that thymocytes could develop into double-positive cells. Specifically, IL-7 inhibits transcription factors that are essential for this transition.

Regarding the homeostasis of naïve CD4$^+$(helper) and CD8$^+$(killer) T cells, IL-7 is necessary, but not sufficient for proliferation, because they necessitate the signals from the TCR engagement with $-$/MHC ligand. (Here, the minus sign in "$-$/MHC" describes a somewhat strange condition, in which a peptide is not required to be present in the cleft of MHC molecules, despite the high probability that some kind of "flat" peptide might be anchored there; however, in such a way that it does not disturb the TCR-MHC binding.)

In contrast to naïve helper and killer T cells, homeostatic proliferation of resting memory killer CD8$^+$ T cells can be induced by a very high, but unfortunately, non-physiological dosage of IL-7 (which is in this instance sufficient to make them divide without the TCR signal). A physiological concentration of IL-15 is, on the other hand, quite sufficient to let them undergo homeostatic proliferation (see *Other features of IL-15*), suggesting it might be more relevant *in vivo* for this population of cells than the former cytokine.

Another interleukin, namely, IL-2, negatively regulates the expression of IL-7R chain on T cells, probably through the PI3 kinase pathway. This causes the ligand competition by the IL-2- and IL-7R-receptor chains as they are using the same additional chain (IL-2R common γ) in their assembly at the cell surface. In contrast, glucocorticoids increase the expression of IL-7R on T cells, and thus play a role in survival (homeostasis) of peripheral (resting) T lymphocytes.

Studies in mice injected with monoclonal antibodies against the IL-7 cytokine inhibit development of B-lymphocytes at the pro-B stage, and reduce cellularity of thymus.

If the gene encoding IL-7 is inserted into tumor cells' genome, and injected into a mouse, the result is an increase of "*defensive immune-cell-mediated activity against*" (immunity to) tumors and tumor rejection.

Associated with Human Diseases

Effector CD8$^+$ (killer) T cells in people infected with the HIV virus generate a population that is CD127-negative with absent IL-7R. It is likely that this reflects the reduced potential of homeostatic recovery of the remaining T cell pool in such patients, and thus contributes to the pathogenesis of AIDS.

Increased plasma concentration of IL-7 was found in *cutaneous T lymphoma* (and no increase in IL-2, 4, 12, 13, and 15 levels).

In *breast cancer* tissue of the most aggressive form, a significantly increased expression of IL-7R and all factors in the IL-7 signal transduction were found (with the exception of STAT-5). Association also exists between serum IL-7 levels and the worst prognosis in this disease. It has been proposed to take aberrant expression of IL-7 for diagnostic and prognostic purposes.

Naturally occurring absence of IL-7R (a defect in the gene) is a rare mutation that presents with symptoms matching *SCID* (and it is similar to cases with congenital lack of the IL2RG gene, see "*IL-2*", p. 151). IL-7R deficiency has recently been found in some patients with *RA*.

Research studying associations of several SNPs in the gene for the IL-7 receptor found only a trend for predisposition to an autoimmune disease such as *multiple sclerosis*. Otherwise, genome-wide analysis identified the chromosomal region on chromosome 5 as one of many candidates for the increased hereditary risk in this polygenic disease.

Therapeutic Options

A hybrid construct with IL-7 covalently attached to the Fc portion of antibody molecule, when injected with γδT lymphocytes has shown beneficial therapeutic activity in a mouse model of *disseminated neuroblastoma*.

Another hybrid molecule utilizing IL-7 that is associated with a portion of diphtheria toxin (DAB389-IL-7 immunotoxin; see "*IL-2: Therapeutic options,*" p. 17, for information on a similar type of hybrid protein) could be a means for targeted therapy of some malignancies whose cells express the IL-7R receptor like *cutaneous T lymphoma, acute T cell leukemia, acute* and *chronic* B cell malignancies, *Burkitt's lymphoma*, and *Hodgkin's disease*.

Therapeutic options are also its use in HIV-infected persons.

After allogenic stem cell transplant, IL-7 could improve the immune system recovery.

IL-7 receptor blockade seems to reverse *autoimmune diabetes* by inhibiting effector and memory T cells.

IL-8

IL-8 is an older name of chemokine CXCL1, described with other CXC-related molecules (see Chapter 7 on chemokines).

IL-9

IL-9 was initially annotated with many different names like "T-cell growth factor p40"; "a homolog of mouse T cell and mast cell growth factor 40"; "p40 T-cell and mast cell growth factor"; "cytokine p40"; or "p40 protein."

Structure

IL-9 is a protein of 32–39 kDa. The gene encoding IL9 (alias: HP40, IL-9, P40) is on chromosome 5q31.

Source

It is secreted by activated Th9 cells.

Function

IL-9 is a pleiotropic cytokine with anti-inflammatory effects. It was discovered because it stimulates the growth of some T cell clones *in vitro*. Besides acting on T cells at specific stages of development and growth, IL-9 has a synergistic effect with IL-2 on thymocytes *in vivo*. Furthermore, IL-9 increases the secretion of IL-4-induced production of IgE and IgG1 antibodies in plasma cells.

IL-9 induces proliferation of mast cells from the bone marrow (alone, in combination with IL-3, or with SCF) and their differentiation (by stimulating the production of IL-6). It also stimulates the growth of erythroid progenitor. It has a synergistic effect on the stimulation of growth of megakaryocytes together with erythropoietin and SCF.

It acts on the epithelium lining the airways. On monocytes activated with LPS, it has a calming effect (reduces the secretion of TNF-α and IL-10) and increases the secretion of TGF-β.

Receptor

The receptor for IL-9 has two chains (Figure 6-9). The first is a glycoprotein IL-9R *in strictu senso*, called α chain (alias: CD129). It has 64 kDa in the mouse. The human gene (IL9R) is located on pseudo-autosomal parts of chromosomes Xq28 and Yq12. The second part of the IL-9 receptor is the IL-2R common γ_c chain, found also in IL-4R, IL-7R, IL-15R, and IL-21R (*see* description of the IL-2R, for more information on common γ_c, p. 10). Signal into the cell is transmitted through Jak1 and Jak3 kinases, engaging STAT-1, STAT-3, and STAT-5 transcription factors. In addition, signal transduction might activate some MAP kinases.

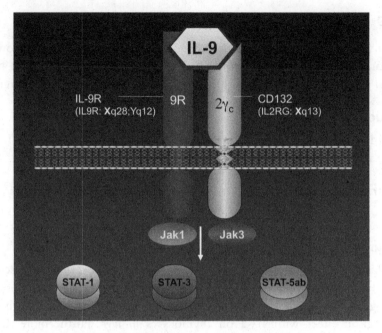

Figure 6-9 The IL-9 receptor and its signaling factors.

Association with Human Diseases

It is believed that by increasing the secretion of Th2 cytokines, mobilization of mast cells and the effect on the respiratory epithelium plays a role in *allergic* diseases (i.e., *allergic contact dermatitis*) and *asthma*. Genetic studies have suggested an association between IL-9R with *asthma*.

In addition, increased systemic and local levels of IL-9 were found in patients with carotid and coronary *atherosclerosis*.[56]

Interestingly, 5% of mice transgenic for IL9 get *thymic lymphomas*. Deregulated production of IL-9 may have a role in oncogenesis of T lineage tumors.

There is an association between the production of IL-9 with *Hodgkin's disease* and infection with HTLV I virus. *Nasal NK/T-cell lymphomas* produce IL-9, which serves as an autocrine growth factor that is considered to play a role in the development of this tumor.

In mice deficient for Th17 subset (with gene knockouts encoding RORγ and IL-23R proteins), Th9 cells producing IL-9 provide robust activity against *melanoma* cancer cells.[57]

IL-10

IL-10 has other names like *Cytokine synthesis inhibitory factor* and T-cell growth inhibition factor.

Structure

It belongs to a group of several related cytokines that can be divided into viral homologs and endogenous cytokines (IL-19, 20, 22, 24, and 26). Human IL-10 is a non-glycosylated protein of 18 kDa (monomer has 160 amino acids), and exists as a non-covalently linked homodimer. The IL10 gene is located on chromosome 1q3-32 near the IL19 and IL20 genes.

Source

It is produced by a wide variety of cells. However, the majority derives from several T cell populations that are inducible upon activation. These are Th_2 (helper $CD4^+$) and Tc_2 (cytotoxic $CD8^+$) cells. Interestingly, another subpopulation, Tr1 lymphocytes (a type of regulatory T cells) also secretes IL-10 as their sole subpopulation identifier (they also produce small amounts of TGF-β). Some B cells also secrete IL-10 in the later stages of activation. Other cell types that produce IL-10 include monocytes/macrophages, mast cells, and keratinocytes. *Cytomegalovirus* (CMV) and *Epstein–Barr* virus (EBV) have IL10 gene paralogs, and upon infection produce viral homologs of this cytokine.

Function

IL-10 is a cytokine with multiple roles in immunoregulation and inflammation. It reduces the secretion of Th1-type cytokines, MHC class II molecules, and costimulatory molecules (CD80/86) on macrophages. IL-10 boosts the survival of B cells, their proliferation, and production of antibodies. Under the influence of IL-10 (in the presence of IL-4), activation of naïve CD4 and CD8 T lymphocytes skews into Th2 and Tc2 subpopulations. IL-10 inhibits the development of Th1 (or Tc1) subpopulation of T lymphocytes (see *Further development of immune cells upon activation*, Chapter 3, p. 83).

Other Features

KO studies in mice suggested that IL-10 functions as an essential immunoregulator in the intestinal tract.

IL-10 inhibits the secretion of LPS- or IFN-γ-induced secretion of proinflammatory cytokines (IL-1α, IL-1β, IL-6, TNF-α), chemokines

(IL-8), and factors of growth and development (GM-CSF and G-CSF) by macrophages. It also inhibits the maturation of DCs. IL-10 in combination with other cytokines can have a stimulating effect on megakaryocytes, erythroid lineage cells, and primitive hematopoietic cells.

Interaction of ICOS molecule (on T cell) and ICOS-ligand (on DC) stimulates (effector) T cells to secrete IL-10, whereas CD28 interaction (on T cell) and CD80/86 (on DC) is a powerful inhibitor of IL-10 production. In human monocytes, IL-10 induces a set of 19 genes, including *interleukin-1-receptor antagonist* (IL-1Ra) and SOCS-3 (see *"IL-6: Regulatory feedback loops in signal transduction,"* p. 170).

Some viral genomes have a viral copy of the IL-10 gene (that is very similar), including EBV and CMV. This viral IL-10 (vIL-10) exerts an activity similar to the endogenous IL-10. Therefore, vIL-10 can inhibit development of defensive cellular immunity facilitating infectivity and survival of the virus that encodes it. However, viral homolog of EBV has a weaker effect than human IL-10.

IL-10 is an inhibitory factor in wound healing.

Receptor

IL-10R is composed of two chains (RA and RB). The signal is transduced into the cell via phosphokinases Jak1 and Tyk2, under whose influence they recruit transcription factors STAT-1 and STAT-3 (Figure 6-10). The latter act in the nucleus as transcriptional regulators and are responsible for the action of IL-10. The signal can be inhibited by negative feedback via SOCS1 and SOCS3 (see *"IL-6: Regulatory feedback loops in signal transduction,"* p. 28, for more on SOCS molecules).

IL-10 receptor chains belong to a family of receptor chains that participate in various combinations in the formation of receptors for related cytokines like IL-19, IL-20, IL-22, IL-24, and IL-26. Furthermore, the IL-10R2 receptor chain participates in the formation of shared receptor for IL-28 and IL-29 cytokines.

Another name for the IL10RA gene is IL-10R1 (alias: CDW210A; IL10R; HIL-10R) and it is located on chromosome 11q23. The IL10RB gene is alternatively called IL-10R2 (synonyms: CDW210B; CRFB4; CRF2-4, D21S58, D21S66) and is located on chromosome 21q22, near the genes IFNAR1, IFNAR2, and IFNGR2.

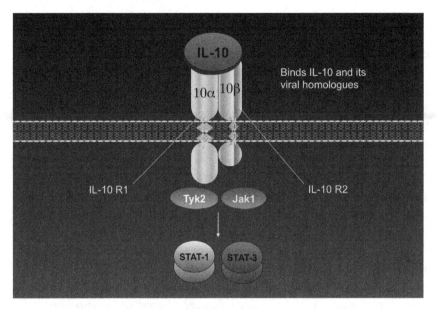

Figure 6-10 The IL-10 receptor and signal transduction factors.

Association with Human Diseases

Mutations in the IL10 gene are associated with an increased susceptibility to HIV-1 infection. In detail, IL-10, as part of the Th2-type immune response may limit the replication of HIV-1 *in vivo,* possibly through inhibition of macrophage division, reduction of Th1 lymphocytes proliferation, and reduced secretion of proinflammatory cytokines. SNP in the promoter of the IL10 gene at position −592 (rs1800872) has high (C) and low (A) production alleles. Carriers of A alleles have likely increased risk of infection with HIV-1 infection, and those who are already ill, progress faster to AIDS than those who were homozygous for high producer allele (C/C). Approximately 25–30% of people who have a long latency in the progression of AIDS (over 10 years) have the C/C genotype.

Another SNP in the promoter of the IL10 gene is also associated with the production of IL-10: A-1082G (rs1800896). Carriers of the G allele have a high producer phenotype. The G alleles were significantly more frequent in people who live more than 100 years, and may protect against *myocardial infarction.* On the other hand, the G allele shows a higher prevalence in patients with *small cell lung cancer.*

SNPs in the IL10 gene were associated with risk for *NHL* and in some instances with a specific histologic subtype (together with IL4, IL5, and IL6 gene polymorphisms). Analysis of four SNPs in the IL10 promoter −3575T>A, −1082A>G (rs1800896), −819C>T (rs3021097), and −592C>A (rs1800872) revealed that both the AGCC haplotype and the TATA haplotype were associated with increased risk for B-cell *lymphomas*. Interestingly, the IL4 gene −1098G allele was additionally linked with increased susceptibility to developing T-cell *lymphomas*.[58]

Furthermore, three SNP genotypes in the promoter of the IL10 gene A-1082G (rs1800896), T-819C (rs3021097), and A-592C (rs1800872) were associated with predisposition to *oral cancer* in Taiwanese.[59] Another genotype with the phenotype of high producer of IL-10 was significantly associated with risk of *gastric cancer* (in *cardia*) in the Taiwanese population.

Polymorphism in the IL10 gene promoter (G-1082; wrongly annotated as −1087) is associated with *RA* in women of the Swedish population. A genotype of IL10 locus (using haplotype analysis of several SNPs and microsatellite markers) that has high producer phenotype is associated with *systemic lupus erythematosus* in Chinese.

In mice with defective IL10 gene (IL10-gene KO transgenic strain), *irreversible septic shock* after ligation of *caecum* and *colon* occurs much earlier than in those with a functional gene. It is believed that IL-10 might regulate the transition and the beginning of irreversible stages of shock. The IL-10 KO mice exhibit severe alveolar bone loss.[60]

Therapeutic Options

Because of the potential to reduce inflammation and inhibit the Th1 responses, IL-10 may be used for therapeutic purposes to control autoimmune diseases. Some argue that it may be useful in the treatment of chronic inflammations as well as certain types of cancer.

IL-11

IL-11 is known as the "adipogenesis inhibitory factor" and "oprelvekin" (alias: AGIF).

Structure

IL-11 is a cytokine of 19–21 kDa and a member of a family of cytokines that also includes IL-6, IL-31, LIF, CNTF, CTF1, BSF3, and OSM. The IL11 gene is located on human chromosome 19q13.

Source

IL-11 is produced by bone marrow stroma and endothelium, as well as endometrial stroma.

Function

The biological activity can be classified as anti-inflammatory, hematopoietic, osteoclastogenic, neurogenic. It also has an influence on women's fertility and promotes development of T-cell-stimulated Ig-producing B cells.

Receptor

IL-11 receptor (Figure 6-11) has two chains: IL-11RA (the gene is on chromosome 9p13), and IL-6ST. IL-11RA is similar to the CNTF factor. IL-6ST (gp130) is a member of a group of related receptors (see *IL-6: Receptor*). Expression of IL-11 receptor is spread on many cells throughout the body.

Other Features

IL-11 polarizes naïve CD4$^+$ T cells into Th2-type immunity, and inhibits the secretion of IL-12 by macrophages. Thus it has an anti-inflammatory effect. It works on a wide variety of cells of hematopoietic origin including

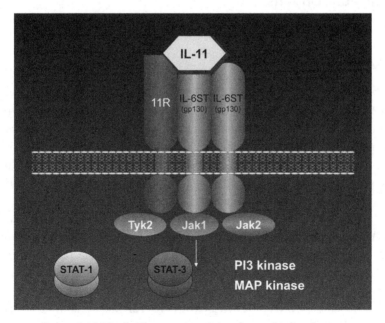

Figure 6-11 The IL-11 receptor and signal transduction factors.

primitive, erythroid, and megakaryocytic progenitors. It also induces the synthesis of acute phase proteins, inhibits the development of adipocytes, and has an impact on the regeneration of intestinal epithelium. Additionally, IL-11 induces the generation of osteoclasts from monocytes. In uterus, it plays an important role in generating the decidua and placenta, and its secretion is regulated by local growth factors (like *heparin binding epidermal growth factor*, HB-EGF).

Association with Human Diseases

In *Hodgkin lymphoma,* increased expression of IL-11RA was found in Reed–Sternberg's cells.

IL-11 and IL-11RA was found in the cytoplasm of some tumors, such as *colorectal adenocarcinoma.*

IL-11 (the lack of) may be associated with infertility, because it is dysregulated in infertile women (like LIF).

IL-11 is (together with IL-6) important in bone remodeling, but it is not associated with estrogen-related bone loss.

Interestingly, increased expression of IL-11 is associated with bone metastasis of *breast cancer* and may be useful in its prediction.[61]

Therapeutic Options

IL-11 is used in the treatment of chemotherapy-induced *thrombocytopenia.*

IL-12

Structure

IL-12 is a heterodimeric protein with two subunits, one a bit smaller than the other (p35/p40), and is referred to as IL-12p70 (Figure 6-12). However, a homodimer comprising only larger subunit (p40/p40) also exists, sometimes termed IL-12p40^2. The heterodimeric form IL-12p70 (p35/p40) makes together with IL-23 (p19/p40), IL-27 (EBI3/p28), and IL-35 (EBI3/p35) a related group of cytokines.

The smaller subunit has 35 kDa and is called IL-12A, but often just as p35. The p35 subunit resembles the cytokines of the IL-6 group including IL-23p19 and IL27p28 (see "*IL-6*"). Other names for the IL-12A subunit are: *interleukin 12A, natural killer cell stimulatory factor 1, cytotoxic lymphocyte maturation factor 1,* and *p35.* The IL12A gene is located on chromosome 3p12-13.2 (alias: CLMF; NFSK; NKSF1, IL-12A). This subunit is shared with IL-35 (p35/EBI3).

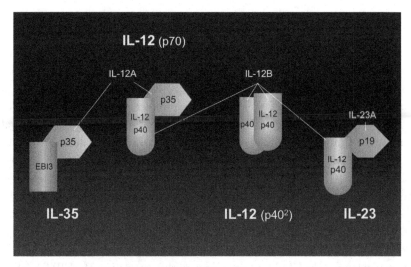

Figure 6-12 IL-12 shares its subunits with IL-23 and IL-35 cytokines. The homodimer p40 has been also implicated in signaling.

The second subunit has molecular weight of 40 kDa (IL-12B; p40 resembles the extracellular part of IL-6-receptor α-chain, see "*IL-6 Receptor*"). Other names for the IL-12B subunit are: *interleukin 12B, natural killer cell stimulatory factor 2, cytotoxic lymphocyte maturation factor 2,* and *p40*. The IL12B gene is located on chromosome 5q31-33 (alias: CLMF; NKSF; CLMF2; NKSF2, IL-12B). This subunit is shared with IL-23 (p19/p40).

Source

The main source of IL-12 is *peripheral blood mononuclear cells* stimulated by bacteria, intracellular parasites, or their products. Of tissue cells, which are the source of IL-12, it is important to mention dendritic cells type 1 (DC1, $CD11c^+$), the epithelium and endothelium.

Function

It has an important proinflammatory role in innate immunity, and plays a fundamental role in the initiation of the protective immune response. Many actions and functions of IL-12, like for example the generation of Th1-type response, have been credited to IL-12 (as researchers measured only one of the subunits, namely p40), while they could be perhaps attributed to IL-23 (p19/p40). Only after the discovery of IL-23, research has started to clear this issue. A similar issue happened with the discovery of IL-35 cytokine that shares the p35 subunit with IL-12p70. Therefore, one should be still cautious when reading the following paragraphs. In general, if not specified differently, IL-12 refers to heterodimeric cytokine detected by its p40 subunit.

The biological activity of IL-12 includes stimulation of IFN-γ production by NK and activated Th1 (and Tc1) cells. IL-12 is a key factor in the development of Th1 and inhibition of Th2 lines (and thus indirectly in diminishing the production of IgE). These actions result with stimulation of cellular adaptive immunity (Th1,Tc1), and inhibition of (a part of) humoral immunity (inhibition of Th2). IL-12 enhances the defensive action of T and B cells (adaptive immunity) by displaying anti-viral, anti-bacterial (for those that live intracellularly), and anti-tumor activity. IL-12 might participate in the pathogenesis of some autoimmune diseases, or may increase the frequency of exacerbations.

Receptor

The receptor for IL-12 is a heterodimer with two chains: IL-12Rβ1 (alias: CD212; gene: IL12RB, IL-12R-BETA) and IL-12Rβ2 (gene: IL12RB2). The receptor lacks α chain, but only in the name, as two beta chains form a fully functional cell surface receptor. Perhaps the receptor chains are called betas in order to stress the relationship of this cytokine to IL-6 family. Namely, the ligand subunit IL-12B (p40) is homologous to the α-chain of the IL-6 receptor (IL-6R), and the other subunit IL-12A (p35) is homologous to IL-6 cytokine. Signal transduction in the cell involves Jak2 and Tyk2 kinases (Figure 6-13). They phosphorylate intracellular portions of receptor chains that recruit mainly STAT-4 molecules, which subsequently also get phosphorylated. STAT-3 can also be activated in a similar way. Phosphorylation of STAT-3 and STAT-4 causes conformational changes in them, and increase the affinity for building homodimeric STAT molecules. As homodimers, they exhibit increased affinity for the nucleus. They move and transfer into the nucleus, binding to specific sites in DNA where they regulate transcription of IL-12-controlled genes.

Receptors for IL-12 are expressed only in NK and activated T cells. IL12RB2 is transcribed in Th1 cells by the action of IFN-γ.

Other Features

It was suggested that p40 (IL-12B) is secreted as the first response of an organism upon encounter with microbes, and p35 (IL-12A) or p19 (IL23A, see "IL-23") in answer to immunomodulatory stimuli from the microenvironment of T cells during their activation, which would result in different types of the immune response.

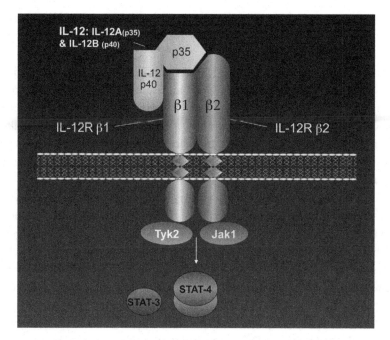

Figure 6-13 The IL-12 receptor and signal transduction factors.

IL-12 induces perforin in NK cells. IL-12 can cause the secretion of IFN-γ by NK cells, which is not related to activation of T cells.

IL-12 has an anti-tumor and anti-metastatic effect against murine tumors.[62]

Association with Human Diseases

Excessive IL-12 production was found in several organ-specific autoimmune diseases, including *RA*,[63] *type I diabetes mellitus*,[64] *multiple sclerosis*,[65] and *Crohn's disease*.[66] Increased production of IL-12B (p40) that was observed in the CNS of patients with *multiple sclerosis* is thought to play a role in the pathogenesis of the disease.

The IL12B gene promoter polymorphism is associated with the intensity of atopic and non-atopic *asthma* in children.

Furthermore, SNP (A+1188C, rs3212227), which controls the expression of mRNA for IL-12B is associated with a tendency for people to suffer from *atopic dermatitis* and *psoriasis vulgaris*. The same SNP in combination with high-risk HLA haplotypes is an additional risk factor for *type I diabetes mellitus* in Japanese population.

Genetic polymorphisms in the intron of the IL12B gene and genotypic analyses of similar markers provided the basis for the association with a predilection for *tuberculosis* in Chinese.

The IL12B gene SNP (A>C +1188, rs3212227) was found associated with occurrence of *breast cancer* in Croatian Caucasians.[67] It has been found associated with *cervical cancers* in Chinese (in combination with IL12A polymorphism)[68] and Korean populations,[69] *nasopharyngeal cancers in Tunisians*,[70] *gliomas* and *NHL*,[71] but interestingly also with autoimmune diseases like *ankylosing spondylitis*,[72] *insulin-dependent diabetes mellitus type 1*,[64] and *multiple sclerosis*.[65]

In addition, regarding IL12A, polymorphisms in several susceptibility loci that associate with *Sjögren's syndrome* have been recently identified, including the MHC region, IRF5, STAT4, IL12A, FAM167A/BLK, and TNIP1 genes.

The receptor for IL-12 has also been linked to several diseases. Lack of expression of the IL12RB1 gene is associated with resilient *mycobacterioses* and *salmonelloses*. Natural IL12RB1 gene deficiency is rare, and these children get the lethal infection with BCG (instead of being protected by such vaccination). A polymorphism in the IL12RB1 gene is associated with risk for *tuberculosis* in Japanese. Decreased expression of this chain can predispose to *allergies* and *atopies*.

Overexpression of the IL12RB2 gene is observed in a number of infectious diseases, and in patients with *Crohn's disease* and *leprosy*.

Therapeutic Options

Targeted inhibition of IL-12B (p40) subunit by neutralizing it with various methods (also part of the IL-23 cytokine) proves effective in the treatment of *autoimmune* diseases. And IL-12 could be used to enhance Th1 response in some infectious diseases or as anti-cancer therapy.

Systemic administration of IL-12 prevented occurrence of *mammary carcinomas*, in mice transgenic for the rat HER2/neu oncogene. IL12 strongly increased the effects of tumor cell vaccination in this model.[73] Furthermore, IL-12 shows anti-angiogenic properties in the *murine breast cancer* model.[74] Unfortunately, administering IL-12 systemically might also increase the chance of developing autoimmunity.

IL-13

Structure

IL-13 is a cytokine of 14–40 kDa (depending on glycosylation). Primary protein structure has 25–30% similarity with IL-4 cytokine. The gene is located on chromosome 5q31 in the vicinity of genes encoding IL–3, IL–4, IL–5, and GM–CSF.

Source

Activated Th2 cell population secretes IL–13. Eosinophil granulocytes secrete IL–13 under the influence of IL–5 and GM–CSF (also secreted by Th2-type response). Innate helper type 2 cells secrete IL–13 upon stimulus from IL–25 and IL–33.

Function

IL–13 is an immunoregulatory cytokine. It regulates the function of human B cells and monocytes (but only macrophages in the mouse). In general, the activity of IL–13 resembles that of IL–4. IL–13 can activate monocyte cell lines and inhibit the production of inflammatory cytokines (IL–1α, IL–1β, IL–6, IL–8, G–CSF, and IFN–α), for example, from macrophages activated with LPS. IL–13 causes the Ig isotype switch in B lymphocytes into IgE, and thus has a role in development of *allergies*. IL–13 is a powerful inducer of *fibrosis* in many *inflammatory* and *autoimmune* diseases.

Receptor

There are two receptors for IL–13: IL–13R1 and IL–13R2 (Figure 6-14).

The first receptor for IL–13 is composed of two chains: IL–13Rα1 (alias: CD213A1, IL–13Ra; the gene is located on chromosome Xq24) and IL–4Rα (see *"IL-4 receptor"*). Both chains have intermediate affinity, and high affinity for IL–13 has only a heterodimer composed of IL–13Rα1/ IL–4Rα chains that transduces the signal into the cell via Jak2–Tyk2 kinases and STAT-1, STAT-3, STAT-5ab, and STAT-6 transcription factors in monocytes. In lung myofibroblasts, however, the signal transduction includes different tyrosine kinase combination: Jak3–Tyk2 (instead of Jak2–Tyk2) and only STAT-3 nuclear factor (Figure 6-14).

The second IL–13 receptor has a single chain—IL–13Rα2 (alias: CD213A2; IL13BP; the gene is located on chromosome Xq13-28), which was until recently considered to be a decoy receptor, because it lacks cytosolic part (Figure 6-14). However, it has a high affinity for the ligand and signaling through it induces TGF-β1 secretion from macrophages. (TGF-β1 can cause tissue *fibrosis*, with collagen deposition.) IFN-γ causes the upregulation of IL–13Rα2 on the cell membrane and thereby modulates the effect of IL–13. Furthermore, SOCS-1 has been identified as a factor in the negative feedback loop of signal transduction in the cell (see *"IL-6 receptor,"* p. 168, for more on SOCS molecules).

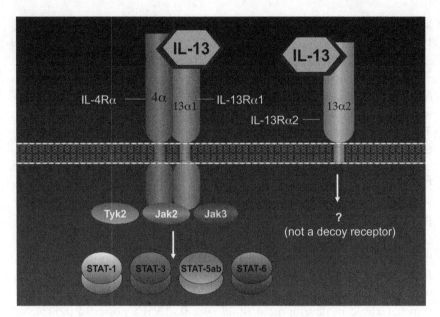

Figure 6-14 The IL-13 receptors and their signal transduction factors.

Association with Human Diseases

A combination of genetic polymorphisms in the IL13 gene and IL4 gene is correlated with the level of IgE antibodies and the development of childhood *asthma*. Furthermore, in *allergic rhinitis*, there is a significant correlation between the Arg130Gln SNP of the IL13 gene with total IgE levels in the blood. Patients with Gln/Gln genotype have much higher levels of total IgE levels than those with the Arg/Arg genotype in adult Chinese population.

In *Hodgkin's disease*, Reed–Sternberg cells produce a multitude of cytokines including IL-13.

IL-13 is correlated with the immune response to the parasite *Schistosoma hematobium*, and genetic risk study of the SNP (G-1055T) in the IL13 gene showed an association with the infection in Mali's population.

Some IL13RA1 alleles are associated with rapid deterioration of lungs in smokers.

Therapeutic Options

IL-13 antagonists could be useful in the treatment of *asthma* and *allergies* (perhaps along with antagonists of IL-4).

IL-14 (IL-14 DOES NOT EXIST IN DATABASES)

IL-14 was a name for a cytokine of 50–60 kDa that was found in experiments causing proliferation of activated B lymphocytes. It is no longer mentioned in the databases (Entrez: *nucleotide;* Genebank).

IL-15

Structure

IL-15 is a cytokine with two forms: a trans-membrane and a secretory; the latter form has 14–15 kDa.

Source

IL-15 is secreted by monocytes, macrophages, DCs, follicular dendritic cells, stromal cells, T cells, and some *cancer* cells (prostate, ovary).

Function

IL-15 is bi-directional cytokine with a wide variety of functions. It drives homeostatic (lymphopenic) division of human $CD8^+$ and $CD4^+$ memory T cells, and NK cells. The effect resembles somewhat that of the IL-2 cytokine. However, the main difference is that IL-15 inhibits IL-2-induced apoptosis of T cells. The latter usually occurs as a result of activation in the periphery. Membrane form of IL-15 (mIL-15) has a reverse signal transduction, by which it participates in the production of proinflammatory cytokines and exerts immunomodulatory effects (Figure 6-15).

Secretory form of IL-15 also has proinflammatory and immunoregulatory effects like IL-2 (via autocrine and juxtacrine mechanisms). It is important in homeostatic proliferation of T and NK cells (see *T lymphocyte Homeostasis,* Chapter 3, p. 93). It has anti-apoptotic effect on $CD8^+$ memory T cells, probably also on naïve $CD8^+$ T cells, and on B cells in the germinal centers. In addition to being hematopoietic, IL-15 affects the somatic tissues (e.g., it has anabolic effects on muscle tissue).

Receptor

The IL-15 receptor consists of three subunits (α, β, and γc). IL-15R α and β chains are associated with the common γ_C chain (which is also part of the IL-2R, IL-4R, IL-7R, IL-9R, and IL-21R). The alpha chain of the receptor (IL-15RA) has a particularly high affinity for the ligand in comparison with all other cytokine receptors. This is due to an unusual structure of the

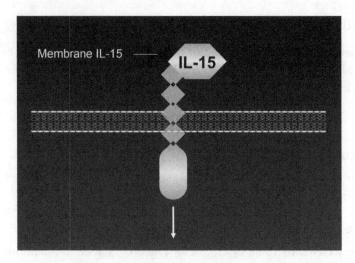

Figure 6-15 Membrane IL-15 and reverse signaling.

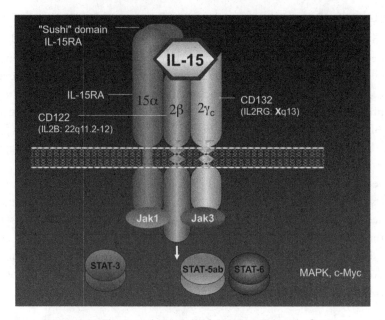

Figure 6-16 The IL-15 receptor and signal transduction factors.

IL-15RA chain that has an additional region, which is called the *sushi* domain (Figure 6-16).

The IL-15Rβ chain is actually the same as for the IL-2 receptor—IL-2Rβ (CD122) chain.

The action on the *sushi*-domain receptor is transduced into the cell via the Jak1 and Jak3 kinases that phosphorylate STAT-3, STAT-5, and STAT-6 nuclear factors. With the help of some *mitogen-activated kinase* (MAPK) these factors enhance the transcription of IL-15-dependent genes in the nucleus.

Reverse signaling is an interesting form of feedback communication between cells: the signal carrier cell, which has for example a membrane form of IL-15, receives signals that it come in contact with a cell that expresses the IL-15 receptor. Similarly, the cell expressing the membrane form of IL-15 can receive another type of the signal by soluble part of the receptor (sIL-15RA) that has been enzymatically peeled from the membrane by a sheddase. The sIL-15RA action on the membrane bound IL-15 causes signal transduction into the cell by MAP kinases (ERK and p38). This can facilitate induction and secretion of proinflammatory cytokines such as IL-6, IL-8, and TNF-α in monocytes.

The soluble form of IL-15RA has 42 kDa, and is spontaneously released probably by metalloproteinase activity. It can have significant immunoregulatory effects because soluble receptors can act on distant target cells. Release of metalloproteinases (sheddases) is significantly increased during cell activation, and moderately with IL-1 and TNF-α.

Other Features

1. IL-15 stabilizes *telomerase* enzyme in CD8$^+$ T cells, and thus extends the life of the respective clones (*telomerase* shortens telomeres of chromosomes. Telomere length is directly proportional to cell division ability, e.g., in tissue regeneration).
2. In humans, IL-15 affects by autocrine and paracrine mechanisms homeostatic growth of CD4$^+$ T memory cells without the need for interaction with MHC class II molecules, and without the need for IL-7 cytokine.
3. By its effect it resembles the influence of IL-2 on naïve T cells (in the sense of division and growth). The difference is that IL-15 has less influence on *de novo* protein synthesis in T cells than IL-2. A further difference is that IL-2 acts apoptotically on memory T cells, while IL-15 has an anti-apoptotic effect on CD8 memory T cells. Furthermore, IL-15 enhances apoptosis of activated CD4$^+$ T lymphocytes (effectors).
4. In the endometrium, in its secretory phase, IL-15 plays a central role in the post-ovulatory stage by attracting NK cells from the blood into the tissue.

5. After 10 weeks of daily muscle training, the level of IL-15 increases in plasma. It is probably an important factor in the regulation of muscle mass under workout.

6. IL-15 and IL-15 receptor mRNAs were found in all examined structures of the fetal brain, suggesting their potential role in normal development and physiology of the brain.

7. In the mouse, IL-15 may increase the expression of BCL2 (inhibitor of apoptosis). It is believed that this reduces the incidence of *diabetes mellitus* like condition in mice genetically predisposed to the disease (NOD).

8. Mice with genetically engineered absence of the IL15 gene (IL-15 KO) have a phenotype in which there is an increased apoptosis of CD8$^+$ T effectors after infection, and this can be prevented by injecting IL-15 cytokine.

9. IL-15 KO mice have almost no NK cells. Interestingly, IL-15 is a dominant factor in the early development of NK cells in the mouse, because KO mice of genes encoding IL-2, IL-4, IL-7, IL-9, or IL-21 cytokines have NK cells.

10. IL-15 stops chemokine signaling between fractalkine (FKN) and its receptor CX3CR1 (see *Chemokines* in Chapter 7). The latter participates in atherogenesis by promoting the proliferation of smooth muscle cells in vessel walls.

11. It is possible that during signaling the receptor molecule IL-15RA binds with Axl receptor tyrosine kinase (RTK) and thereby contributes to the specificity of the signal in the nucleus.

Association with Human Diseases

Systemic inflammatory reaction with IL-15 may play a role in the occurrence of cardiovascular disease in essential hypertension.

In *diabetes mellitus* (type I) there are increased concentrations of IL-15 in serum.

In *IBD*, IL-15 and IL-15R can play an important role in the activation and development of B cells in the *lamina propria*, especially in *ulcerative colitis*.

In *RA*, IL-15 secreted by synovial T cells (with IL-17, TNF-α, and IL-1β) promotes development of osteoclasts (osteoclastogenesis) from monocytes (*ex vivo*). Osteoclastogenesis is not observed in samples from patients in remission (after treatment). This suggests a role for IL-15 in the pathogenesis of *RA*.

In *polymyositis* and *dermatomyositis*, increased production of IL-15 was detected in muscle cells, suggesting the role of IL-15 in their pathogenesis.

Muscular hypertrophy that occurs after training in healthy populations is associated with genetic polymorphisms in the IL15RA gene.

The IL-15 gene polymorphisms might be associated with some *allergic* and *atopic* conditions.

Therapeutic Options

According to a study of adoptive cellular immunotherapy of *cancer*, short treatment with (autologous) CD56$^+$ cells (presumably NK and *lymphokine activated killer* LAK cells) with IL-15 in combination with IL-12 or IL-18 at intervals of 8 days offer a potential for better clinical outcome.

Knowledge about the increased serum levels of IL-15 in *diabetes mellitus* (type I) can be perhaps used in the prevention of *pre-diabetic condition* or late diabetic complications by treatment that inhibits IL-15 effects. However, there is no correlation between hyperglycemic episodes and levels of IL-15, and it is questionable whether there is a causal relationship at all.

IL-15 reduces intimal thickening of carotid arteries after experimentally induced atherogenetic changes in experimental mice. Maybe this is an opportunity for the development of a novel treatment of atherosclerotic changes.

IL-16

Structure

Interleukin-16 is synthesized as a larger precursor and is found in the nucleus and cytoplasm. After cleavage of the C-terminal 14-kDa end, the remainder of the molecule forms tetramers and becomes bioactive (alias: *lymphocyte chemoattractant factor*, LCF). The gene coding for IL-16 is located on chromosome 15q26.

Source

IL-16 is constitutively produced by peripheral blood monocytes, epithelial cells, epidermal *Langerhans* cells, mast cells, macrophages, DCs, CD8$^+$T, CD4$^+$T, and eosinophils. The amount of secreted IL-16 is directly proportional to the amount of infiltration with CD4$^+$ T lymphocytes.

Function

The name that originally described IL-16, LCF, already suggests a chemotactic role similar to chemokines, but in fact it is indirect (see below, *IL-16:*

Other features). Furthermore, IL-16 also plays a role in cell adhesion, fusion, migration, *epidermal growth factor* (EGF) signal transduction, and tumor suppression. The precursor (pro-IL-16) in the nucleus is linked to the arrest in G0/G1 cell cycle stage.

Receptor

There are two IL-16 receptors: CD4 and CD9 molecules (Figure 6-17). CD4 is also the coreceptor for MHC class II molecules expressed on T helper cells. CD4 is also expressed on some other hematopoietic cells, but in lesser quantities than on T cells.

CD9 molecule is tetraspanin, a protein that is embedded in the cell membrane by palmitoylation (the covalent attachment of fatty acids, in this case palmitic acid, to cysteine, serine, or threonine residues of a protein). CD9 has four transmembrane domains. It belongs to the superfamily of TM4SF molecules that also includes CD63, CD81, and CD151. They are all associated with c-kit (SCF receptor) tyrosine kinase. Although their role is not yet fully understood, it is known that tetraspanins are involved in antigen presentation, and in the interaction between sperm and egg cells. The CD9 gene is located on chromosome 12p13.

Signal transduction in cells attracted by IL-16 is transmitted through PI4 kinase, PKC, and influx of calcium ions.

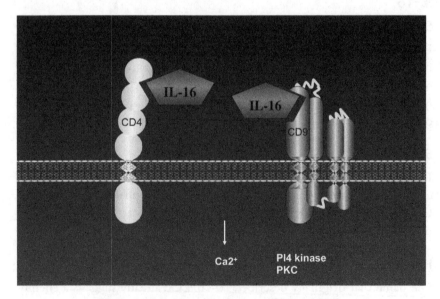

Figure 6-17 IL-16 and its receptors (CD4 and CD9).

Other Features

Chemotaxis of cells by IL-16 is initiated through activation of components of the extracellular matrix. This starts by binding of IL-16 to CD4 and is maintained by secreting CCR3-binding chemokines (see *Chemokines,* Chapter 7).

IL-16 causes an increase in the expression of IL-2R and the human MHC class II molecules (HLA-DR), reversible inhibition of T lymphocyte activation (if induced via TCR and CD3), and induction of the transcription repressor of HIV-1 virus.

CD9 has a function in adhesion to and transmigration through endothelium, as it probably binds integrins such as ICAM-1 and (to a lesser extent) VCAM-1. Palmitic acid parts are likely affecting the homogenization of the same tetraspanin molecules in the cell membrane.

Association with Human Diseases

IL-16 is associated (together with IL-12) in the pathogenesis of *periodontitis,* with perhaps higher risk in severity of the disease in alcoholics and smokers.

Furthermore, there may be a role in the development of *alopecia areata.*

In peritoneal fluid, it is possible that IL-16 participates in the pathogenesis of *endometriosis,* because of its initial or permanent proinflammatory effects in the peritoneal cavity.

Increased IL-16 concentrations are associated with *hemophagocytic lymphohistiocytosis.*

It is also possible that it has a role in the process of joint destruction in *RA.*

One IL16 genotype is associated with *contact dermatitis* caused by *para*-substituted *aryl* substances.

In *asthmatics,* IL-16 is a prominent source of chemotactic activity that attracts lymphocytes after sensitization with the antigen.

CD9 molecule expression is inversely correlated with *metastasis* to lymph nodes. It is possible to monitor the level of expression CD9 on tumor cells by monoclonal antibodies, and thus perhaps recognize their metastatic potential.

Therapeutic Options

Potential therapeutic use lies in taking an inhibitor of IL-16 in *asthma.* Likewise, the agonist could be useful in the $CD4^+$ T cell immune reconstitution in patients with AIDS after chemotherapy.

IL-17

ALIAS (IL17A): CTLA-8, cytotoxic T-lymphocyte-associated antigen 8; cytotoxic T-lymphocyte-associated serine esterase 8.

Structure

IL-17 makes a group of *homodimeric cytokines* of approximately 32 kDa. Proteomic and genomic analysis revealed six similar proteins that are classified in IL-17 family (IL-17A-F). However, it has been observed soon that 1 of these molecules is special, and thus IL-17E became IL-25. Human IL-17A monomer has ~15 kDa with 155 amino acids. The IL17A and IL17F genes are located very close to each other on chromosome 6p12. The IL17B gene is located on chromosome 5q32-34. The IL17C gene is located on chromosome 16q24. The IL17D gene is on chromosome 13q11.

Source

IL-17A and IL-17F are mainly secreted by subgroup of effector (activated) helper T cells (proinflammatory) called Th17. In the mouse, IL-17 is secreted by double positive thymocytes in the thymic cortex with $\alpha\beta$T-cell receptor ($\alpha\beta$TCR$^+$CD4$^+$CD8$^+$). On the other hand, IL-17B was found only in the cell body of neurons. IL-17C is produced by epithelial cells.

Function

IL-17 is a group of proinflammatory cytokines. IL-17A/F causes neutrophilia. IL-17A/F mobilizes granulocytes by granulopoesis, causes migration with CXC chemokines, and prolongs their lives in target tissues. It stimulates cyclooxygenase-2 (COX-2), as well as the production of nitric oxide (NO) and IL-6 in some target cells. Even IL-17B (neuronal) acts proinflammatory (stimulates release of TNF and IL-1 by monocytic cell line). IL-17C is produced by keratinocytes, and respiratory epithelia by ligands to TLR3 (i.e., double-stranded RNA) or TLR5 (flagellin). IL-17C is involved in epithelial innate immunity in autocrine manner. It binds to a complex made of receptors IL-17RA and IL-17-RE. IL-17E is renamed IL-25.

Receptor

There are several IL-17 receptors. The IL17RA (CD217) (Figure 6-18) gene is located on chromosome 22q11.1. The IL-17RA protein binds IL-17A and F subtypes. It is expressed on various types of cells. Other IL-17 cytokine subtypes IL-17B and IL-17E (now called—IL-25) bind to

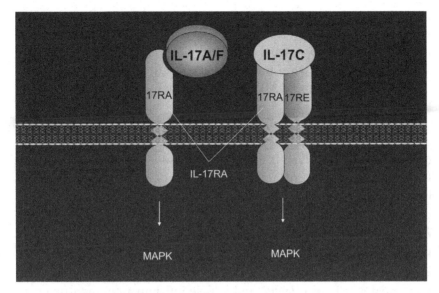

Figure 6-18 The IL-17RA receptor. The IL-17C receptor (IL-17RA/IL-17RE).

IL-17RB. IL-25 (IL-17E) influences activation of IL-17RB and signaling via NF-κB pathway with IL-8 production. IL-17RB is highly expressed in rat model of intestinal inflammation. IL-17 signaling system has been found in various tissues such as articular cartilage, bones, meniscus, brain, hematopoietic tissues, kidneys, lungs, skin, and intestine. IL-17RA and IL-17RE chains are expressed on epithelial cells (i.e., of a respiratory system).

Other Features

IL-17 (A or F) binds to *Herpesvirus saimiri*, which is lymphotropic for T cells. Furthermore, IL-17 induces the secretion of IL-6, IL-8, PGE2, MCP-1, and G-CSF by adherent cells like fibroblasts, keratinocytes, epithelial, and endothelial cells.

In vitro, IL-17 acts synergistically with other proinflammatory signals via TNF-α for induction of GM-CSF, and with CD40-ligand for secretion of IL-6, IL-8, CCL5 (RANTES), and CCL2 (MCP-1) from kidney epithelial cells.

In vivo, injection of IL-17 induces neutrophilia, except in IL-6-KO mice. IL-17 also has a role in the rejection of transplanted kidneys.

In the lungs, IL-17 (A or F) has a dual role. During sensitization with antigen, IL-17 enhances *allergic* type reaction and the development of *asthma.* However, in established disease, IL-17 has opposite effects. For example, the exogenous application of IL-17 reduces the migration of eosinophils, negatively regulates the eosinophil chemokine eotaxin (CCL11) and *thymus and activation regulated chemokine* (TARC; CCL17) after re-stimulation with antigen *in vitro* and *in vivo*. *In vitro*, IL-17 decreases production of TARC in DCs, which are the main source of this chemokine. (DCs are beside macrophages main collectors of phago-cytosed tissue antigens that are presented later in the lymph nodes to T cells.) Furthermore, IL-17 causes a decrease in IL-5 and IL-13 produc-tion in the regional lymph nodes. Also, these effects are controlled by IL-4. All this seems to reduce the symptoms of *asthma* in already estab-lished disease.

Association with Diseases

High values have been found in chronic *inflammation*, including *RA* (RA resistant to anti-TNF therapy), *psoriasis*, and *multiple sclerosis*. Also, it has a potential role in *periodontitis* and muscle inflammation. Increased con-centrations of IL-17 are also associated with *cutaneous T lymphoma*.

Polymorphisms in the IL17RB gene (a receptor for IL-17E, see "*IL-25*") has been associated with *asthma*.

Therapeutic Options

Anti-IL-17A treatment could prove to be (along with inhibition of IL-23) effective in *organ-specific autoimmune diseases,* because it would reduce the risk of infections that would otherwise occur as a complication of treatment with general immunosuppressive agents.

Although it is associated with the sensitization during development of *allergic asthma*, in already established forms of the disease it may have the opposite role and attenuate symptoms, if it were added exogenously.

IL-18

Alias

IL1F4, IGIF, IL-1g.

Structure

IL-18 is a cytokine of ~22 kDa similar to IL-1. This human protein has 193 amino acids, and the IL18 gene is located on chromosome 11q22. The antago-nists to IL-18 are IL-18BP ("IL-18 *binding protein*") and IL-1F7, and both of

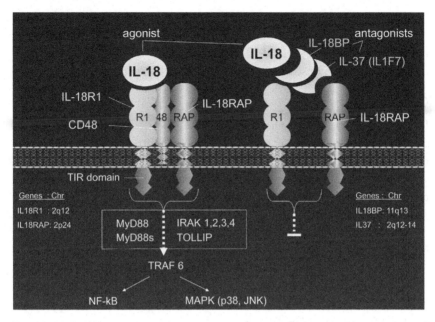

Figure 6-19 IL-18 versus IL-37 as agonist versus antagonist. IL-18 receptor and signal transduction.

them are also similar to IL-1 cytokine antagonists system (Figure 6-19). Signal transduction into the cell goes through IL-1/TLR receptor superfamily, with the predominant activation of MAPK (p38). Human IL-18BP has 24–25 kDa, 219 amino acids, and the gene (IL18BP) is located on chromosome 11q13.

Source

IL-18 is mainly secreted by activated monocytes, macrophages, and DCs.

Function

IL-18 is a proinflammatory cytokine with immunomodulatory functions; it stimulates the development of Th1 and inhibits development of Th2. IL-18 is a cytokine that increases the secretion of IFN-γ by activated T cells and NK cells, and is reminiscent of the IL-12 effect.

Receptor

IL-18 receptor (Figure 6-19) has three chains: the two of them have TIR domains (IL-18R1 and IL18RAP; *receptor acceptor protein*) and the third is linked is embedded in the cell membrane, because it is without the cytoplasmic region (CD48). Signal transduction in target cells is transmitted through NF-κB and MAP kinases. Antagonists like IL-18 binding protein (IL-18BP) and IL-37 (previously IL-1F7) inhibit association of the receptor chains, and thus prevent signal transduction.

Other Features

IL-18 has the effect that, generally (based on the results of so far published studies), resembles the effect of IL-12. It is possible that the reason for this is the fact that it acts with the latter one in synergy.

Among other properties it is important to note that, although belonging to the IL-1 family, it does not cause fever.

TNF induces production of IL-18 in *synovium*.

Phenotype of mice with targeted disruption of the IL-18 gene (KO) indicates that IL-18 KO cannot develop *collagen-induced arthritis*. This indirectly indicates the role of IL-18 in the development of this disease.

IL-18, similar to IL-12, stimulates the repair of DNA after UV radiation. Thereby it has influence on the decrease of photo-immunosuppression resulting from UV radiation.

Association with Diseases

It is believed that IL-18 is associated with autoimmune diseases such as RA, then with the pathogenesis of *atherosclerosis*, as well as *endometriosis*. In the *congestive heart disease* it seems that it has a pro-hypertrophic effect. In *ischemic and dilated cardiomyopathy* it is considered to have a pro-*atherosclerotic* effect. In a study with *cardiovascular disease* patients, comparison between the dead and the survivors revealed that the former had increased levels of mRNA for IL-18 and IL-18RA in cardiomyocytes, and reduced IL-18BP levels in serum. Values of IL-18 in serum could be a prognostic sign for progression of *diabetic nephropathy* as well as *cardiovascular disease*.

The presence of A-607C allele (SNP in the IL18 gene promoter) correlates with infection with the AIDS virus (HIV-1) and represent an increased risk for infection in those people who are carriers of this polymorphism in the genome. The same polymorphism does not influence the risk for development of *RA*. (However, some other genotypic polymorphisms are associated with *juvenile RA* in Japanese.)

A genetic susceptibility to both *type 1 diabetes* and *celiac disease* is complex. It involves an unknown number of various genetic elements that could be either allelic variants of expressed genes or their regulatory elements. The risk of developing these two diseases shares common alleles, in addition to distinct genetic variants for each disease. Data from a large case–control study (involving over 16,000 individuals) suggest that common biologic mechanisms, such as autoimmunity-related tissue damage and intolerance to dietary antigens, could be causing both diseases.[75] The authors identified seven shared genetic variants in *type 1 diabetes* and *celiac disease*, as follows: (1) IL18RAP on chromosome 2q12; (2) RGS1 on chromosome 1q31; and (3) TAGAP on chromosome 6q25; (4) the 32-bp insertion-deletion variant on chromosome 3p21; (5) PTPN2 on chromosome 18p11; (6) CTLA4 on chromosome 2q33; and (7) SH2B3 on chromosome 12q24. The effects of the IL18RAP and TAGAP alleles confer protection in *type 1 diabetes* and susceptibility in *celiac disease*. Loci with distinct effects in the two diseases included INS on chromosome 11p15, IL2RA on chromosome 10p15, and PTPN22 on chromosome 1p13 in *type 1 diabetes* and IL12A on 3q25 and LPP on 3q28 in *celiac disease*.

IL-18 production is increased in the pulmonary and pleural *tuberculosis*. Levels of IL-18 and osteopontin (OPN) in the circulation correlate with the activity of *tuberculosis* in patients before and after tuberculostatic therapy in a study from Japan. (IFN-γ and IL-12 does not correlate with the disease in the same study.)

Furthermore, the increased values of IL-18 concentrations were found in *cutaneous T-lymphoma*. IL-18 production was increased in keratinocytes after exposure to UVB rays, and the level of IL-18 correlates with an increased risk of developing skin malignancies such as *melanoma*.

Therapeutic Options

Inhibitors of IL-18 action (mAb) might be able to reduce the specified immune-pathogeneses. Measurement of IL-18 in the circulation could be used in diagnostic and preventive counseling purposes in situations where there is a correlation with diseases.

IL-19

Alias

IL-10C, MDA1, NG.1, ZMDA1.

Structure

Human IL-19 has about 18 kDa molecular weight. It is made by processing larger precursors. The larger precursor (pre-IL-19) has 215 amino acids; the IL19 gene is located on chromosome 1q32. IL-19 belongs to the IL-10 family of cytokines (including IL-20, 22, 24, and 26).

Source

IL-19 is secreted by activated T cells and monocytes, and a distinct type of keratinocytes (induced by IL-1β).

Function

Its role is in communication between hematopoietic and non-hematopoietic tissues (especially in the areas of inflammation). IL-19 stimulates the development of Th2-type CD4 T lymphocytes. Together with IL-20 and IL-24, it promotes growth of keratinocytes.

Receptor

The receptor for IL-19 (Figure 6-20) is called differently, the IL-20 receptor, because IL-20 also binds to it. IL-20 receptor has two subunits, IL-20R1 (α or chain) and IL-20R2 (or β chain). Receptor chains are weakly expressed in

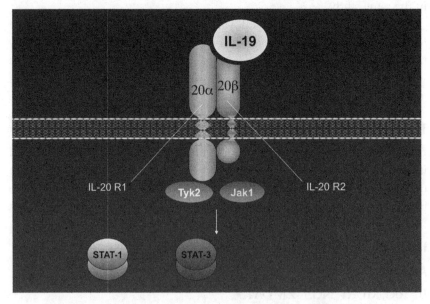

Figure 6-20 The IL-19 (and IL-20) receptor and signal transduction factors.

hematopoietic cells (R1 chain is absent in immunocytes) and strongly expressed in epithelial and stromal cells (e.g., fibroblasts) of skin, respiratory and reproductive systems, and some paracrine glands. The signal is transduced into the interior of the cell via the Jak-STAT system: Jak1, Tyk2, STAT-1, and STAT-3.

Other Features

IL-19 has a role in apoptosis and inflammation (pyroptosis), and probably in other immune responses.

Its regulation involves IL-10, which inhibits secretion of IL-19.

The gene coding for IL-19 is located near the IL15 gene (20 kB upstream). Regulation of expression of IL-19 is probably more complex than in other cytokine genes. Namely, as IL-10, IL-19 is induced by the LPS-stimulated monocytes, but in contrast to IL-10, it is not expressed by stimulated T lymphocytes. IL-19 may participate in peripheral development of T cells (after activation). IL-4 increases the possibility of LPS to induce IL-19 mRNA, whereas IFN-γ acts in the opposite direction—it inhibits its transcription. Thus, IL-19 can be a factor of development of Th2 type of immune response. Furthermore, in cultures of human cells, long-term incubation with IL-19 induces IL-4, IL-5, IL-10, and IL-13 cytokine secretion during the activation of naïve T cells (CD45RA$^+$). This result is a hallmark of Th2 type of cytokine response (this feature of IL-19 is shared with other cytokines of the IL-10 family—IL-20 and IL-22, but not with IL-10). Interestingly, in the mouse, IL-19 induces IL-4 and TNF-α.

Association with Human Diseases

IL-19 has a possible role in the development of *asthma*. Genetic linkage studies suggest a possible association of genetic region on chromosome 1q32 (containing other genes of the IL10 family including IL10 and IL20) with clearance of hepatitis C virus (HCV) in African-Americans, but not in Europeans (the study included 54 SNP).

IL-20

Alias

IL10D, ZCYTO10, four alpha helix cytokine, interleukin 20 short form.

Structure

IL-20 is a protein of about 20 kDa (176 amino acids). IL-20 is IL-10 homolog, detected by bioinformatics tool in screening transcriptome data making use of an algorithm based on structural similarities among cytokines. Chromosomal localization of IL-20 is at 1q32. Its discovery later on served to detect other homologs of the IL-10 family (which includes IL-19, IL-22, IL-24, and IL-26).

Source

IL-20 is secreted by monocytes and T cells.

Function

Generally, IL-20 is important for the communication between the hemato-poietic and non-hematopoietic tissues, particularly in *inflammation*. IL-20 stimulates Th2 type of the immune response.

Receptor

IL-20 can bind to two different heterodimeric receptors (Figure 6-21) comprising:
(a) IL-20R and IL-20R2 (also binds IL-19 and IL-24); and
(b) IL-22R1 and IL-20R2 (also binds IL-24).

The receptors are expressed in the skin (keratinocytes), and in stromal cells of respiratory and reproductive tracts. Signal transduction sets in

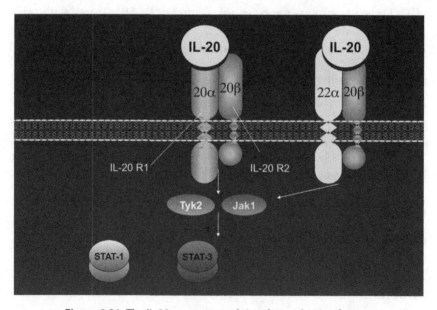

Figure 6-21 The IL-20 receptors and signal transduction factors.

motion a cascade of phosphorylation events from the cytosolic portions of the receptors to the nucleus, and employs the Jak-STAT tyrosine kinase–nuclear factor mechanism to drive transcription of IL-20-regulated genes. Particularly, Jak1, Tyk2, STAT-1, and STAT-3 molecules are involved.

Other Features

Overexpression of IL-20 in transgenic mice causes neonatal lethality with skin abnormalities and aberrant differentiation of the epidermis. IL-20 acts on keratinocytes (and includes STAT-3 nuclear factor). The IL-20 receptor (IL-20R1 and R2) is expressed in normal skin; however, its expression is dramatically increased in *psoriatic* skin.

Receptor chains IL-20R1, 20R2, and 22R1 are mostly expressed on epithelial and stromal cells (fibroblasts), but their expression is very low on hematopoietic cells.

IL-20 is a negative regulator of COX-2/PGE2 enzymes. Its effects include the inhibition of angiogenesis.

In human T cell cultures, IL-20 induces IL-4 and IL-13 (and inhibits IFN-γ) secretion during activation of naïve T cells (CD45RA$^+$), which is an indication of the Th2 type of the response (IL-20 shares this feature with IL-19 and IL-22, but not with IL-10).

Association with Human Diseases

IL-20 has a probable role in *psoriasis*. As for IL19, the IL20 gene is located in the genetic region on chromosome 1q32 (containing the other IL10 gene family loci, the IL10 and IL19 genes), and it is possible that the IL20 gene is associated with clearance of HCV in African-Americans, but not in Europeans (the study included 54 SNPs).

IL-21

Structure

IL-21 is a cytokine similar to IL-2. The gene coding for IL-21 is located on chromosome 4q26-27, in the vicinity of the gene encoding IL-2.

Source

IL-21 is secreted by the activated T cells.

Function

IL-21 is pleiotropic cytokine that has an impact on development, activation, survival, and migration of T, B, and NK cells. It is necessary for the survival and migration of Th2 cells in the periphery. IL-21 can cause contradictory effects, such as proliferation or growth inhibition (and sometimes apoptosis) of immunocytes, which are puzzling. For example, IL-21 inhibits proliferation of IgE⁺ B cells, but it can induce some B cells to become cytotoxic. These actions probably depend on the stage of the peripheral development of T or B cells (which are most likely due to preceding actions of a number of other cytokines; for theoretical possibilities, see *Theories about the function of the immune system*, Chapter 9, pp. 283–301).

Receptor

Interleukin-21 receptor (IL-21R) is composed of two chains: IL-21R α chain (RA) and the IL-2Rγ_C common chain (with receptors for IL-2, 4, 7, 9, 15). Signal transduction involves Jak1, Jak3 kinases, STAT-1, STAT-3, and STAT-5 factors (Figure 6-22).

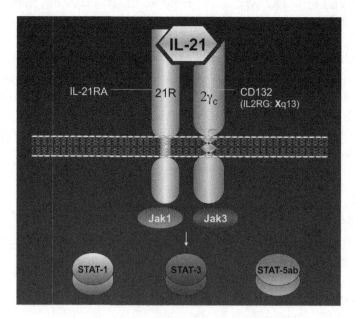

Figure 6-22 The IL-21 receptor and signal transduction.

Other Features

IL-21 enhances the proliferation of T and B cells, and the development of B lymphocytes (in the plasma cells) and facilitates isotype switch into the IgG1 and IgG3 (typical for the Th2 type response). On the other hand, IL-21 inhibits B cells that have previously (with IL-4) switched the isotype in IgE.

It enhances the expression of costimulatory molecules (CD28) on naïve $CD8^+$ T cells after homeostatic proliferation by IL-15 cytokine. This is an important feature of IL-21 that deserves more consideration. Namely, human naïve CD8 T cells can respond (divide) in an antigen-independent manner (e.g., without recognizing peptide/MHC ligand) by the actions of IL-7 and IL-15 cytokines. While IL-7 mostly maintains $CD8^+$ T cells in the naïve phenotype, IL-15 stimulates them to develop into an effector phenotype that is characterized among other things by a reduction in the expression of CD28. In the latter case, IL-21 can inhibit IL-15-induced reduction of CD28 molecules at the transcriptional level. Consequently, in functional terms, the IL-15/IL-21 pretreated $CD8^+$ T cells activated by antigenic-peptide/MHC-ligand mimicry (e.g., artificial generation of the "first" and "second" signals by stimulation with antibodies against TCR/CD3 and CD28) can produce greater amounts of IL-2 and IFN-γ cytokines than those $CD8^+$ T cells pretreated only with IL-15. We conclude that IL-21 contributes to restoring the homeostatically amplified $CD8^+$ T lymphocytes after effects of IL-15 in the naïve state. In other words, since the CD28 molecules transduce the "second" signal during the activation of naïve T cells, their re-expression represents re-gained readiness of $CD8^+$ T cells to respond to antigens.

IL-21R-induced CD40 molecules (that bind CD40L on T cells) can deliver a pro-apoptotic signal in B-cell *chronic lymphocytic leukemia*.

Furthermore, IL-21 promotes the production of NK in the bone marrow. Then, IL-21 enhances NK-cell lysis of target cells devoid of self-MHC antigens. IL-21 stimulates the expansion of particular T and B cell subpopulations.

B cells acquire cytotoxicity by induction of granzyme B as a consequence of their stimulation with IL-21 cytokine.

Mice deficient in the IL-21 receptor (IL-21R KO) lack Th2 type of immunity, whereas Th1 and Th17 types are not affected.

Association with Human Diseases

IL-21 has a possible role in the pathogenesis of *allergic asthma*.

In synovial membranes in patients with *RA* an increased amount of the IL-21R molecules was found.

Therapeutic Options

In DNA vaccinations (e.g., against HIV-1), using the gene encoding immunizing antigen (e.g., the *Env* gene) in combination with the genes for IL-21 and IL-15 prolongs the duration of protective immunity and boosts immunity.

IL-21 is being tested as a treatment for cancer because of its anti-tumor activity in many types of *cancer* (e.g., from low immunogenic *melanoma*, until very immunogenic *fibrosarcoma*). Compared to IL-2 and IL-15, IL-21 is minimally toxic (in mouse).

IL-22

Alias

IL-D110, IL-TIF, IL21, ILTIF, TIFIL-23, TIFA, zcyto18, *IL-10-related T cell-derived inducible factor.*

Structure

IL-22 belongs to the IL-10 family of cytokines with IL-19, -20, -24, and IL-26. Its protein has about 20 kDa (179 amino acids) in humans; the gene is located on chromosome 12q15.

Source

IL-22 is solely produced, so far, by activated T cells under particular conditions.

Function

IL-22 has proinflammatory role in the skin, and digestive and respiratory systems. In the skin, it inhibits differentiation of keratinocytes, and stimulates the migration. In humans, during activation of naïve T cells (CD45RA$^+$) in cell cultures, prolonged exposure to IL-22 induces IL-4 and IL-13 (and inhibits IFN-γ), which are hallmarks of Th2 type response (IL-22 shares this feature with IL-19 and IL-20, but not with IL-10 cytokine). IL-22 binding protein (BP) inhibits the formation of Th2 type response.

Receptor

IL-22 binds to two receptors, one with a single chain and another with two:[1] IL-22BP that is attached to cell membrane without the intracellular portion (and thus probably does not transduce signal); and[2] a heterodimeric

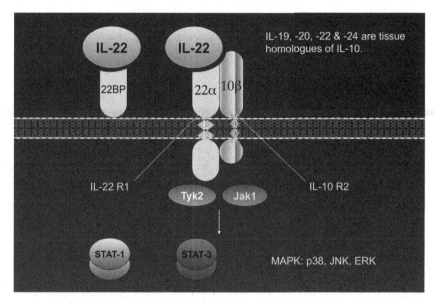

Figure 6-23 The IL-22 receptor and signal transduction factors.

IL-22R1 and IL-10R2 (β chain) receptor that signals inside the cell. Signal transduction employs Jak1/Tyk2, STAT-1 and STAT-3 molecules, and MAP kinases (p38, JNK, and ERK) (Figure 6-23).

Other Features

IL-22 acts on subepithelial miofibroblasts of colon to secrete proinflammatory cytokines and enzymes that can remodel mucosa in inflammatory processes. It induces acute phase proteins (its proinflammatory role).

It can cause *neonatal death* from skin lesions similar to *psoriasis*.

IL-22 receptor chain IL-10R2 has ubiquitous (widespread) expression.

However, IL-22R1 chains are mainly expressed in epithelial and stromal cells (fibroblasts), while IL-22BP is expressed solely on DCs.

Association with Human Diseases

IL-22 is associated with proinflammatory processes in the gastrointestinal tract such as the inflammatory diseases of autoimmune character—IBD and *Crohn's disease*.

Association with *psoriasis* is possible, because in psoriatic lesions, IL-22 receptor is very strongly expressed.

IL-22 seems to have a protective role in hepatocytes.

Furthermore, the genetic region encompassing the genes IL-22–IL-26 –IFNG on the chromosome 12q15 is associated with gender differences in the predisposition to developing *RA* and *multiple sclerosis*.

Therapeutic Options

In obese mice, as a result of IL-22 inhibition of induction, they become susceptible to infection with *Citrobacter rodentium*. Metabolic disorders have been observed in IL-22 receptor-deficient mice that were fed with a high-fat diet. The symptoms of these disorders (hypoglycemia and insulin resistance) can be rescued by adding exogenous IL-22 to their diets. It is likely that IL-22 might be beneficent in treating metabolic disease and/or GI-tract inflammation.

IL-23

Alias

(IL23A/p19): P19; SGRF, IL-23A; IL23P19; JKA3 induced upon T-cell activation, interleukin-23 p19 subunit.

Structure

IL-23 is a heterodimer composed of two subunits: IL-23A (p19) and IL-12B (p40). It has about 60 kDa. The genes for the two subunits of human IL-23 are differently located: the IL23A gene (coding for p19) is on chromosome 5q31-33, whereas the IL12B gene (encoding p40) is on chromosome 12q13.

Source

The expression of p40 is described under section for IL-12 (see, *Source*—of IL-12p40 expression), whereas p19 is secreted by DCs, epithelial cells of the intestine, and probably by other epithelial cells.

Function

IL-23 has immunoregulatory and proinflammatory roles that were based on many reports in the past as p40 was considered part of only the IL-12 action. Due to mistaken identity, all results related only to p40 were automatically attributed to IL-12. These now should be reproduced and confirmed, and probably not all experiments have been completed yet. IL-23 stimulates the production of IL-17 in the subpopulation of CD4 helper (Th) cells, called Th17. (Th17 development can be stopped with IL-12p70.) Furthermore, IL-23 promotes tumor growth (mice with defective gene for

IL-23 or IL-23R (KO) have an increased incidence of tumors induced by chemical mutagenesis). IL-23 promotes inflammation by activation of matrix metalloproteinase MM9 and angiogenesis, but (unlike IL-12) reduces the infiltration of CD8 cytotoxic T lymphocytes.

Receptor

The receptor for IL-23 is composed of two chains: (a) the first chain is the IL-12β1 and (b) the second chain is the IL-23R (structurally similar to IL-12β2) receptor chain. The signal is transmitted into the cell via Jak1 and Tyk2 kinases and mainly through STAT-3 molecules, although reports indicate involvement of others like STAT-1, -4, and -5 transcription factors (Figure 6-24).

Other Features

Overexpression of IL-23A (p19) causes a systemic inflammatory response in mice (reduction in body size, infertility, death at 3 months of age; infiltration of many tissue cells).

The finding of p40 in ovarian follicles suggests a role of IL-23 in reproduction.

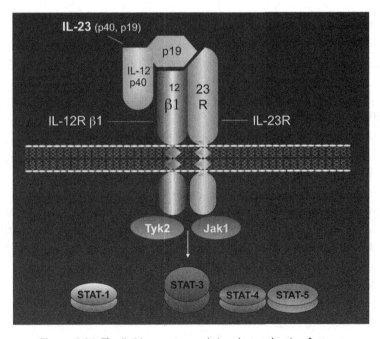

Figure 6-24 The IL-23 receptor and signal transduction factors.

Association with Human Diseases

IL–23 is associated with the generation of pathogenic T cells in an experimental model of *multiple sclerosis* in mice. In this, an anti–IL–23 enhances *experimental acute encephalomyelitis*.

Increased secretion of IL–23 in keratinocytes of *psoriatic* lesions suggests association with *psoriasis* (Th1-associated disease) and seems to have a more dominant role than IL–12.

Therapeutic Options

Anti–IL–23 therapy could be used in organ-specific autoimmune diseases, because they may reduce complications from infections that accompany general *immunosuppression* (with e.g., cyclosporine).

IL-24

Alias

MDA7; C49A; FISP; IL10B; Mob-5; IL–24 splice variant delE3/delE5; *melanoma differentiation association protein 7* (mda-7), *suppression of tumorigenicity 16* (ST16) (melanoma differentiation).

Structure

IL–24 belongs to the IL–10 family of cytokines (IL–19, -20, -22, and IL–26). It has about 18 kD; the IL–24 gene is located on chromosome 1q32. There are several isoforms with about 200 amino acids.

Source

IL–24 is produced by activated monocytes and T cells.

Function

IL–24 has a role in communication between hematopoietic and non-hematopoietic tissues. It has a role in apoptosis and immune responses of the Th2-type. IL–24 can selectively induce cell death in cancer cells without affecting normal cells.

Receptor

IL–24 binds to two heterodimeric receptors (Figure 6-25):
1. IL–20R1 and IL–20R2; and
2. IL–22R1 and IL–20R2.

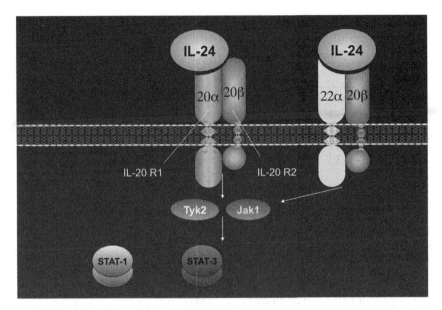

Figure 6-25 Two receptors for IL-24 and their signal transduction.

Receptors are expressed in cells of the skin and the respiratory and reproductive systems as well as in some exocrine glands. The signal from the membrane is transmitted through Jak-STAT system to the nucleus by Jak1 and Tyk2 kinases, and STAT-1 and STAT-3 nuclear factors.

Other Features

IL-20R1, -20R2, and -22R1 receptor chains are poorly expressed on hematopoietic tissue, and are mainly found in epithelial cells and stromal (fibroblast) cells.

Association with Human Diseases

Paralogs of the IL-10 family cytokines are produced by some *Herpes* and *Pox* viruses.

It is found secreted in the last stage of differentiation of *melanoma* cells.

Overexpression induces apoptosis selectively in cells of some cancers.

Therapeutic Options

IL-24 is a candidate therapy for *various cancer* types as a killing cytokine. IL-24 has proven efficacious in a Phase I/II clinical trial in humans with multiple advanced cancers.

Judging by the association with the apoptosis of cancer cells, there may be a new way of therapy in many tumors like *breast cancer* and *melanoma*.

IL-25

Structure

IL-25 belongs to the IL-17 family of cytokines; human protein has about 17 kDa, and 177 amino acids (its alternative name is also the former one, known as IL-17E).

Source

IL-25 is secreted by (non-T/non-B) cell populations, as well as by eosinophils, mast cells, and alveolar macrophages.

Function

IL-25 is a cytokine with immunomodulatory functions; stimulates the development of Th2-type immune response.

Receptor

IL-25 acts via the IL-17RB receptor (single chain), and signal transduction involves the activation of MAPK (p38, JNK, ERK) and NF-KB pathways (Figure 6-26).

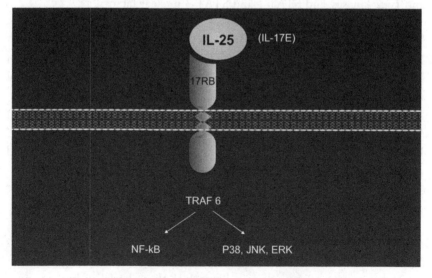

Figure 6-26 Receptor for IL-25 (IL-17RB).

Other Features

IL-25 induces IL-4, IL-5, and IL-13 in (non-T/non-B) cells, eosinophilia in the lung and in the bronchio-alveolar tissue sample *in vitro.*

Furthermore, in cell culture, it increased secretion of IL-6, IL-8, MCP-1, and MIP1-α from activated eosinophils and thus resembles the effects of IL-4 and IL-13 cytokines.

In the embryonic fibroblasts it increases the formation of IL-6, TGF-β and G-CSF factors, chemokines and TARC chemokine.

Alveolar macrophages (in rodents) stimulated by tiny particles secrete IL-13 and also IL-25.

Intranasal administration of IL-25 in mice causes *hyperplasia* and increased mucus secretion in the respiratory system, as well as the hyper-reaction of the respiratory epithelium.

IL-25 KO mice have no defense against the parasite *Nippostrongylus brasiliensis.* They lack (non-T/non-B) cell populations that secrete IL-25, and have delayed Th2 responses. Also the phenotype includes the aggravation of *chronic inflammatory* processes in the gastrointestinal tract.

Association with Disease

IL-25 is associated with amplification of *allergic* inflammation of the airways, but has no role in its generation.

Some SNP polymorphisms in the IL-25 gene carry a possible tendency towards increased risk of parasitic infection.

It is believed that IL-25 may play a role in limiting (reducing) the extent of *chronic inflammation* of the digestive tract (*IBD* and *Crohn's disease*). However, there are no associations of genetic polymorphisms with these diseases.

Therapeutic Options

They are still unknown, but studies are in progress with agonists and inhibitors of the effects of IL-25 (such as monoclonal antibodies).

IL-26

Alias

AK155.

Structure

IL-26 belongs to the IL-10 family of cytokines (IL-19, -20, -22, and IL-24). Human IL-26 protein has about 18 kDa, and 171 amino acids and is a homodimer. The IL26 gene is located on chromosome 12q15.

Source

It is produced by memory T cells, induced after infection with the *Herpes virus Saimiri*, and monocytes.

Function

It has a function in communication between hematopoietic and non-hematopoietic tissues. Its role is likely in local mucous and skin immunity.

Receptor

The receptor for IL-26, IL-26R is a heterodimer consisting of IL-20R1 and IL-10R2. The signal transduction involves tyrosine kinases Jak1 and Tyk2 and transcription factors STAT-1 and STAT-3 (Figure 6-27).

Other Features

IL-26 stimulates the T cells to secrete IL-10, IL-8, and the expression of CD54.

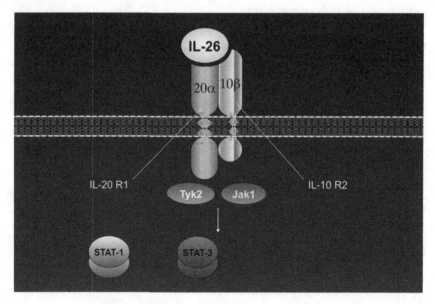

Figure 6-27 Receptor for IL-26 and its signal transduction.

The target cells by IL-26 are also *colon cancer* cells and keratinocytes.

Receptor for IL-26 is variably expressed in human tissues. Although the expression of the IL-10R2 chain is widespread, IL-20R1 chains are faintly expressed in hematopoietic cells, whereas they are mostly detectable in epithelial and stromal cells such as fibroblasts. Therefore the distribution of IL-26 action is limited to the target cells expressing IL-20R1 chains, and it probably does not work by autocrine mechanism.

Association with Human Diseases

Genetic regions IL-22–IL-26–IFNG that are located on chromosome 12q15 are associated with gender differences in the predisposition to developing *RA*, and *multiple sclerosis* (IFNG is a prime candidate). In particular, one haplotype is associated with protection in male population from developing these diseases. This indicates that this region has a role in the susceptibility to these diseases, although probably only partially.

Therapeutic Options

IL-26's therapeutic potential is still unexplored, and probably lies in the anti-microbial humoral response, inter-cellular signaling, and the cellular immune response.

IL-27

Alias

IL27p28; IL30 (*wrong name*), p28; IL-17D (*wrong name*).

Structure

Human IL-27 is a heterodimer of about 70 kDa, composed of two subunits: (1) EBI3 (*Epstein–Barr-like 3*); and (2) the p28 subunit. IL-27 resembles IL-12 and IL-23 in structure. The IL27 gene (IL27P28) is located on chromosome 16p11, whereas the other subunit's gene (EBl3) is on chromosome 19p13.

Source

IL-27 is produced by "activated" macrophages and DCs (antigen presenting cells).

Function

It has an immunoregulatory function in cellular immunity. It promotes generation of the Th0 activated T cells from naïve stage together with IL-2, that would eventually, together with IL-12 (IL-18 or IFN-γ), develop into Th1 type immune response. IL-27 can also promote development of Tregs together with TGF-β and IL-10.

Receptor

IL-27 receptor is a heterodimer made of IL-27RA (alias: WSX1) and IL-6ST (alias: gp130) chains. Signal transduction involves Jak1 and Tyk2 kinases and STAT-1, -3, -4, and STAT-5 transcription factors (Figure 6-28).

Other Features

IL-27 can stimulate isotype switching to IgG2a, and simultaneously inhibit the switch to IgG1, in germinal centers during B lymphocyte activation.

IL-27 has anti-angiogenic and anti-tumor effect (in a mouse model of *melanoma*).

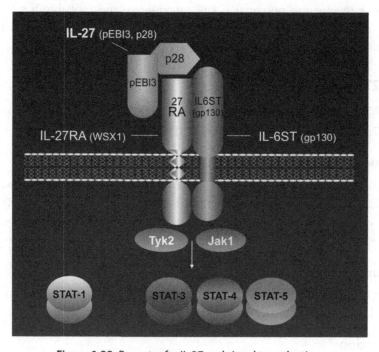

Figure 6-28 Receptor for IL-27 and signal transduction.

It has been observed that the lack of effect of IL-27 causes autoimmune lethal infection (e.g., with *Toxoplasma gondii*) or/and enhanced expulsion of parasites in the gastrointestinal tract.

That is similar to what happens in models of *autoimmune arthritis*, where vaccination and inducing antibodies against the small subunit (p28) can cause a lack of action of IL-27. This can alleviate the symptoms of arthritis in these experimental animals. It seems that the inhibition of secretion of IL-2 is also important, and the mechanism of inhibition involves SOCS molecule, SOCS-3 (for details, see *IL-6*, p. 168).

Mice lacking one subunit of the receptor, IL-27R KO (WSX-1 −/−), infection with *T. gondii* causes *lethal inflammation* that can be mitigated by providing IL-2. Furthermore, response to helminth *Trichuris muris* causes hyper-reaction of Th2-type immune responses, increased expulsion of parasites, mastocytosis, and goblet cell *hyperplasia*.

If CD4⁺ T cells from these KO mice (IL-27R−/−) were transferred into culture, they secrete strikingly more IL-2 during activation *in vitro* than normal. Addition of IL-27 during the activation decreases production of IL-2 in the IL-27R−/− T cells. The addition of IL-12 has a synergistic effect in the similar setting, which was not observed by adding IL-6 or IL-23 cytokines in such experiments.

In a cross between parent mouse strain deficient in receptors for IL-27 (IL-27R KO) and a strain that spontaneously develops *autoimmune colitis*, the F1 generation becomes resistant to disease. In addition, they have lower than normal production of IFN-γ, IL-6, and TNF cytokines in mononuclear immunocompetent cells in *lamina propria* (as well as the absence of T-bet factors that are important for the development of Th1-type immune response).

Association with Human Diseases

In the mouse, IL-27 may cause the complete regression of primary or metastatic *neuroblastoma* or *melanoma*. Neutralization of the small subunit (p28) of IL-27 leads to withdrawal of autoimmune *encephalitis*.

Therapeutic Options

This cytokine is a candidate for the treatment of chronic bowel diseases like *IBD*, *Crohn's disease*, and *ulcerative colitis*, and possibly against some types of *cancer*.

IL-28 AND IL-29 (TYPE III INTERFERON, λ1–3)

Structure

The human IL-28/29 cytokine family has three members: IL-28A, IL-28B, and IL-29. Structurally, they are distant cousins of type I interferons (α/β). Previously they were called interferon *lambda* 1–3. Proteins are about 22 kDa, or about 200 amino acids. The genes encoding IL28A, IL28B, and IL29 are aligned in sequence in a locus on chromosome 19q13.

Source

They are induced by viral infections (in *intestinal epithelium*).

Function

They have antiviral activity similar to all interferons, and additional ones with immunomodulatory effects. For example, they can induce tolerogenic DCs (which can generate suppressive T cells (Tregs), see *Further development of immune cells upon activation*, Chapter 3, p. 83).

Receptor

The receptor for IL-28A, IL-28B, and IL-29 resembles the IL-10 receptor family, and it comprises two polypeptide chains. The first is a ligand-binding specific one called IL-28R1 (IL-28α-chain) and the second chain is that of the IL-10R2. Signal transduction engages Jak1 and Tyk2 kinases and STAT-1,-2,-3,-4,-5 transcription factors (Figure 6-29).

Other Features

IL-28s and IL-29 induce MxA protein and 2′,5′-oligo-adenylate synthase in the cell (and therefore antiviral activity).

They can influence monocyte differentiation and maturation of DCs. This can result in the generation of antigen presenting cells, which, as such, help the development of regulatory T cells—CD4$^+$ CD25$^+$ Foxp3$^+$ Tregs.

Furthermore, they induce anti-viral and anti-proliferative signals in intestinal epithelial cells.

While IL-10R2 expression is ubiquitous, IL-28R is expressed only in some tissues where, it seems, it is inducible.

Therapeutic Options

It is assumed that the use of these cytokines may be useful for antiviral activity in fighting off particular viral infections. Therefore perhaps it might be

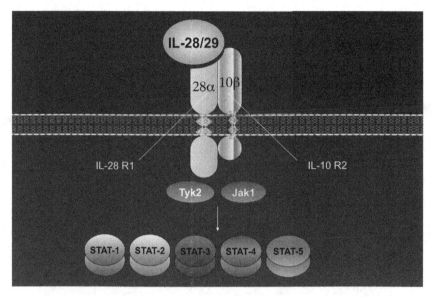

Figure 6-29 Receptor for IL-28 or IL-29, and signal transduction.

useful against some types of *cancer*, and finally in immunoregulation (e.g., Tregs induction).

IL-30

(DOES NOT EXIST)

IL-31

Structure

IL-31 is a member of the large IL-6 family of cytokines (LIF, CNTF, OSM, etc.). Human protein is about 18 kDa. The IL31 gene is located on chromosome 12q24.

Source

It is secreted by activated Th2 cells.

Function

IL-31 has an immunoregulatory role, which is still not well understood. It seems to play a role in *allergic* skin reactions. It promotes Th2 type adaptive immunity.

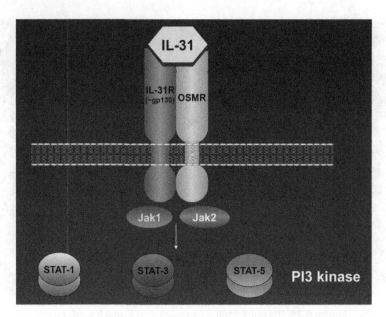

Figure 6-30 Receptor for IL-31 and signal transduction.

Receptor

The IL-31 receptor has two subunits: one resembles the IL-6ST (gp130) and the other is OSMR. Signal from the receptor upon binding the ligand travels into the cell through Jak1 and Jak2 kinases, engage transcription factors STAT-1, -3, -5, and phosphoinositol-3 kinase to promote transcription of the IL-31 sensitive genes (Figure 6-30).

Other Features

IL-31 acts on keratinocytes and epithelial skin cells, which have a constitutively expressed receptor. The IL-31R receptor can be induced in monocytes after their activation.

Association with Human Diseases

Secretion of large amounts of IL-31 in the skin by CLA⁺ T cells causes itching and *contact atopic dermatitis*. In experimentally induced *contact dermatitis* in mice, it was found that the expression of IL-31R increased beyond the normal value.

It is assumed that it may participate in the regulation of other types of *allergies* or perhaps *asthma*.

Therapeutic options are being explored.

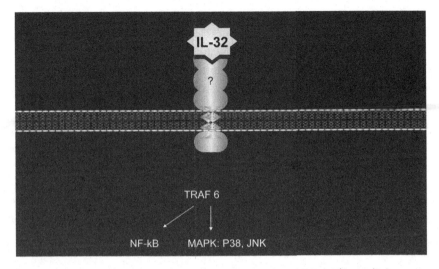

Figure 6-31 IL-32 and signal transduction (receptor—unknown).

IL-32

Alias

IL-32alpha, IL-32beta, IL-32delta, IL-32gamma, NK4, TAIF, TAIFb, TAIFc, TAIFd, natural killer cell transcript 4, natural killer cells protein 4, tumor necrosis factor alpha-inducing factor.

Structure

The human protein has about 22 kDa, and the IL-32 gene is located on chromosome 16p13.3 (Figure 6-31). IL-32 has no similarity with any other cytokine.

Source

Cells of the immune system (lymphocytes, NK, monocytes) and epithelial cells produce IL-32.

Function

IL-32 has a proinflammatory role. Its expression is increased after the activation of T-cells or NK cells. IL-32 also promotes angiogenesis.

Other Features

IL-32 induces the secretion of TNF-α and IL-8 in monocytes (THP-1 line), and in macrophages *in vitro*.

IL–32 was first found in activated NK cells by stimulation with a combination of IL–12 and IL–18 cytokines. Later it was found that it could be induced in other cells, such as epithelial cells by IFN-γ.

Interestingly, apoptosis of T cells induces IL–32, especially after activation, and it is assumed that IL–32 has a role in it.

Association with Human Diseases

IL–32 has a possible role in autoimmune and inflammatory processes where TNF plays a role in the pathogenesis (perhaps *Crohn's disease*).

IL–32 plays a role in the tumor-associated inflammatory microenvironment. Its overexpression was found to contribute to invasion and metastasis in *primary lung adenocarcinoma*. It also has a role in *cutaneous T-cell lymphoma* lesions.

Therapeutic Options

Therapeutic options are being explored.

IL-33

Alias

C9orf26; DVS27, NF-HEV; NFEHEV; DVS27-related protein, nuclear factor from high endothelial venules.

Structure

IL–33 belongs to the IL-1 family of cytokines. It is formed from the precursor and activated by caspase 1/5 (similarly to IL-1 and IL-18). Human IL–33 has about 31 kDa, and the IL33 gene is located on chromosome 9p24.1.

Source

The endothelium of vessels in the lymphatic secondary tissues "High endothelial venules" (HEV) produces IL-33.

Function

It promotes the development of Th2 responses and secretion of IL-4, IL-5, and IL-13 in mucosa. *In vitro* it stimulates the secretion of these cytokines from Th2 effector cells. IL-33 is also a nuclear factor in specialized endothelial venules (HEV).

Receptor

IL-33 receptor has a single chain, which is also related to the IL-1 receptor (*interleukin-1 receptor-like 1*, IL-1RL1). Signal transduction upon ligand binding involves the Toll-like receptor (TIR) domain of the receptor chain and resembles that of IL-1 and IL-18, and TLRs. These activities include activation of NF-κB and MAP kinase (JNK and p38) (Figure 6-32).

(Receptor aliases: DER4; FIT-1, ST2; ST2L; ST2V; T1; homolog of mouse growth stimulation-expressed genes, interleukin-1 receptor-related protein.)

Association with Human Diseases

It is associated presumably with *allergies*, because of the role in generating the Th2 type immune response.

Therapeutic Options

IL-33 could be used against inflammation caused by Th1 response, and antagonists perhaps might be developed as anti-allergic compounds.

IL-34

Alias

C16orf77.

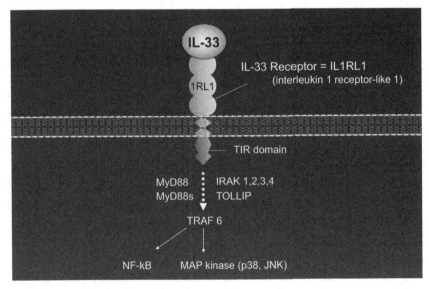

Figure 6-32 Receptor for IL-33 and signal transduction.

Structure

IL-34 forms homodimers. It was found by large-scale screening of secreted proteins. It has 241 amino acids (39 kDa, in mass).

Source

Secreted by fibroblast like cells in various tissues including synovia. IL-34 mRNA was found in many tissues. The most abundant expression was found in spleen, but it is also detected in heart, brain, thymus, lung, kidney, liver, small intestine, colon, testes, ovary, and prostate.

Receptor

The colony-stimulating factor-1 receptor CSF-1R is the binding moiety for IL-34.

Function

IL-34 promotes the differentiation and viability of monocytes and macrophages through the colony-stimulating factor-1 (CSF-1) receptor. It also steers development of Langerhans DCs in skin. It is thus a crucial factor for differentiation and maintenance of macrophages and Langerhans DCs in tissues.

Association with Disease

IL-34 is associated with *synovitis* severity in *RA*.

IL-35

Structure

IL-35 is a heterodimer of about 75 kDa, composed of EBI3 (*Epstein–Barr-like 3, the subunit of the IL-27*) and p35 (IL-12p35; IL12A) subunits. It resembles the structure of IL-12, IL-23, and IL-27.

Source

Anti-CD3/CD28-stimulated pan T cells produced high concentrations of IL-35 in 3-day cell-culture supernatants as well as $CD4^+CD8^+$ and $CD4^+CD25^-$ T cell subpopulations. IL-35 is produced and secreted by a regulatory T cell ($CD4^+FoxP3^-$) subset iTr35 that can suppress T cell proliferation and convert conventional naïve T cells ($CD4^+CD25^-CD45RB^{hi}$) into iTr35 cells. The IL35-producing Treg cells are a separate subpopulation distinct from $FOXP3^+$ Tregs as they do not express FOXP3.

The mRNAs for EBI3 and p35 subunits were also found in γδT cells, CD8⁺ T cells and placental trophoblast.

Receptor

The receptor of IL-35 (IL-35R) is a heterodimeric protein: the first chain is IL-12Rβ2 and the second one is the IL-6R (gp130). The signal transduction into the cell is transduced via Jak-STAT pathway, which includes Jak1, STAT1, and STAT4 factors (Figure 6-33).

Function

It is suggested that it has anti-inflammatory role, probably by inhibition of proliferation of proinflammatory effector Th cells.

Association with Disease

This is being explored as well as therapeutic options. The regulatory effects of IL-35 might be beneficent for treatment of autoimmune diseases or alternatively, its inhibitors might be helpful in potential cancer therapies.

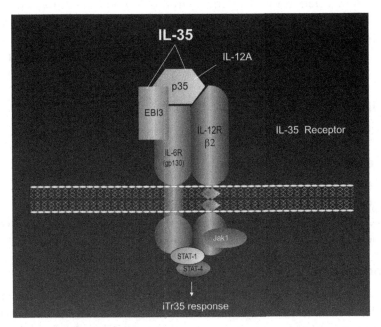

Figure 6-33 Receptor for IL-35 and signal transduction. iTr35 response involves regulatory T cells induced by the IL-35, different from (CD4 CD25 Foxp3) + Tregs.

IL-36

Aliases

IL-36α, IL-36β, and IL-36γ were previously known as IL-1F6, IL1-F8, and IL-1F9, respectively. IL-36RN was previously known as IL-1F5.

IL-36α encoding gene (IL36A) aliases are: FIL1; FIL1E; IL1F6; IL-1F6; IL1(EPSILON); FIL1(EPSILON).

IL-36β encoding gene (IL36B) aliases are: FIL1, FIL1-(ETA), FIL1H, FILI-(ETA), IL-1F8, IL-1H2, IL1-ETA, IL1F8, IL1H2.

IL-36γ encoding gene (IL36G) aliases are: UNQ2456/PRO5737, IL-1F9, IL-1H1, IL-1RP2, IL1E, IL1F9, IL1H1, IL1RP2.

IL-36RN encoded by the gene (IL36RN) has the following aliases: FIL1; FIL1D; IL1F5; IL1L1; PSORP; IL1HY1; IL1RP3; IL36RA; FIL1(DELTA).

Structure

The IL-36 system includes IL-36α, IL-36β, IL-36γ, and IL-36 receptor antagonist (IL-36RN). They are members of the IL-1 cytokine family. Their genes are located in the IL1 gene locus on chromosome 2 (together with five other genes). It closely resembles IL-1α/β IL-1Ra and receptor assembly. In addition, IL-38 (IL-1F10), a cytokine that belongs to IL-1 superfamily (and encoded by the IL1 gene locus) is another antagonist of the IL-36 system (Figure 6-34).

Source

Secreted by epithelial cells in respiratory system and skin (in mice).

Receptor

IL-36 receptor is a heterodimer formed by the IL-36R chain, which is also known as IL1RL2 (alias: IL1RRP2; IL-1Rrp2; IL1R-rp2). The other chain is the RACp (alias: IL-1RacP) protein (Figure 6-34). The IL-36 receptor cannot bind IL-1α or IL-1β with high affinity.

Function

The IL-36 cytokine system (α,β,γ and RN with IL-38) has an important effect on skin and lungs immunity and mediate inflammation. IL-36α can induce keratinocytes to secrete chemokines (CXCL1, CXCL8, CCL3, CCL5, and CCL20) that results with leukocyte infiltration and *acanthosis*. IL-36 can

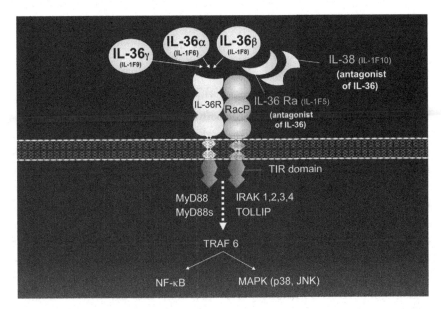

Figure 6-34 IL-36 and its receptor (IL-1 homolog). IL-38 and IL-36Ra are antagonists.

stimulate maturation of monocyte-derived DCs and indirectly drive T cell proliferation.

Other Effects

Myeloid DCs and blood monocytes express IL-36 receptor. However, no direct effects on T cells or neutrophils were found.

Association with Diseases

IL-36 might be associated with *generalized pustular psoriasis.*

IL-37

Alias

IL-1F7; IL-1H; IL-1H4; IL-1RP1; FIL1(ZETA).

Structure

IL-37 is a member of the interleukin-1 cytokine family.

Source

It is secreted by macrophages or epithelial cells (i.e., skin).

Receptor

IL-37 binds to IL-18 receptor (IL18R1/IL-1Rrp) (Figure 6-19).

Function

IL-37 is IL-18 antagonist (Figure 6-19). By binding to IL-18 receptor (IL18R1/IL-1Rrp) it can inhibit the activity of IL-18. It can do it by forming a complex with interleukin-18 binding protein (IL18BP), which is in itself also an inhibitory binding protein of IL-18 (through binding to IL-18 receptor beta subunit).

IL-37 is a natural inhibitor of proinflammatory cytokines, and a fundamental inhibitor of innate immunity.[76] For example, experiments with human blood cells in which expression of IL-37 in macrophages or epithelial cells was induced resulted in almost complete inhibition of proinflammatory cytokine production. On the other hand, the abundance of proinflammatory cytokines was augmented with silencing of endogenous IL-37, without perturbation in the expression of anti-inflammatory cytokines.

The IL37 gene (together with eight other genes) is located in IL-1 gene cluster on chromosome 2. There are five alternatively spliced transcript variants encoding distinct isoforms of the IL-37.

Association with Diseases

It is thought that IL-37 can ameliorate inflammation in *psoriasis* by inhibiting proinflammatory cytokine production.

In patients with *Guillain–Barré syndrome*, IL-37 was found in elevated levels in their cerebrospinal fluid and plasma.

IL-37 was also found elevated in patients with *atopic dermatitis*.

IL-38

Alias

IL-1F10, FKSG75; IL-1HY2; IL1-theta; FIL1-theta.

Structure

IL-38 belongs to IL-1 family of cytokines.

Source

It can be secreted by memory T-lymphocytes (from freshly isolated human PBMC) when stimulated by that is, heat-killed *Candida albicans*.

Receptor

IL-38 binds only to the IL-36 receptor (Figure 6-34), as does IL-36RN (receptor antagonist). IL-38 binds to the IL-36 receptor and has biological effects on immune cells similar to IL-36 receptor antagonist.[77]

Function

The functional role of IL-38 seems to be in skin immunity, as it acts similarly as IL-36 receptor antagonist.

Association with Disease

In a case–control study, an IL38 SNP (IL1F10.3; rs3811058) was found associated with spondylopathies, namely, with non-*ankylosing spondylitis* phenotype of *spondyloarthritis*, whereas the IL1A locus was strongly associated with *ankylosing spondylitis* phenotype.[11]

REFERENCES

1. Ramadas RA, et al. Interleukin-1R antagonist gene and pre-natal smoke exposure are associated with childhood asthma. *Eur Respir J* Mar, 2007;**29**:502.
2. Moxley G, et al. Interleukin-1 region meta-analysis with osteoarthritis phenotypes. *Osteoarthritis Cartilage* Feb, 2010;**18**:200.
3. Kerkhof HJ, et al. Large-scale meta-analysis of interleukin-1 beta and interleukin-1 receptor antagonist polymorphisms on risk of radiographic hip and knee osteoarthritis and severity of knee osteoarthritis. *Osteoarthritis Cartilage* Mar, 2011;**19**:265.
4. Wu X, et al. IL-1 receptor antagonist gene as a predictive biomarker of progression of knee osteoarthritis in a population cohort. *Osteoarthritis Cartilage* Jul, 2013;**21**:930.
5. Nakki A, et al. Allelic variants of IL1R1 gene associate with severe hand osteoarthritis. *BMC Med Genet* 2010;**11**:50.
6. Solovieva S, et al. Association between interleukin 1 gene cluster polymorphisms and bilateral distal interphalangeal osteoarthritis. *J Rheumatol* Sep, 2009;**36**:1977.
7. Stock CJ, et al. Comprehensive association study of genetic variants in the IL-1 gene family in systemic juvenile idiopathic arthritis. *Genes Immun* Jun, 2008;**9**:349.
8. Sims AM, et al. Prospective meta-analysis of interleukin 1 gene complex polymorphisms confirms associations with ankylosing spondylitis. *Ann Rheum Dis* Sep, 2008;**67**:1305.
9. Wu Z, Gu JR. A meta-analysis on interleukin-1 gene cluster polymorphism and genetic susceptibility for ankylosing spondylitis. *Zhonghua yi xue za zhi* Feb 13, 2007;**87**:433.
10. Lea WI, Lee YH. The associations between interleukin-1 polymorphisms and susceptibility to ankylosing spondylitis: a meta-analysis. *Joint Bone Spine* Jul, 2012;**79**:370.
11. Monnet D, et al. Association between the IL-1 family gene cluster and spondyloarthritis. *Ann Rheum Dis* Jun, 2012;**71**:885.
12. Rahman P, et al. Association between the interleukin-1 family gene cluster and psoriatic arthritis. *Arthritis Rheum* Jul, 2006;**54**:2321.
13. Harrison P, Pointon JJ, Chapman K, Roddam A, Wordsworth BP. Interleukin-1 promoter region polymorphism role in rheumatoid arthritis: a meta-analysis of IL-1B-511A/G variant reveals association with rheumatoid arthritis. *Rheumatology* Dec, 2008;**47**:1768.

14. Mamyrova G, et al. Cytokine gene polymorphisms as risk and severity factors for juvenile dermatomyositis. *Arthritis Rheum* Dec, 2008;**58**:3941.
15. Liu N, et al. The association of interleukin-1alpha and interleukin-1beta polymorphisms with the risk of Graves' disease in a case–control study and meta-analysis. *Hum Immunol* Apr, 2010;**71**:397.
16. Borzani I, et al. The interleukin-1 cluster gene region is associated with multiple sclerosis in an Italian Caucasian population. *Eur J Neurol* Jul, 2010;**17**:930.
17. Hahn WH, Cho BS, Kim SD, Kim SK, Kang S. Interleukin-1 cluster gene polymorphisms in childhood IgA nephropathy. *Pediatr Nephrol* Jul, 2009;**24**:1329.
18. Lu D, et al. A functional polymorphism in interleukin-1alpha (IL1A) gene is associated with risk of alopecia areata in Chinese populations. *Gene* Jun 1, 2013;**521**:282.
19. Zeng XF, Li J, Li SB. A functional polymorphism in IL-1A gene is associated with a reduced risk of gastric cancer. *Tumour Biol* Jan, 2014;**35**:265.
20. Luotola K, et al. Associations between interleukin-1 (IL-1) gene variations or IL-1 receptor antagonist levels and the development of type 2 diabetes. *J Intern Med* Mar, 2011;**269**:322.
21. Pontillo A, et al. Polymorphisms in inflammasome' genes and susceptibility to HIV-1 infection. *J Acquir Immune Defic Syndr* Feb 1, 2012;**59**:121.
22. Sudenga SL, et al. Variants in interleukin family of cytokines genes influence clearance of high risk HPV in HIV-1 coinfected African-American adolescents. *Hum Immunol* Dec, 2013;**74**:1696.
23. Carrol ED, et al. The IL1RN promoter rs4251961 correlates with IL-1 receptor antagonist concentrations in human infection and is differentially regulated by GATA-1. *J Immunol* Feb 15, 2011;**186**:2329.
24. Wu X, et al. Association of interleukin-1 gene variations with moderate to severe chronic periodontitis in multiple ethnicities. *J Periodontal Res* Apr 2, 2014.
25. Mfuna Endam L, Cormier C, Bosse Y, Filali-Mouhim A, Desrosiers M. Association of IL1A, IL1B, and TNF gene polymorphisms with chronic rhinosinusitis with and without nasal polyposis: a replication study. *Arch Otolaryngol Head Neck Surg* Feb, 2010;**136**:187.
26. Levy H, et al. IL1B polymorphisms modulate cystic fibrosis lung disease. *Pediatr Pulmonol* Jun, 2009;**44**:580.
27. Olsson S, et al. Genetic variation within the interleukin-1 gene cluster and ischemic stroke. *Stroke* Sep, 2012;**43**:2278.
28. Zee RY, et al. An evaluation of candidate genes of inflammation and thrombosis in relation to the risk of venous thromboembolism: The Women's Genome Health Study. Circulation. *Cardiovasc Genet* Feb, 2009;**2**:57.
29. White KL, et al. Ovarian cancer risk associated with inherited inflammation-related variants. *Cancer Res* Mar 1, 2012;**72**:1064.
30. Charbonneau B, et al. Risk of ovarian cancer and the NF-kappaB pathway: genetic association with IL1A and TNFSF10. *Cancer Res* Feb 1, 2014;**74**:852.
31. Pooja S, et al. Polymorphic variations in IL-1beta, IL-6 and IL-10 genes, their circulating serum levels and breast cancer risk in Indian women. *Cytokine* Oct, 2012;**60**:122.
32. Kiyohara C, Horiuchi T, Takayama K, Nakanishi Y. IL1B rs1143634 polymorphism, cigarette smoking, alcohol use, and lung cancer risk in a Japanese population. *J Thorac Oncol* Mar, 2010;**5**:299.
33. Hosgood 3rd HD, et al. A pooled analysis of three studies evaluating genetic variation in innate immunity genes and non-Hodgkin lymphoma risk. *Br J Haematol* Mar, 2011;**152**:721.
34. Martino A, et al. Genetic variants and multiple myeloma risk: IMMEnSE validation of the best reported associations—an extensive replication of the associations from the candidate gene era. *Cancer Epidemiol Biomarkers Prev* Apr, 2014;**23**:670.

35. Korthagen NM, van Moorsel CH, Kazemier KM, Ruven HJ, Grutters JC. IL1RN genetic variations and risk of IPF: a meta-analysis and mRNA expression study. *Immunogenetics* May, 2012;**64**:371.
36. Lee KA, et al. Cytokine polymorphisms are associated with poor sleep maintenance in adults living with human immunodeficiency virus/acquired immunodeficiency syndrome. *Sleep* Mar, 2014;**37**:453.
37. Tsai SJ, et al. Interleukin-1 beta (C-511T) genetic polymorphism is associated with cognitive performance in elderly males without dementia. *Neurobiol Aging* Nov, 2010;**31**:1950.
38. Antony PA, et al. Interleukin-2-dependent mechanisms of tolerance and immunity in vivo. *J Immunol* May 1, 2006;**176**:5255.
39. Howson JM, et al. Evidence of gene-gene interaction and age-at-diagnosis effects in type 1 diabetes. *Diabetes* Nov, 2012;**61**:3012.
40. Fichna M, et al. Polymorphic variant at the IL2 region is associated with type 1 diabetes and may affect serum levels of interleukin-2. *Mol Biol Rep* Dec, 2013;**40**:6957.
41. Fedetz M, et al. Multiple sclerosis association study with the TENR-IL2-IL21 region in a Spanish population. *Tissue Antigens* Sep, 2009;**74**:244.
42. Diaz-Gallo LM, et al. Implication of IL-2/IL-21 region in systemic sclerosis genetic susceptibility. *Ann Rheum Dis* Jul, 2013;**72**:1233.
43. Christensen U, et al. Family based association analysis of the IL2 and IL15 genes in allergic disorders. *Eur J Hum Genet* Feb, 2006;**14**:227.
44. Wu J, et al. Promoter polymorphisms of IL2, IL4, and risk of gastric cancer in a high-risk Chinese population. *Mol Carcinog* Jul, 2009;**48**:626.
45. Sim GC, Radvanyi L. The IL-2 cytokine family in cancer immunotherapy. *Cytokine Growth Factor Rev* Aug 1, 2014;**25**(4):377–90.
46. Mendez-Lagares G, et al. HIV infection deregulates the balance between regulatory T cells and IL-2-producing CD4 T cells by decreasing the expression of the IL-2 receptor in Treg. *J Acquir Immune Defic Syndr* Mar 1, 2014;**65**:278.
47. Luo XJ, et al. The interleukin 3 gene (IL3) contributes to human brain volume variation by regulating proliferation and survival of neural progenitors. *PloS one* 2012;**7**:e50375.
48. Miyake Y, Tanaka K, Arakawa M. IL3 rs40401 polymorphism and interaction with smoking in risk of asthma in Japanese women: the Kyushu Okinawa Maternal and Child Health study. *Scand J Immunol* Jun, 2014;**79**:410.
49. Miyake Y, Tanaka K, Arakawa M. IL3 SNP rs40401 variant is a risk factor for rhinoconjunctivitis in Japanese women: the Kyushu Okinawa maternal and child health study. *Cytokine* Oct, 2013;**64**:86.
50. Zheng L, et al. Interleukin 1B rs16944 G>A polymorphism was associated with a decreased risk of esophageal cancer in a Chinese population. *Clin Biochem* Oct, 2013;**46**:1469.
51. Meyer CG, et al. IL3 variant on chromosomal region 5q31-33 and protection from recurrent malaria attacks. *Hum Mol Genet* Mar 15, 2011;**20**:1173.
52. Molfino NA, Gossage D, Kolbeck R, Parker JM, Geba GP. Molecular and clinical rationale for therapeutic targeting of interleukin-5 and its receptor. *Clin Exp Allergy* May, 2012;**42**:712.
53. Scheller J, Ohnesorge N, Rose-John S. Interleukin-6 trans-signalling in chronic inflammation and cancer. *Scand J Immunol* May, 2006;**63**:321.
54. Fragoso JM, et al. The interleukin 6 -572 G>C (rs1800796) polymorphism is associated with the risk of developing acute coronary syndrome. *Genet Test Mol Biomark* Dec, 2010;**14**:759.
55. Totaro F, et al. Impact of interleukin-6 -174 G>C gene promoter polymorphism on neuroblastoma. *PloS one* 2013;**8**:e76810.

56. Gregersen I, et al. Increased systemic and local interleukin 9 levels in patients with carotid and coronary atherosclerosis. *PloS one* 2013;**8**:e72769.
57. Purwar R, et al. Robust tumor immunity to melanoma mediated by interleukin-9-producing T cells. *Nat Med* Aug, 2012;**18**:1248.
58. Lan Q, et al. Cytokine polymorphisms in the Th1/Th2 pathway and susceptibility to non-Hodgkin lymphoma. *Blood* May 15, 2006;**107**:4101.
59. Tsai CW, et al. Significant association of Interleukin-10 genotypes and oral cancer susceptibility in Taiwan. *Anticancer Res* Jul, 2014;**34**:3731.
60. Sasaki H, et al. The interleukin-10 knockout mouse is highly susceptible to Porphyromonas gingivalis-induced alveolar bone loss. *J Periodontal Res* Dec, 2004;**39**:432.
61. Ren L, Wang X, Dong Z, Liu J, Zhang S. Bone metastasis from breast cancer involves elevated IL-11 expression and the gp130/STAT3 pathway. *Med Oncol* 2013;**30**:634.
62. Brunda MJ, et al. Antitumor and antimetastatic activity of interleukin 12 against murine tumors. *J Exp Med* Oct 1, 1993;**178**:1223.
63. Morita Y, et al. Expression of interleukin-12 in synovial tissue from patients with rheumatoid arthritis. *Arthritis Rheum* Feb, 1998;**41**:306.
64. Morahan G, et al. Linkage disequilibrium of a type 1 diabetes susceptibility locus with a regulatory IL12B allele. *Nat Gen* Feb, 2001;**27**:218.
65. van Veen T, et al. Interleukin-12p40 genotype plays a role in the susceptibility to multiple sclerosis. *Ann Neurol* Aug, 2001;**50**:275.
66. Monteleone G, et al. Interleukin 12 is expressed and actively released by Crohn's disease intestinal lamina propria mononuclear cells. *Gastroenterology* Apr, 1997;**112**:1169.
67. Kaarvatn MH, et al. Single nucleotide polymorphism in the interleukin 12B gene is associated with risk for breast cancer development. *Scand J Immunol* Sep, 2012;**76**:329.
68. Chen X, et al. Interactions of IL-12A and IL-12B polymorphisms on the risk of cervical cancer in Chinese women. *Clin Cancer Res* Jan 1, 2009;**15**:400.
69. Han SS, et al. Interleukin-12 p40 gene (IL12B) polymorphisms and the risk of cervical cancer in Korean women. *Eur J Obstet Gynecol Reprod Biol* Sep, 2008;**140**:71.
70. Ben Chaaben A, et al. Association of IL-12p40 +1188 A/C polymorphism with nasopharyngeal cancer risk and tumor extension. *Tissue Antigens* Aug, 2011;**78**:148.
71. Cerhan JR, et al. Genetic variation in 1253 immune and inflammation genes and risk of non-Hodgkin lymphoma. *Blood* Dec 15, 2007;**110**:4455.
72. Wong RH, et al. Association of IL-12B genetic polymorphism with the susceptibility and disease severity of ankylosing spondylitis. *J Rheumatol* Jan, 2012;**39**:135.
73. Nanni P, et al. Combined allogeneic tumor cell vaccination and systemic interleukin 12 prevents mammary carcinogenesis in HER-2/neu transgenic mice. *J Exp Med* Nov 5, 2001;**194**:1195.
74. Dias S, Boyd R, Balkwill F. IL-12 regulates VEGF and MMPs in a murine breast cancer model. *Int J Cancer* Oct 29, 1998;**78**:361.
75. Smyth DJ, et al. Shared and distinct genetic variants in type 1 diabetes and celiac disease. *N Engl J Med* Dec 25, 2008;**359**:2767.
76. Nold MF, et al. IL-37 is a fundamental inhibitor of innate immunity. *Nat Immunol* Nov, 2010;**11**:1014.
77. van de Veerdonk FL, et al. IL-38 binds to the IL-36 receptor and has biological effects on immune cells similar to IL-36 receptor antagonist. *Proc Natl Acad Sci U S A* Feb 21, 2012;**109**:3001.

FURTHER READING

Abdi K. IL-12: the role of p40 versus p75. *Scand J Immunol* Jul, 2002;**56**:1.
Arend WP. The balance between IL-1 and IL-1Ra in disease. *Cytokine Growth Factor Rev* Aug-Oct, 2002;**13**:323.

Aspinall R, Henson S, Pido-Lopez J, Ngom PT. Interleukin-7: an interleukin for rejuvenating the immune system. *Ann NY Acad Sci* Jun, 2004;**1019**:116.

Bowman EP, Chackerian AA, Cua DJ. Rationale and safety of anti-interleukin-23 and anti-interleukin-17A therapy. *Curr Opin Infect Dis* Jun, 2006;**19**:245.

Celestin J, et al. IL-3 induces B7.2 (CD86) expression and costimulatory activity in human eosinophils. *J Immunol* Dec 1, 2001;**167**:6097.

Groux H, Cottrez F. The complex role of interleukin-10 in autoimmunity. *J Autoimmun* Jun, 2003;**20**:281.

Guimond M, Fry TJ, Mackall CL. Cytokine signals in T-cell homeostasis. *J Immunother* Jul-Aug, 2005;**28**:289.

Heinrich PC, et al. Principles of interleukin (IL)-6-type cytokine signalling and its regulation. *Biochem J* Aug 15, 2003;**374**:1.

Izuhara K, Arima K, Yasunaga S. IL-4 and IL-13: their pathological roles in allergic diseases and their potential in developing new therapies. *Curr Drug Targets Inflamm Allergy* Sep, 2002;**1**:263.

Knoops L, Renauld JC. IL-9 and its receptor: from signal transduction to tumorigenesis. *Growth Factors* Dec, 2004;**22**:207.

Liu YJ. Thymic stromal lymphopoietin: master switch for allergic inflammation. *J Exp Med* Feb 20, 2006;**203**:269.

Martinez-Moczygemba M, Huston DP. Biology of common beta receptor-signaling cytokines: IL-3, IL-5, and GM-CSF. *J Allergy Clin Immunol* Oct, 2003;**112**:653.

Shulga-Morskoy S, Rich BE. Bioactive IL7-diphtheria fusion toxin secreted by mammalian cells. *Protein Eng Des Sel* Jan, 2005;**18**:25.

Watanabe N, et al. Hassall's corpuscles instruct dendritic cells to induce CD4+CD25+ regulatory T cells in human thymus. *Nature* Aug 25, 2005;**436**:1181.

CHAPTER 7

Cytokines of the Immune System: Chemokines

ABOUT CHEMOKINES

Chemokines are cytokines that stimulate the migration of cells that are attracted to the sites with higher concentration of ligands. The ligands can attach themselves to the extracellular matrix and form gradients of varying expanses in any tissue. The concentration gradient is sensed by cells with the chemokine receptors.

Chemokines are a large group of molecules that are fairly homogeneous in terms of structure and basic functions. The group, so far, has nearly 50 similar proteins from 8 to 10 kDa in molecular weight. They are divided into four subgroups, with respect to the position of the first two cysteine residues in the molecule, which are either adjacent (CC) or separated by one amino acid (CXC). Beside these there are groups without first cysteine (XC) and a group that has two cysteines separated by three amino acids (CX_3C). The names of chemokines and their receptors are made using this feature; namely, chemokines add the letter L, and receptors R, followed by the number after the CC, CXC, CX_3C, or XC group designations. This principle avoids confusion, first, because there were too many previous names that were rather uninformative although descriptive, and second, because ligands and receptors interact rather promiscuously with each other.

The chemokines' main function is in the regulation of migration of various cells in an organism. The word chemokine stems from chemotaxis, which is a movement of cells or microorganisms provoked by a chemical stimulus (*taxis*, in *Ancient Greek* τάξις means "arrangement"). This stimulus attracts cells toward chemicals (chemoattractants including chemokines), which are arranged in criss-crossing gradients in the microenvironment. Chemokines pose beacons towards which source a cell would move in order to reach its final destination. Migrating cells are relocated from one site to another of the body, and can colonize (infiltrate) various tissues or recirculate via blood or lymph. In the complex process of infiltration, besides

The Cytokines of the Immune System
http://dx.doi.org/10.1016/B978-0-12-419998-9.00007-9

241

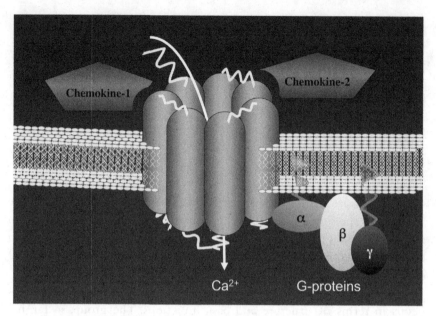

Figure 7-1 Chemokine receptors: basic structure and signal transduction.

chemokines and their receptors, there are other important molecules like *homing* receptors, *integrins*, and *selectins* that are necessary in colonization.

The homing receptors are like addresses of particular tissues of the body. Migrating cells in their continuous pressure to reach their destinations detect them on endothelium of blood or lymph vessels. Leukocytes can exit any vessel even during a fast flow rate. They characteristically roll along the endothelium of blood vessels. This is caused by the interaction of integrins and selectin receptors on endothelial cells on the one side, and their binding counterparts on leukocytes on the other side, which are also integrins or selectins. The effect of chemokines on leukocytes begins by binding to its receptors (Figure 7-1), which can anchor them at the site of highest chemokine concentrations even at fast blood flow (Figure 7-2). This allows diapedesis or migration out of the blood vessels by sneaking or squeezing in between adjacent endothelial cells. Leukocytes change shape within a few seconds after binding to chemokine receptors and change the expression of a number of genes. Actin polymerization and decomposition lead to the formation and retraction of lamellipodia, which function as legs and arms of migrating cells. Increased expression of integrins allows tighter binding to the endothelium, diapedesis, and relocation into tissues. In addition to these, fluctuations can be observed in the transient increase of intracellular

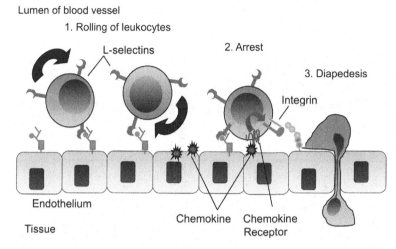

Figure 7-2 Function of chemokine receptors in arresting leukocytes during rolling on endothelium in blood vessels.

Ca^{2+}, and production of microbiocidal reactive oxygen species and bioactive lipids. These could be accompanied by the release of proteins deposited in various granules such as proteases in neutrophils, histamine in basophils, and cytotoxic proteins in eosinophils.

Some chemokines such as CCL27 can exist in a dual conformation, one attached to the cell membrane, and other that is soluble like most of the other chemokines. Interestingly, and especially for CCL27, it can be internalized in the cell and transferred to the nucleus where it acts as a transcription factor.

Chemokines maintain the traffic of lymphocytes in physiological conditions, during the immune response, as well as in inflammation and infection. In addition, they have a role in the development of white blood cells in the bone marrow and in peripheral mechanisms of renewal of leukocyte populations (homeostasis). They are produced in many pathological conditions, not only by infiltrating leukocytes, but also from various tissue cells.

Receptors for chemokines are divided by subgroups of chemokines that they bind: there are ten (10) receptors for CCLs (CCR1-10), six (6) for CXCLs (CXCR1-6), and one for CX3CL (CXC3R) and XCL (XCR) groups. Common features are that they have seven transmembrane regions, and in signaling they bind GTP-binding proteins (G-proteins). Many chemokines can bind to several receptors.

Two tables show lists of all chemokines and their receptors expressed by the cells of the immune system (Tables 7-1 and 7-2).

244 The Cytokines of the Immune System

Table 7-1 Chemokine receptors expressed by human leukocytes

Neutrophils	Monocytes	Eosinophils	Basophils
CXCR1	CCR1	CCR1	CCR1
CXCR2	CCR2	CCR3	CCR2
CXCR4	CCR5		CCR3
	CXCR5		

Resting T-lymphocytes	In vitro activated T-cells (with IL-2)
CCR7	CCR1
CXCR4	CCR2
	CCR3
	CCR5
	CXCR3
	CXCR4

Th1 cells	Th2 cells	Th17	Th22
CCR5	CCR3	CCR4	CCR4
CXCR3	CCR4	CCR6	CCR6
	CCR8		CCR10
	CXCR4		

Resting B cells	Plasma cells
CCR2	CCR5
CCR7	
CXCR5	

Immature dendritic cells	Mature dendritic cells
CCR1	CCR4
CCR2	CCR7
CCR5	CXCR4
CXCR1	
CXCR4	
CX3CR1	

Table 7-2 Important human receptors for chemokines on immune cells

Receptor	(Expressed by)	Ligands
CXCR1 (CD181)	T, DC	CXCL8 (IL-8), CXCL6 (GCP-2)
CXCR2 (CD182)	T	CXCL1,-2,-3 (GRO-α,-β,-γ), CXCL5 (ENA-78), CXCL6,-7 (NAP-2), -8
CXCR3 (CD183)	Th1, B?	CXCL9,-10, -11 (MIG, IP-10, I-TAC)
CXCR4 (CD184)	Naïve Th, Th2, T★, B, DC	CXCL12 (SDF-1-α /SDF-1-β)
CXCR5 (CD185)	T subgroups, B	CXCL13 (BCA-1/BLC)
CXCR6 (CD186)		CXCL16
CCR1 (CD191)	T★, DC	CCL5 (RANTES), CCL3 (MIP-1α), CCL15 (MIP-5), MCP-1, MCP-2
CCR2A/B (CD192)	T★, DC	CCL2, -8,-7, -13, -12 (MCP-1,-2,-3, -4,-5)
CCR3 (CD193)	Th2	CCL11 (Eotaxin), CCL24 (Eotaxin-2), RANTES, MIP-5, MCP-2,-3,-4
CCR4 (CD194)	Th2, Th17, Th22, DC	CCL5 (RANTES), CCL17 (TARC), MIP-1α, MCP-1, MDC/STCP-1
CCR5 (CD195)	Th1, Th22, DC	CCL5 (RANTES), CCL3,-4 (MIP-1α, -β), CCL8 (MCP-2)
CCR6 (CD196)	Th17, B, DC	CCL20 (MIP-3α/LARC/Exodus-1)
CCR7 (CD197)	Naïve Th, Th2, B★, DC★	CCL19 (MIP-3β/ELC/Exodus-3), CCL21 (SLC/6Ckine/Exodus-2)
CCR8 (CD198)	Th2	CCL17, CCL4, CCL1 (Tarc, MIP-1β, I-309/TCA-3)
CCR9 (CD199)	Pre T	CCL25 (RANTES, Eotaxin, MIP-1α, MIP-1β-1, MCP-1, -2,-3,-4)
CCR10	T, Th22	CCL27, -28 (CTACK, MEC)
CX3CR1	T★, DC	CX3CL1 (Fractalkine/neurotactine)
XCR1	Unknown	XCL1-2 (Lymphotactine; SCM-1b)

DC: dendritic cells.
★Receptors on activated or mature cells.

THE ROLE OF CHEMOKINES IN THE IMMUNE SYSTEM

Chemokines play an important role in the immune response. They guide migration of dendritic cells to lymph nodes, which is important in the beginning of the adaptive immune response. DCs in tissues express CCR5 (Figure 7-3). It is believed that mature DC (laden with antigens phagocytosed at the sites of tissue damage, such as infections or wounds) induce the expression of CCR7, and are thus attracted by the chemotactic ligand CCL19 (ELC; Epstein–Barr virus-induced molecule 1 Ligand Chemokine), which is secreted by endothelial cells of lymph vessels. When DCs arrive in afferent lymph vessels, they travel passively by lymphatic flow into the draining lymph nodes. In the lymph nodes (Figure 7-4), the second phase of migration starts, with DCs being attracted to areas of paracortex that is filled with resting T cells via CCL21 (SLC; Secondary Lymphoid-tissue-derived Cytokine) chemokine (*see* section on dendritic cells in *Cellular innate immunity*, Chapter 2, p. 30). It seems that the DCs can cause tolerance to antigens if they were "poorly" activated or "immature," or if they are mature and secrete a particular combination of cytokines and cell-surface molecules that are co-inhibitory. This is still a controversial area of research and the rules of the origin of tolerance are still not completely known. Conversely, if DCs are "strongly" activated, then DCs can start the immune response by the activation of CD4 T cells in draining lymph nodes (or T-cell areas in spleen). Mature DCs in the lymph nodes secrete CCL21 (SLC),

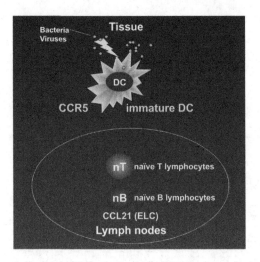

Figure 7-3 Function of chemokine receptors in initiation of the immune response.

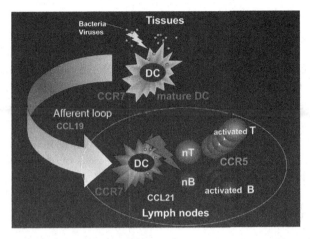

Figure 7-4 CCR7 causes migration of DC in afferent lymphatics, and later from lymph sinusoids into paracortex of lymph nodes.

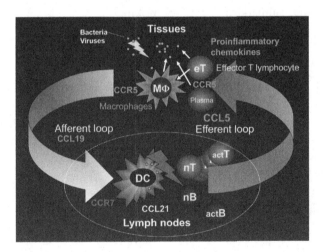

Figure 7-5 CCR5 causes migration of B and T effector cells from lymph nodes.

CCL17 (TARC; Thymus and Activation Regulated chemokine), and CCL22 (MDC; Macrophage-derived chemokine) that attract new incoming DCs and activated T cells that express CCR7 and CCR4 to move into the same compartment of the lymph node.

First ligands that have been found to attract T cells to sites of inflammation (Figure 7-5) are CCL5 (RANTES) and some other proinflammatory chemokines including CCL3 (MIP-1α) and CCL4 (MIP-1β).

Furthermore, CCL2, -7, -8, and-13 (MCP-1 to -4) are potent chemotactic factors for colonization of inflamed target tissues not only for T cells but also for NK cells as well as immature dendritic cells. In addition, to these CC chemokines, some CXC chemokines attract T cells and they are very specific. Namely, CXCL10 (IP-10) and CXCL9 (MIG) act via CXCR3 receptor on T cells activated by IL-2. CXCL10 and CXCL9 are induced by the action of IFN-γ (that normally inhibits the expression of most other chemokines). In viral infections, IFN-γ, which is produced locally at the site of infection by effector Th1 cells or NK cells, is responsible for the creation of CXCL10 and CXCL9 chemokines, and these then attract effector cytotoxic T lymphocytes (or those cells that express CXCR3) (Tables 7-1 and 7-2).

CCL CHEMOKINES (CCL1–CCL28)

The structure of these chemokines includes four highly conserved cysteines, which are the hallmark of all CC chemokines.

CCL1

(I-309; TCA-3)

CCL1 is secreted by T cells, monocytes, and mast cells. It attracts immature dendritic cells (monocytes) and activated Th2 type cells. It does not attract neutrophils or granulocytes. The biologically active form is monomeric (74 amino acids), and can react cross-species (human–mouse).

Receptor

CCL1 binds to CCR8 receptor.

CCL2

(Monocyte chemoattractant protein-1 [MCP-1]; MCAF, JE)

CCL2 attracts monocytes and activates them. It also attracts basophils, activated T cells, NK cells, and immature dendritic cells. These proteins can react with cells from another species. The human mature protein has 76 amino acids (the rodent protein is 49 amino acids longer).

Receptor

CCL2 binds to CCR2 receptor.

CCL3

(Macrophage inflammatory protein-1α [MIP-1α]; LD78α)

CCL3 is a potent chemoattractant for eosinophils, monocytes, B cells, and immature dendritic cells. It can contribute to activation of macrophages. CCL3 selectively attracts CD8 T lymphocytes.

There is a variant of this chemokine known as LD78β (due to gene duplication).

Receptor

CCL3 binds to CCR1 and CCR5 receptors.

CCL4

(Macrophage inflammatory protein-1β [MIP-1β]; ACT-2)

CCL4 is a potent chemoattractant for eosinophils, monocytes, B cells, and immature dendritic cells. It can contribute to activation of macrophages. CCL3 selectively attracts CD4 T lymphocytes.

There is a variant of this chemokine known as LAG-1 (due to gene duplication).

Receptor

CCL4 binds to CCR5 receptor.

CCL5

(Regulated upon Activation Normal T cell Express Sequence [RANTES], SIS-delta)

CCL5 is a potent chemoattractant for eosinophils, basophils, monocytes, effector memory T cells (CD4$^+$/CD45RO$^+$), B cells, NK cells, and immature dendritic cells. The protein has 68 amino acids. It can inhibit T-tropic types of HIV-1 and HIV-2 viruses (and simian immunodeficiency virus [SIV]).

Receptor

CCL5 binds to CCR1, CCR3, and CCR5 receptors, and also to cyto-megalovirus receptor (US28).

CCL6

(C10; MRP-1)

CCL6 is a chemoattractant for CD4$^+$ T cells, B cells, monocytes, and NK cells. The protein has 95 amino acids. It is expressed in cultures of myelopoetic bone marrow cells stimulated by GM-CSF, M-CSF IL-3 and IL-4.

Receptor

CCL6 binds to CCR1, CCR2, and CCR3 receptors.

CCL7

(Monocyte chemoattractant protein-3 [MCP-3]; MARC)

CCL7 attracts eosinophils, basophils, monocytes, activated T cells, NK cells, and immature dendritic cells. This protein can react with cells from another species. The human mature protein has 76 amino acids.

Receptor

CCL7 binds to CCR1, CCR2, and CCR3 receptor.

CCL8

(Monocyte chemoattractant protein-2 [MCP-2]; HC14)

CCL8 attracts basophils, monocytes, activated T cells, NK cells, and immature dendritic cells. These proteins can react with cells from another species. The human mature protein has 76 amino acids.

Receptor

CCL8 binds to CCR2, CCR3, and CCR5 receptor.

CCL9/10

(Macrophage Inflammatory Protein-gamma [MIP-1γ]; MRP-2; CCF18)

CCL9/10 has no known human homolog and is described in murine blood. Its murine protein contains 101 amino acid. It attracts neutrophils (and activated T cells). However, it has inhibitory action on the formation of colonies of bone marrow myeloid immature progenitors.

Receptor

CCL9/10 binds to CCR1 receptor.

CCL11

(Eotaxin-1)

CCL11 attracts eosinophils, and together with eotaxin -2 and -3 plays a role in regulation of eosinophil recruitment in the asthmatic lung and allergic reactions. It is produced by TNF-stimulated monocytes and IFN-γ-stimulated endothelial cells. Protein has 74 amino acids.

Receptor

CCL11 binds to CCR3 receptor.

CCL12

(Monocyte chemoattractant protein-5 [MCP-5])

CCL12 attracts basophils, monocytes, activated T cells, NK cells, and immature dendritic cells. These proteins can react with cells from another species. The human mature protein has 76 amino acids.

Receptor

CCL12 binds to CCR2 receptor.

CCL13

(Monocyte chemoattractant protein-4 [MCP-4]; NCC-1)

CCL13 attracts eosinophils, basophils, monocytes, activated T cells, NK cells, and immature dendritic cells. This protein can react with cells from another species. The human mature protein has 75 amino acids.

Receptor

CCL13 binds to CCR1, CCR2, and CCR3 receptor.

CCL14

(HCC-1)

CCL14 attracts monocytes and eosinophils. It has 72 amino acids. It is secreted by various tissues including spleen, bone marrow, liver, heart, and skeletal muscle.

Receptor

CCL14 binds to CCR1 receptor.

CCL15

(Macrophage Inflammatory Protein-5[MIP-5]; HCC-2; Lkn-1)

CCL15 attracts T cells and monocytes. It is found in various tissues including adrenal gland, heart, and skeletal muscle. It has 92 amino acids.

Receptor

CCL15 binds to CCR1 and CCR3 receptors.

CCL16

(Liver Expressed Chemokine [LEC]; HCC-4; NCC-4; LCC-1; MTN-1; IL-10-inducible chemokine)

CCL16 attracts lymphocytes (activated Th1 cells) and monocytes, but not neutrophils. It contains 97 amino acids. It is expressed in thymus, spleen, and liver.

Receptor

CCL16 binds to CCR1 and CCR8 receptors.

CCL17

(Thymus and Activation Regulated chemokine [TARC]; ABCD-2)

CCL17 attracts T cells. It is predominantly expressed by dendritic cells. Mature DCs in the paracortex of lymph nodes secrete CCL17 (TARC), CCL21 (ELC), and CCL22 (MDC) that can attract new DCs and T cells (Th2). The protein contain 71 amino acids.

Receptor

CCL17 binds to CCR4 receptor.

CCL18

(Macrophage Inflammatory Protein-4 [MIP-4]; PARC; DC-CK1; AMAC-1)

CCL18 attracts T lymphocytes and immature dendritic cells. It has 69 amino acids. It is expressed in lymph nodes, bone marrow, lungs, and placenta.

Receptor

CCL18 binds to unknown receptor.

CCL19

(Macrophage Inflammatory Protein-3β [MIP-3β]; Epstein–Barr virus-induced molecule 1 Ligand Chemokine [ELC]; Exodus-3)

CCL19 attracts all cells expressing CCR7 like mature dendritic cells, B cells, naïve (or activated) T cells, and myeloid progenitor cells. It is secreted by endothelial cells of lymph vessels. It is also expressed in thymus and activated bone marrow cells. The human protein has 77 amino acids and acts on murine cells also.

Receptor

CCL19 binds to CCR7 receptor.

CCL20

(Macrophage Inflammatory Protein-3α [MIP-3α]; LARC; Exodus-1)

CCL20 attracts lymphocytes and immature dendritic cells. It promotes adhesion of memory CD4 T cells, but inhibits colony formation of immature myeloid progenitors. It has 70 amino acids. It is expressed in lymph nodes, liver, and appendix.

Receptor
CCL20 binds to CCR6 receptor.

CCL21
(**S**econdary **L**ymphoid-tissue-derived **C**ytokine [SLC]; 6CKine; Exodus-2)

CCL21 attracts T cells and mature dendritic cells. It is produced by endothelium of high endothelial venules in lymph nodes, spleen, and appendix. When DCs arrive in afferent lymph vessels, they travel passively by lymphatic flow into the draining lymph nodes. In the lymph nodes (Figure 4-4), DCs migrate into areas of paracortex that is filled with resting T cells being attracted by CCL21 chemokine. There, DCs secrete CCL19 (ELC) and CCL21 that attract additional mature DCs. Other activities include inhibition of hematopoiesis. The protein has 111 amino acids.

Receptor
CCL21 binds to CCR7 receptor.

CCL22
(Macrophage-derived chemokine [MDC]; STCP-1; ABCD-1)

CCL22 attracts monocytes, dendritic cells, NK cells, and activated Th2 cells. It is produced by B cells, macrophages, monocyte-derived dendritic cells, activated NK and CD4 T cells. The human protein contains 69 amino acids. It exerts a suppressive HIV activity (on T tropic virus).

Receptor
CCL22 binds to CCR4 receptor.

CCL23
(Macrophage Inflammatory Protein-3 [MIP-3]; MPIF-1; CKβ-8)

CCL23 attracts monocytes, resting T cells, and neutrophils. It inhibits colony formation of bone marrow myeloid progenitors. The human protein has 99 amino acids.

Receptor
CCL23 binds to CCR1 receptor.

CCL24

(MPFIF-2; CkB-6; Eotaxin-2)

CCL24 attracts eosinophils, basophils, Th2 T cells, mast cells, and subsets of (immature) dendritic cells. It inhibits proliferation of multipotential hematopoietic progenitor cells. It has 78 amino acids. It is produced by activated monocytes and T cells.

Receptor

CCL24 binds to CCR3 receptor.

CCL25

(Thymus Expressed-Chemokine [TECK])

CCL25 attracts activated macrophages, dendritic cells, thymocytes, and common lymphoid precursors. It is expressed by thymic stromal cells. This is important during colonization of thymus and for T cell development. It contains 127 amino acids and it is cross-species active (human–murine).

Receptor

CCL25 binds to CCR9 receptor.

CCL26

(Eotaxin-3)

CCL26 attracts eosinophils, basophils, T cells, and monocytes similarly to other eotaxin activities. It has 71 amino acids and is produced by endothelial cells stimulated with IL-4 or IL-13.

Receptor

CCL26 binds to CCR3 receptor.

CCL27

(ALP; Skinkine; Eskine)

CCL27 selectively attracts CLA+ (activated) T cells into the skin. Keratinocytes in normal and irritated epithelia express CCL27 as well as its CCR10 receptor. CCL27 has 88 amino acids.

Receptor

CCL27 binds to CCR2, CCR3, and CCR10 receptors.

CCL28

(Mucosae-associated Epithelial Chemokine [MEC])

CCL28 attracts resting $CD4^+$, $CD8^+$ T cells, and eosinophils. The mature protein has 105 amino acids. It is produced by epithelial cells of the bronchioles, salivary and mammary glands, and colon.

Receptor

CCL28 binds to CCR10 receptor.

CXCL CHEMOKINES (1–16)

The CXC cytokines have one amino acid between the first and the second cysteine residue of the conserved chemokine domains that are defined by four Cs as their hallmark.

CXCL1

(Growth Regulated Protein-α [GRO-α]; Melanoma Growth Stimulatory Activity-α [MGSA-α]; Macrophage Inflammatory Protein-2α [MIP-2α]; mKC; NAP-3; GRO-1; rCINC)

CXCL1 attracts and activates neutrophils and basophils. It belongs to a family of chemokines together with CXCL2 and CXCL3. Human CXCL1 has 73 amino acids (approx. 7.9 kDa).

Receptor

CXCL1 acts via CXCR1 or CXCR2 receptors.

CXCR2 receptors are implicated in neutrophil infiltration of the pancreas during autoimmune diabetes that is orchestrated by macrophages and pancreatic β-cells.

CXCL2

(Growth Regulated Protein-β [GRO-β]; Melanoma Growth Stimulatory Activity-β [MGSA-β]; Macrophage Inflammatory Protein-2β [MIP-2β]; mKC; NAP-3; GRO-1; rCINC)

CXCL2 is a chemoattractant and activator of neutrophils and basophils. It belongs to a family of chemokines together with CXCL1 and -3.

Through CXCL2 in epithelia, helper macrophages and TNF seem to be critical regulators in innate immunity against bacterial infections.

Receptor

CXCL2 signals via CXCR1 or CXCR2 receptors.

CXCL3

(Growth Regulated Protein-γ [GRO-γ]; Melanoma Growth Stimulatory Activity-γ [MGSA-γ]; MIP-2α; mKC; NAP-3; GRO-1; rCINC)

CXCL3 chemoattracts and activates neutrophils and basophils. It belongs to a family of chemokines together with CXCL1 and -2.

Receptor

CXCL3 action is directed through CXCR1 or CXCR2 receptors.

CXCL4

(Platelet Factor-4 [PF-4]; Oncostatin A, Iroplact)

CXCL4 is produced in megakaryocytes and stored in the α granules of platelets. It is chemoattractant for neutrophils and monocytes, and can inhibit angiogenesis. It has 70 amino acids.

CXCL5

(Epithelial Neutrophil Activating Peptide 78 [ENA-78]; LIX [murine])

CXCL5 is expressed in monocytes and mast cells. It has also been found in endothelial cells and platelets. There are three naturally existing variants of this chemokine: ENA 5-78, 9-78, and 10-78 with 74, 70, and 69 amino acids, respectively, that share the same biologic activity. CXCL5 attracts and activates neutrophils.

Receptor

CXCL5 can bind to CXCR1 and CXCR2 receptors.

CXCL6

(Granulocyte Chemotactic Protein-2 [GCP-2])

CXCL6 selectively attracts neutrophilic polymorphonuclear granulocytes. It has also anti-angiogenic activity. Mature CXCL6 has four different forms due to different truncation of the N-terminal of the protein thus having 69, 72, 75, and 77 amino acid residues (7.8-8.8 kDa).

Receptor

CXCL6 can bind to CXCR1 and CXCR2 receptors.

CXCL7

(Neutrophil Activating Protein-2 [NAP-2]; Platelet Basic Protein [PBP]; CTAP-III, precursor)

CXCL7 attracts neutrophils and activates them. It is produced in leukocytes, and the active form is made by proteolytic cleavage of the Platelet Basic Protein precursor. The mature protein has 70 amino acid residues (down from 128 aa of the PGP precursor).

Receptor

CXCL7 can bind to CXCR1 and CXCR2 receptors.

CXCL8

(IL-8; Monocyte-Derived Neutrophil Chemotactic Factor [MDNCF]; Neutrophil-Activating Factor [NAF]; NAP-1)

CXCL8 is secreted by monocytes, activated macrophages, and endothelial cells. It attracts and activates neutrophils. It has 72 amino acids (8.4 kDa). The endothelial form has five more amino acids.

Receptor

CXCL8 binds CXCR1 and CXCR2 receptors. Both receptors have a high affinity for IL-8 and transfer the signal into the cell. They are found in many cells, including neutrophils, monocytes, fibroblasts, and lymphocytes. There is a decoy receptor for IL-8/CXCL8 (with a lower affinity) on human erythrocytes (also known as *Duffy* antigen, or DARC), endothelial cells, post-capillary venules, and on *Purkinje* cells in *cerebellum*, which also binds CCL2 (MCP-1) and CCL5 (RANTES), but does not transduce the signal, having an uncleared role. DARC is the receptor for *malaria* parasite *Plasmodium vivax*.

CXCL9

(Monokine-Induced by Interferon-γ [MIG])

CXCL9 is produced by IFN-γ stimulated monocytes, macrophages, and endothelial cells. It attracts Th1 effector cells. It has other activities including inhibition of angiogenesis, tumor growth, and inhibition of colony formation of hematopoietic progenitors.

Receptor

CXCL9 acts through CXCR3.

CXCL10

(γ–interferon Inducible Protein 10 [IP-10])

CXCL10 attracts Th1 subset of T cells and monocytes. It is produced in macrophages, as the older name implies, by the action of IFN-γ. It has other activities that include inhibition of cytokine-stimulated hematopoietic progenitor cell proliferation, anti-angiogenetic effect. It is mitogenic for vascular smooth muscle cells. The protein has 77 amino acids (8.5 kDa).

Receptor

CXCL10 signals through CXCR3.

CXCL11

(Interferon Inducible T-cell α Chemokine [I-TAC])

CXCL11 attracts IL-2 stimulated T cells. It has no activity on resting T cells, neutrophils or monocytes. It has 73 amino acids (8.3 kDa).

Receptor

CXCL11 acts via CXCR3.

CXCL12

(Stromal cell Derived Factor-1 [SDF-1α/β])

CXCL12 attracts T and B cells, and can induce migration of CD34+ stem cells. Human and mouse proteins have a cross-species activity. The two variants of CXCL12, SDF-1α, and SDF-1β have 68 or 72 amino acids, respectively, due to alternative splicing of the CXCL12 gene.

Receptor

CXCL12 acts via CXCR4.

HIV carriers injected with CXCL12 can show HIV suppressive activity in cells expressing CXCR4.

CXCL13

(B cell Attractant Chemokine-1 [BCA-1]; BLC; BLR ligand)

CXCL13 is a potent chemoattractant of B cells. However, it can induce a weak chemotaxis in T cells and macrophages, with no activity towards neutrophils or monocytes. It has 87 amino acids (10.3 kDa). It is expressed in spleen, lymph nodes, liver, gut, and appendix.

Receptor

CXCL13 acts via CXCR5.

CXCL14

(Breast and kidney expressed chemokine [BRAK]; Bolekine)

CXCL14 is a highly selective chemoattractant for monocytes. It is produced in normal tissues without inflammatory stimuli (and also in some cancer cell lines). It has 77 amino acids (9.4 kDa). The function and role is unknown as well as the receptor.

CXCL15

(Lungkine)

CXCL15 so far has no human counterpart. The murine CXCL15 is expressed in lung epithelial cells and in some fetal tissues. Its expression is increased during inflammation in the lungs, when it attracts neutrophils directing them to lung airway system. It has 142 amino acids (16.3 kDa).

Receptor

Murine CXCL15 acts via unknown receptor.

CXCL16

(Small inducible cytokine B6; SRPSOX)

CXCL16 attracts lymphocyte subsets towards sites of inflammation. It facilitates some immune responses. It has 89 amino acids (extracytoplasmic domain).

Receptor

CXCL16 acts via CXCR6 receptor.

CX3CL CHEMOKINE

CX3CL1

(Fractalkine; neurotactin; FKN)

CXCL1 is a potent attractant for monocytes, activated T cells, NK cells, and microglia cells. The structure of this chemokine includes three amino acids between the first and the second cysteine of the domain that is highly conserved in chemokines. The extracellular domain contains 76 amino acids, which are embedded (as a precursor) in the cell membrane via transmembrane region and a C-terminal cytoplasmic tail.

Receptor

CX3CL1 binds to CX3CR1 receptor.

XCL CHEMOKINES (1–2)

XCL1

(Lymphotactin; SCM-1a; ATAC)

XCL1 is a chemoattractant for T cells (and not to monocytes or neutrophils). The spleen is the highest producer in comparison to lung, intestines, and peripheral leukocytes. It has 92 amino acids.

Receptor

XCL1 binds to XCR1 receptor (GPR5).

XCL2

(SCM-1b)

XCL2 is a potent attractant for T cells.

Receptor

XCL2 binds to XCR1 receptor.

OTHER FEATURES OF CHEMOKINES

It is important to mention the difference in expression of receptors for chemokines in activated T-lymphocytes: T cells incubated with IL-2 increase the expression of CCR1, 2, and 5 receptor, and those activated with antibodies to CD3 and/or CD28 molecules reduce the expression of the above-mentioned chemokine receptors and reduce chemotaxis. This means that effector T cells can migrate towards the source of chemotaxis after stimulation with IL-2, but not after activation induced by antigen.

Furthermore, during differentiation into Th1 and Th2 subsets, Th1 subpopulation expresses CCR5 and CXCR3, whereas Th2 type cells have CCR3 and CCR4 receptors on their surface. These markers can be used to study better the role of individual T cell subpopulations in various pathological conditions.

It was observed that CCL5 (RANTES) and CCL7 (MCP-3) could activate eosinophils and basophils, in addition to causing their chemotaxis and release of histamine and leukotrienes. Therefore, it is assumed that these chemokines play an important role in *allergy*. After the discovery of CCL11 (eotaxin), also strong chemotactic factor for eosinophils, the focus of interest focused on the exploration of its role in *asthma*. Receptor for eotaxin, CCR3 is expressed not only in eosinophils, but also on basophils and the

Th2 type subpopulation of T-lymphocytes. For example, in *asthma*, basophils and eosinophils release mediators for muscle contraction, increase vascular permeability, mucus secretion, and airway hyperresponsiveness. Th2-lymphocytes involved in that case secrete cytokines such as IL-4 (increases the production of IgE) and IL-5 (sensitizes and activates eosinophils and basophils). They all have the expression of CCR3 and thus may be "invited" to sites of *allergic inflammation* by the same chemokines.

CCR10 is also important for chemokines that may have a role in a mouse model of *asthma*.

CCR10 is also associated with the generation of Th22 type of cells and some regulatory T cells (CD4$^+$ CD25$^+$ Foxp3$^+$).

Chemokines are not only important for hematopoiesis and immune processes; their role is growing, which raises the interest of many researchers. Furthermore, chemokines play an important role in morphogenesis during embryonic development, particularly for the formation of new blood vessels in the gastrointestinal tract as well as the arrangement of neurons. Some chemokine receptors are associated with the metastatic potential of various *cancers*: CCR6 with metastases to the liver, most likely by all tumors that express it, and CXCR4 in the metastatic spread of *breast cancer*, *melanoma*, and *osteosarcoma*.

Summary

1. Chemokines attract migrating cells by chemotaxis.
2. High affinity receptors for IL-8 (CXCL8) transfer the signal into the cell, whereas a decoy receptor (with lower affinity) does not transduce the signal. The latter is known as *Duffy* antigen, or DARC, when expressed on human erythrocytes. DARC is the receptor for *malaria* parasite *Plasmodium vivax*.
3. In T lymphocyte development, the expression of CCR9 receptor on common lymphoid precursors lead them to colonize the thymus following the expression of the CCL25 ligand in the thymus.
4. CXCR4 and CCR5 are (with CD4) coreceptors for HIV-1 virus that causes AIDS. HIV shows a predilection for infection of macrophages and CD4 T lymphocytes depending on the amount of co-receptors, because both cells have CD4 molecules. CXCR4 is the coreceptor for the T-tropic virus, whereas the CCR5 for the M-tropic one. There is a mutation in the CCR5 gene that protects the carriers of such alleles from disease, as it slows down the spread of the HIV.

Continued

Summary—cont'd

5. Chemokines play an important role in guiding migration of dendritic cells to lymph nodes, which is important in the beginning of the adaptive immune response. DCs in tissues express CCR5. Mature DCs (laden with antigens phagocytosed at the sites of tissue damage, such as infections or wounds) induce the expression of CCR7. They are then attracted by the chemokine CCL19 (SLC) in afferent lymph vessels. DCs travel passively by lymphatic flow into the draining lymph nodes where DCs exit lymphatics. DCs are attracted into paracortex, which is filled with resting T cells via CCL21 (ELC) chemokine.

6. Mature DCs in the lymph nodes secrete CCL21 (ELC), CCL17 (TARC), and CCL22 (MDC) that attract new DCs (and start a new round of migration). DCs also attract activated T cells that express CCR7 and CCR4 to move into the same compartment of the lymph node.

7. Ligands that attract T cells to sites of inflammation are CCL5 (RANTES), CCL3 (MIP-1α), and CCL4 (MIP-1β). Furthermore, CCL2, -7, -8, and -13 (MCP-1 to -4) are potent chemotactic factors for colonization of inflamed target tissues not only for T cells but also for NK cells as well as immature dendritic cells. In addition to these CC chemokines, some CXC chemokines attract T cells like CXCL10 (IP-10) and CXCL9 (MIG) that act via CXCR3 receptor on T cells (activated by IL-2). IFN-γ, which is produced locally at the site of (viral) infection by effector Th1 cells or NK cells, is responsible for the creation of CXCL10 and CXCL9, and these attract effector cytotoxic T lymphocytes (or those cells that express CXCR3).

8. Naïve Th (CD4) cells express CCR7 and CXCR4 receptors. Effector Th1 subpopulation expresses CCR5 and CXCR3, whereas Th2 type cells have CCR3, CCR4, and CCR8, as well as CXCR4 receptors on their cell surface. Th17 cells express CCR4 and CCR6 receptors, and Th22 have additionally CCR10.

CHAPTER 8

Cytokines Important for Growth and/or Development of Cells of the Immune System

TNF-α/β

Structure

Tumor necrosis factor (TNF)-α and TNF-β are very similar in structure and function (Figure 8-1). They belong to the superfamily of tumor necrosis factor (TNFSF, *tumor necrosis factor superfamily*), which has over 20 members and includes molecules such as FasL and CD40L. TNFSF are structurally glycoproteins with the transmembrane regions. By the action of proteases they become soluble, making them the dominant form of existence in the tissues. TNF-α and TNF-β are homotrimers (Figure 8-1), but TNF-α can be associated with another membrane cytokine called Lymphotoxin-β (LT-β) with which it can make heterotrimers.

Source

TNF-α is secreted by activated macrophages, and TNF-β (or lymphotoxin-α) by activated Th1 lymphocytes.

Receptor

TNF-α/β can bind to two receptors, TNFR1 (p55) and TNFR2 (p75), which have different functions. Both TNF receptors are homotrimers (Figure 8-2).

Function

TNF-α/β generally have a proinflammatory role (along with IL-1, which is itself a powerful stimulator of secretion of TNF-α by macrophages). TNFR1 function can be in transmitting apoptotic signals inside cells that can be killed by ligand binding. It is believed that TNF-α/β usually give the signal for cell survival; however due to other signals (probably other factors in the microenvironment) some tumor cells can

The Cytokines of the Immune System
http://dx.doi.org/10.1016/B978-0-12-419998-9.00008-0

263

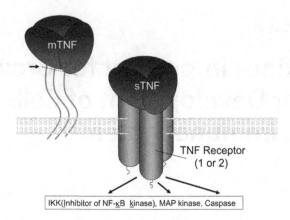

Figure 8-1 Structure (schematic) of tumor necrosis factor (TNF), and receptors TNFR1(p55) and TNFR2 (p75), with signal transduction. mTNF: membrane form and sTNF: soluble tumor necrosis factor.

undergo apoptosis (hence the name of this group). The function of the TNFR2 is less known, however it has a different function according to the second messengers within the cell that are different than those of TNFR1 (Figure 8-2).

Other Features

TNF inhibits the expression of TLR4 on monocytes (while IL-6 increases).

Macrophages secrete TNF as a result of nuclear stress during inability to repair DNA. Such nuclear stress can be experimentally induced in mice deficient in the DNase I gene by *knock-out* technology. Macrophages from (DNase I −/−) mice spontaneously secrete TNF that can then in turn exert its proinflammatory effect and induce changes in tissues. Perhaps due to such effect, tissues exposed to mechanical or chemical stress (i.e., the cells that require enhanced DNA repair) are at higher risk to become damaged by inflammatory action of TNF. The joints are most likely an example of such a mechanical stress, which might result in the subsequent development of arthritis and even *rheumatoid factor* (RF). This RF is similar to the one in autoimmune RF-positive *rheumatoid arthritis* (RA) in humans. Many researchers believe that the RA is an autoimmune disorder of yet unknown initial pathogenetic causative event. According to this assumption, activated T cells and Th1 type response would induce TNF in synovial macrophages, and thereby develop progressive disease.

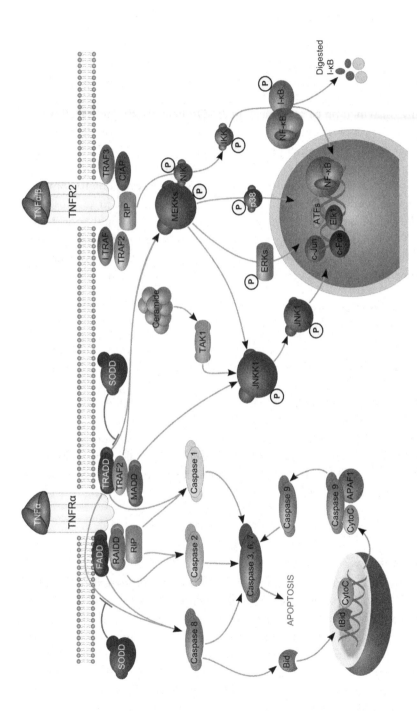

Figure 8-2 Differences in signal transduction between TNFR1(p55) and TNFR2 (p75). c-Jun/c-Fos, Elk1, ATFs, and NFκB are nuclear factors during activation of various genes important for cell survival. JNK, ERK, & p38 are MAP kinases. IκB: inhibitor of NFκB; IKKs: IκB kinase; CytoC: cytochrome P450.

Associations with Disease

The role of TNF in many autoimmune diseases has been amply documented. Many therapeutics against TNF molecules (e.g., antibodies) seem to help reduce the symptoms of some autoimmune diseases, especially *rheumatoid arthritis*. However there is *rheumatoid arthritis* resistant to anti-TNF therapy (in which preparations against IL-6R help, see the next section).

Genetic polymorphisms in the TNFA or TNFB genes have been investigated in parallel with other proinflammatory cytokines like IL-1, IL-6, and IFN-γ. Some of them showed association with susceptibility to many chronic inflammatory and autoimmune diseases. However, due to complex heredity of predisposing factors, they tend to be different in various subpopulations of humans. For example, the single nucleotide polymorphisms (SNPs) in the gene encoding TNF-α (rs1800629 and rs1800630) diseases and the recurrent oral ulceration in Chinese population. However, this could be the only population where such finding was documented.

Therapeutic Options

Infliximab (anti-TNF antibody) is used to treat *rheumatoid arthritis*, although the mechanism of improvement of symptoms and reduction of inflammation is not known. However, long-term use and patient safety is in question, due to the increased incidence of active *tuberculosis* during treatment with anti-TNF antibody, as well as the impossibility of successful therapy in some RA patients. In the resistant RA, inhibition of other cytokines may help in the future (e.g., *Atlizumab* [anti-IL-6R antibody] and, perhaps, soluble IL-6ST that act as inhibitors of IL-6). *Thalidomide* is also an inhibitor of TNF-α, and proved to be very effective in the treatment of experimental *sepsis* with *Escherichia coli*.

TGF-β

Structure

TGF-β is a group of three cytokines with homologous structure (TGFβ1, TGFβ2, and TGFβ3) that act through a common receptor. TGF owes its name to a discovery of being sometimes a factor causing malignant transformation *in vitro*. Later it was found that TGF functions extend to a wide range of activities including the regulation of cell growth and development. Subsequent discoveries of similar factors revealed that the TGF-β superfamily consists of ten members including Anti-Mullerian Hormone (AMH), inhibin A, B, C, and E, *bone morphogenetic factors*

(BMP)-2 and BMP-7, and *growth differentiation factor* (GDF)-5. Effects of TGF-β depend on the type of cell on which it acts, and they can be classified in several categories:

1. The inhibition of proliferation of epithelial, endothelial, and hematopoietic cells in culture.
2. Stimulation of proliferation of cells of mesenchymal origin (some via induction of *platelet derived growth factor* (PDGF)).
3. Chemotaxis of fibroblasts and monocytes, and their activation without proliferation (unlike macrophages, which are also attracted, but become deactivated).
4. The increase in deposition of extracellular matrix.
5. The increase in production of integrins (receptors for extracellular matrix).
6. Decreased synthesis of metalloproteases (enzymes that degrade extracellular matrix).
7. Increased production of metalloprotease inhibitors (which are important in wound healing).
8. The effect of TGF-β on the immune system is inhibitory and immunosuppressive. The inhibition is shown as the reduction in proliferation of B, T, and NK cells, as well as their function, such as, for example, lowering the secretion of some cytokines, and antagonizing the effect of proinflammatory (TNF-like) cytokines. While it strongly attracts macrophages, it calms them (or deactivates).

   TGF-β plays an important role in embryogenesis.

   A large number of tumors secrete TGF-β, and thus probably use TGF-β secretion as one of the mechanisms by which cancer can avoid the immune attack.

Receptor

TGF-β binds the heterodimeric receptor TGFBR, which consists of two chains: TGFBR1 (α) and TGFBR2 (β) (Figure 8-3). Signal transduction into the cell uses the Smad group of factors including Smad-2, -3, -4, and -7 molecules (Figure 8-3). Activation of heterodimeric TGF-β receptor starts with the activation of Smad-3, which joins with the Smad-2 factor making a complex Smad 2/3 that then activates the Smad-4. Activated Smad-4 enters the nucleus together with Smad-2 or Smad-3 and act on TGF-β responsive genes. Smad-4 also activates Smad-7, and the latter works much like transcription factor and also performs activation of TGF-β-stimulated genes. Furthermore, Smad-7 is additionally a regulatory factor. Namely, the

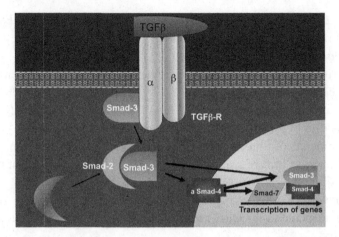

Figure 8-3 TGF-β(1, 2, and 3) bind single heterodimeric receptor, TGFβ-R (α: TGFβ-R1 & β: TGFβ-R2). Signal activates Smad3 that makes heterodimers with Smad-2, and this complex activates Smad-4. aSmad4: activated Smad4. Active Smad4 activates in the nucleus Smad-7 and binds DNA with Smad-3.

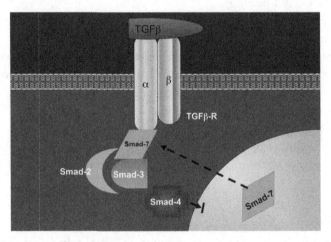

Figure 8-4 The regulation of signal transduction of the TGFβ-R via Smad-2, -3, -4, and -7 factors. Dissociation of Smad-2/Smad-3 complex (by Smad-7) prevents their activation of Smad-4.

regulation of the TGF activation is done via negative feedback loop. The accumulation of activated Smad-7 in the nucleus results in its overflow and release into the cytoplasm, where it can inhibit complex Smad-2/3. Since the dissociation of Smad-2 from Smad-3 reduces the activation of Smad-4, the signal transduction into the nucleus stops (Figure 8-4).

TGF-β is the product of many cells, and is found almost everywhere in the tissues as a larger precursor. Cleavage of the larger precursor produces a smaller active form of TGF-β. Larger amounts of TGF-β2 are secreted by Th3 effector cells. However, regulatory T cells (Treg and Tr1) also secrete intermediate levels of this cytokine with which they can inhibit the immune response of effector cells like Th2 and Th22, or promote the generation of Th9, Th17, and Tregs.

TSLP (THYMIC STROMAL LYMPHOPOIETIN)

Structure

TSLP (thymic stromal lymphopoetin) is a cytokine similar to IL-7.

Source

TSLP is expressed in thymus (*Hassals corpuscles*), mucosa in the gut, parenchymal cells of liver, in heart, and prostate. It is produced by epithelial, stromal, and mast cells. Its production in keratinocytes is strongly increased in *atopic dermatitis*, but not in other skin *inflammations*. In asthmatics, it is also secreted by neutrophils, macrophages, and respiratory epithelium.

Function

Dendritic cells (DCs) stimulated with TSLP produce chemokines CCL17 (TARC), and CCL22 (MDC), which attract naïve T cells. TSLP can polarize the immune response in Th2-type similar ("quasi Th2") response. Quasi-Th2 cells secrete TNF–α instead of IL-10, while producing other Th2-type cytokines (that includes IL-2, -4, -5, and -13). It is associated with the migration of Langerhans cells (one type DC) in the skin.

DCs induced by TSLP have a homeostatic effect on resting quasi-Th2 population (memory cells). In other words, TSLP can cause amplification of memory CD4 Th2 cells without changing its effector phenotype. Th2 cells are considered pro-*allergic* because they are involved in the switch of Ig isotype of B cells into IgE.

Receptor

The receptor is composed of IL-7R and TSLP-R, and the signal is conducted via nuclear factor STAT-5 (Figure 8-5). Interestingly, none of the known Jak kinases were found to partake in it. Negative feedback regulation of the signal transduction is done through SOCS-1 factor.

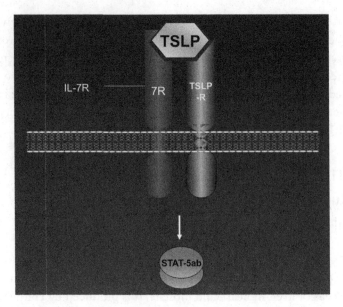

Figure 8-5 The TSLP receptor and signal transduction factors.

Other Features

TSLP from *Hassals* bodies in the thymus stimulates the expression of Foxp3 in CD4$^+$CD25$^-$ thymocytes changing it into the CD4$^+$CD25$^+$CTLA4$^+$ population (in the presence of DCs, IL-2 and costimulatory CD80 and CD86 molecules; see *T-cell development*, Chapter 2, p. 44). There arises another positive selection of T cells in the thymus, and those thymocytes with TCRs having medium to strong affinity (to self) become natural Treg cells, and have a function in the regulation of the immune response, that is, to inhibit activation of T lymphocytes (see *Repertoire and Tolernce*, Chapter 3, p. 94).

   TSLP stimulates early development of B lymphocytes (until immature stage cells that express B220$^+$ IgM$^+$) and can replace IL-7 (it has overlapping functions with IL-7).

Association with Human Diseases

TSLP and some chemokines (produced by its actions) were significantly increased in the airways of *asthmatic* patients and correlate with disease severity. It is thought that TSLP plays a role in the pathogenesis of *allergic* diseases. Specifically, the "quasi-Th2" population that has been stimulated by DCs (induced with TSLP) has the following markers: cystatin A, Charcot–Leyden's crystalline proteins, and prostaglandin D2 synthase.

Genetic polymorphisms in the gene encoding TSLP are being investigated, but might suffer from the similar shortcomings as for the TNF factor. The reason is that many diseases are polygenic in nature, so that susceptibility to them resides in more than a single gene, and probably involves several, if not more genes.

KGF (KERATINOCYTE GROWTH FACTOR)

Keratinocyte growth factor (KGF) has an important immunological activity in developing thymocytes. Its secretion increases with the degree of development of thymocytes and is the strongest at the single positive (SP) stage: in CD4 lymphocytes and CD8 thymocytes. KGF acts on their previous stages in development. It stimulates the production of TSLP (and IL-6) in the thymic epithelium (however, KGF has no effect on IL-7 production). Further, it reduces the expression of MHC class II molecules in thymic epithelium and inhibits the development of CD4 T thymocytes, but it expands its compartment (increases cellularity) in bone marrow (the latter effect caused via FGFRIIIb).

SCF (STEM CELL FACTOR) AND GROWTH FACTORS (CSF, GM-CSF, M-CSF) OF HEMATOPOIETIC LINES

This includes other factors of the development of hematopoietic cell lines such as CSF (colony stimulating factor), G-CSF (granulocyte-CSF), M-CSF (macrophage-CSF), and GM-CSF (granulocyte/macrophage-CSF).

Factors are proteins of approximately 30 kDa. SCF is secreted by bone marrow stroma, endothelium, and fibroblasts. SCF secretion is inhibited by cytokines such as TNF, IL-1, and TGF-β1.

SCF enhances the activity of various CSF to stimulate the production of hematopoietic cells, and mobilizes hematopoietic progenitors from the bone marrow into circulation. SCF acts on hematopoietic cells, melanocytes and stem cells of the germ line and hematopoietic tissue.

Furthermore, it ameliorates *macrocytic anemia*, and induces recovery of hematopoiesis after chemotherapy and radiotherapy.

Receptors

SCF receptor (alias c-kit, KIT, see *Mast cells,* Chapter 2, p. 36) belongs to the type III family of tyrosine kinases. Its expression is increased in *hemoblastoses, testicular,* and *small cell lung cancer.*

GM-CSF receptor: GM-CSFR is similar to those of IL-3 and IL-5 cytokines. It consists of GM-CSFR chain associated with $\beta-$common chain to

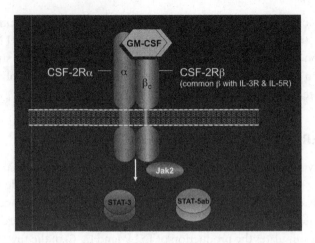

Figure 8-6 The GM-CSF receptor and signal transduction factors.

IL-3R or IL-5R. Signal transduction employs the Jak–STAT system: Jak2 tyrosine kinase and transcription factors STAT-3 and STAT-5ab (Figure 8-6).

SCF—Therapeutic Potential

1. Using SCF for clinical purposes reduces the duration and degree of bone marrow suppression after chemotherapy for *small cell carcinoma* of the *lung, bladder, breast,* and *metastatic melanoma.*
2. SCF induces an increase of hematological reconstitution after bone marrow transplantation in patients with *non-Hodgkin lymphoma* and *Hodgkin's* disease.
3. SCF injection increases the number of stem cells from the bone marrow after burns; and it facilitates their collection before bone marrow transplantation.
4. SCF is used as adjuvant therapy of *leukemia* with cytotoxic agents or toxins in *acute myeloid leukemia.*
5. SCF is a therapy for neutropenic states like *aplastic anemia,* cyclic/congenital *neutropenia, myelodysplastic syndrome,* and the *acquired immunodeficiency syndrome*—AIDS.
6. It can be used to enhance host defense in threatening infections.

LIF—LEUKEMIA INHIBITORY FACTOR

Synonyms

Cholinergic differentiation factor; CDF, D-FACTOR; HILDA.

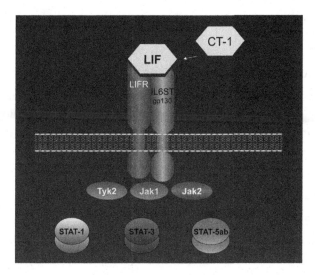

Figure 8-7 The LIF (CTF1) receptor and its signal transduction factors.

Structure

LIF is basic, highly glycosylated protein. It belongs to the family of IL-6 related cytokines with 11 members: IL-6, IL-11, IL-27, IL-31, CNTF, OSM, cardiotrofin-1 (CT-1) and *cardiotrophin-like cytokine* (CLC), NPN (neuropoetin), and viral IL-6 (see *IL-6,* Chapter 6, p. 168). The LIF gene is on chromosome 22q12.2.

Function

One of the first reported functions of pleiotropic cytokine LIF was the inhibition of leukemic cell proliferation, hence the name. It induces differentiation of macrophages, communication between neurons, and chemotaxis of various immunocytes. It has different effects on the hematopoietic cell lines, germline stem cells, and hematopoietic stem cells, the maturation of primary follicles and germ cells, migration of primitive gonadal cells in embryogenesis, and then it has effects on hepatocytes, neurons, adipocytes, myoblasts, and osteoblasts, which are often in cooperation with other cytokines. For example, working in synergy with *Bone morphogenetic protein-2* (BMP-2) LIF can create astrocytes from neural stem cells in culture.

Receptor

LIF receptor consists of two chains: LIFR and IL-6ST (gp130) (Figure 8-7). Signal transduction uses Jak-1, Jak-2, and Tyk2 tyrosine kinases, including

STAT-1, STAT-3, STAT-5ab, and factors such as mitogen-activated protein (MAP) kinase. CT-1 also binds to the LIF receptor.

Association with Human Diseases

Due to the wide spectrum of biological activity *in vitro,* it is assumed that an increase in the secretion of LIF may result with complex pathologies, such as the *wasting syndrome,* or an increase in the number of megakaryocytes and platelets, and, lastly, aberrant accumulation of bone mass.

CNTF—CILIARY NEUROTROPHIC FACTOR

Structure

CNTF is monomeric glycoprotein of 195 amino acids, and belongs to the family of IL-6-related cytokines (see *IL-6,* Chapter 6, p. 168).

Source

CNTF is secreted (a) in the brain by Schwann's cells; (b) skeletal muscle; and (c) in the embryo.

Function

CNTF is pleiotropic cytokine with neural and embryonic component of action. After nerve injury distal Schwann's cells secrete CNTF to regenerate axons of nerve cells of the nerve.

Receptor

CNTF receptor is composed of three chains: LIFR, IL-6ST (gp130), and a specific CNTFR chain (Figure 8-8). Signal transduction is similar to that of LIF receptor.

CNTFR has a soluble form, and as such, upon binding the ligand it acts as an agonist. Furthermore, CNTF can bind to IL-6R (and its soluble form sIL-6R) and that signals (or trans-signals, see *IL-6,* Chapter 6, p. 171) through gp130 and LIF-R chains. The latter may have implications in treatment by CNTF of *neurodegenerative* diseases, or *obesity.*

Other Features

- Among other effects, it is important to mention the effect on survival of neurons, from ciliary, sympathetic, sensory, and motor to hippocampal.

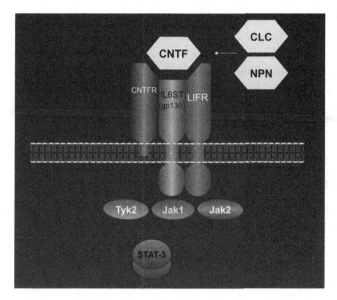

Figure 8-8 The CNTF (CLC & NPN) receptor with signal transduction factors.

- Furthermore, it maintains the embryonic stem cells in a non-differentiated state.
- Then, it promotes the differentiation of neuronal precursors of the sympathetic system, and inhibits their proliferation.
- It promotes cholinergic replacement of mature sympathetic neurons.
- It promotes the development of astrocytes, survival and maturation of oligodendrocytes.

Therapeutic Options

It is being considered in the therapy of *neuro-degenerative* diseases and of excessive weight (*obesitas*).

In the mouse, injection of CNTF can cure progressive motor neuropathy, and thus represents a hope for therapy of *amyotrophic lateral sclerosis*, ALS. Unfortunately, the treatment of ALS was abandoned due to severe peripheral side effects. The latter is surprising because CNTF-R is not too pronounced in tissues outside the CNS. It is more likely that trans-signaling via IL-6R may explain these effects (see above and the section on *IL-6*, Chapter 6, p. 171).

Modification of CNTF into a variant that does not bind IL-6R, but only CNTF-R, is an option that should improve the treatment with CNTF.

It can already be seen in the example of the newer candidates for therapy. These specially designed cytokines are actually ligands fused with their receptor (CNTF–CNTF-R). They would act specifically on cells expressing IL-6ST/LIFR complex (see Figure 8-7). Preliminary results are encouraging because they have a strong neurotrophic effect on cells that are normally negative for CNTF-R.

OSM—ONCOSTATIN M

Structure

OSM is monomeric glycoprotein of 28 kDa, and belongs to the family of the IL-6 related cytokines (see *LIF—Leukemia inhibitory factor,* p. 272).

Source

OSM is secreted by activated monocytes and T lymphocytes.

Function

OSM has many effects from specific induction of differentiation of leukemic cell lines in macrophage-like cells to the function of cells similar to those of the same family of cytokines (see *IL-6,* Chapter 6, p. 168).

Receptor

Human OSM binds two heterodimeric receptors (Figure 8-9), LIF receptor (LIFR, IL-6ST) and Oncostatin-M receptor (OSMR, IL-6ST). Mouse OSM binds only the latter receptor. Signal transduction resembles that of LIF and CNTF (the Jak-STAT pathway and activation of MAPK).

Other Features

- OSM maintains embryonic stem cells in the undifferentiated state. In contrast, it promotes the differentiation of hematopoietic precursors, hepatocytes, fibroblasts, endothelial cells, and neurons.
- It stimulates the growth of fibroblasts and *Kaposi sarcoma.*
- It inhibits cell growth of solid tumors and endothelial cells.
- All this leads to a potentially important role in hematopoiesis, inflammation, cholesterol regulation, and development of the embryo.

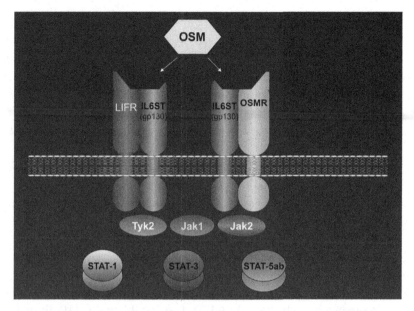

Figure 8-9 The OSM receptors and their signal transduction factors.

A SHORT DESCRIPTION OF OTHER CYTOKINES THAT REGULATE GROWTH AND DEVELOPMENT OF VARIOUS TISSUES

HGF—Leukemia inhibitory factorHepatocyte Growth Factor

HGF is a heterodimer ($\alpha\beta$); its inactive form is secreted by non-parenchymal liver cells, kidney, and lungs. It can make heterodimers with IL-7.

Parenchyma possesses receptors belonging to the family of tyrosine kinases.

It is an embryonic morphogen, and is the main mediator of liver regeneration.

Its inactive precursor is associated with extracellular matrix. The active form of the cytokine is converted by plasminogen activators.

The HGF gene is very large (it has 18 exons, and spans 70 kb) that is located on chromosome 7q21.1.

HGF is mitogen for hepatic cells in culture. In addition, HGF stimulates growth of renal tubular epithelial cells and keratinocytes; it is a potent angiogenetic factor and can act to dissociate layers of the epithelium promoting their invasiveness.

HGF can promote the progression of cancer in *malignant* invasive form.

EGF—Epidermal Growth Factor(s)

EGFs are a family of polypeptide factors including EGF, amphiregulin, β-celulin, TGF-α, HB-EGF, PVGF, lin-3, spitz—all having about 6 kDa in molecular weight. EGF has 53, and TGF-α 50 amino acids.

- Primary products are transmembrane glycoproteins.
- "Heparin Binding-EGF" is a receptor for *diphtheria* toxin.
- EGF is secreted by many tissues—it has effects on non-hematopoietic tissues.
- EGF plays an important role in mitogenesis.
- Many tumors secrete TGF-α, thereby enhancing their growth.
- TGF-α exists in embryo—*tgfa* gene knockout mice have *wave-1* phenotype: abnormal hair follicles and curly fur.
- Some viruses carry genes whose products resemble EGF.

Receptors

One of the receptor for EGF receptor is erbB1. In total, however, there are four receptors, of which all bind EGF, TGF-α, amphiregulin, HB-EGF, VGF, and β-celulin.

EGF receptors belong to the family of tyrosine kinases. Signal transduction involves PI3 kinase, GRB2/SOS/ras, PLC, SHC, and *nck* intracellular messengers and factors.

PDGF—Platelet Derived Growth Factor

PDGF is a protein of 30 kDa—it exists in three homo- or hetero-dimeric variants (α α, β β, α β).

- It stimulates growth and chemotaxis of fibroblasts, and smooth muscle cells.
- It has a role in embryogenesis and wound healing.
- Its overproduction is associated with *atherosclerosis, rheumatoid arthritis, fibrosis*, and *malignant* tumors (β chain is an oncogene).

Receptor

Receptor for PDGF has tyrosine kinase activity. Various isoforms induce different crosslinking of receptor subunits, thereby generating different effects on the target cells.

IGF—Insulin-Like Growth Factor(s)

IGF-I and IGF-II are insulin-like growth factors (somatomedines).

- The main producer is liver (endocrine function), but they are also produced elsewhere, and local autocrine and paracrine mechanisms affect the growth and development of the respective tissues.
- They have many effects and appear in physiological and pathological conditions: regulation of the growth hormone activity in liver, gonadotropic effect in reproductive system, and in bones, they regulate PTH and sex steroids actions.

IGF knockout mouse has a delayed embryonic growth, and postnatal *lethality*.

Receptors

There are two IGF receptors (RI, is a heterotetramer, with tyrosine kinase activity; RII, is a G-coupled protein).

IGFs cause differentiation of myoblasts into myocytes, and fibroblasts into adipocytes. They also cause the production of erythropoietin, and collagen and induce growth of neurites.

There are six IGF binding proteins (1–6), which are found in circulation, which can neutralize IGFs.

Potential clinical use is in wound healing, *osteoporosis*, nerve regeneration, treatment of catabolic states, and in the insulin-resistant *diabetes*.

FGF—Fibroblast Growth Factor(s)

FGFs are a family of 23 single-chain polypeptides having 15–32 kDa.

They are involved in a variety of biological processes as cell growth, development, angiogenesis, wound healing, and transformation.

- They all bind to heparin.
- FGFs play an important role in embryogenesis.
- They are very important in tumor vascularization.
- FGF4 is one of the most representative factors and plays a role in cell growth of the embryonic trophoblast in embryo implantation.
- FGF Receptor-1 and FGFR-2 are increasingly prominent in breast cancer.
- They have a role in *oncogenesis*.
- FGFs stimulate the secretion of collagenase and plasminogen activator.
- They are probably involved in the promotion of tumor invasion.

Receptors

FGFs act through four receptors, which have tyrosine kinase activity, with the exception of FGF1 that can cross the cell membrane and enter the nucleus. This is especially interesting as FGF1 can be a means to assist in the entrance to the cell, for potential therapeutic molecules.

NGF—Nerve Growth Factor(s)—Neurotrophins

NGFs are a family of similar proteins (NGF1-5) having about 120 amino acids.

NGFs have a major role in supporting and survival of embryonic neurons.

They are secreted in the adult individual, probably to maintain and gain the function of neurons.

- Antibodies that neutralize NGFs, completely destroy peripheral sympathetic nerve and cause loss of sensory fibers.
- BDNF (NGF-2) supports the survival of dopaminergic neurons.
- NGF prevents the loss of cholinergic neurons.
  Receptors for NGFs belong to the family of tyrosine kinases.

NDF—Neural Differentiation Factor—Neuregulins

NDF is a protein of 44 kDa.

NDF belongs to the family of neuregulins with EGF motif in the structure.

- It causes growth and development of epithelial cells (breast, lung, stomach), and has an effect on some functions of neurons.
- Neuregulins are primarily secreted by neurons. Fibroblasts secrete NDF after transformation with *ras* oncogene.
- Neuregulins have a potential role in the treatment of nerve injuries and some *adenocarcinomas*.
- The receptor consists of a receptor tyrosine kinase neu/erbB-2.
- The influence of NDF stops growth of some breast tumor cells (epithelial).
- Some of neuregulins (ARIA and GGS) stimulate the proliferation of Schwann cells, or the synthesis of acetylcholine receptor (AChR).

VEGF—Vascular Endothelial Growth Factor(s)

VEGFs comprise a family of three 45 kDa polypeptides: VEGF-a, VEGF-b, and VEGF-c.

They have a major role in angiogenesis, embryo development, and formation of ovarian *corpus luteum*, and they also promote wound healing.

- VEGFs stimulate the growth and migration of endothelial cells of small and large vessels.
- VEGFs are chemotactic for monocytes.
- They have a role in the developing embryo.
- Many tumors secrete VEGFs, enabling angiogenesis and thus their growth. However, endothelium does not produce VEGFs.

Receptor

VEGFs act through VEGF receptors VEGFR-1, VEGFR-2, and VEGFR-3.

VEGFR-3 is expressed only on endothelial cells of lymphatic vessels, whereas VEGFR-1 and -2 are found expressed on blood vessel endothelium.

Endothelins

Endothelin-1, -2, and -3 are 21-kDa polypeptides.

They are secreted by endothelial cells, neurons, and many other cells.

- They have vasoconstrictory, vasodilating, and endocrine effects.
- Endothelins are induced by physical factors (hypoxia), thrombin, angiotensin II, vasopressin (ADH), epinephrine (noradrenaline), and IL-1 cytokine.
- They are inhibited with NO, prostaglandins and a factor from the smooth muscle.
- Endothelins stimulate proliferation of smooth muscle.

Receptors

Endothelin receptors (A and B) are proteins that cross the membrane seven times. The receptors are related to the G-proteins. They transduce signal by causing PI3K activation, and during signaling serve as ion channels thereby increasing the concentration of intracellular Ca^{2+} within the cell.

CHAPTER 9

Theories about the Function of the Immune System

ABOUT SCIENTIFIC THEORIES

Theories and hypotheses are useful explanations of natural phenomena, occurrences, or events. Scientific theories are based on measurable and reproducible facts, highlighting the scientific method. A valid scientific theory should predict events it aims to explain out of proposed rules and laws. Thus, each theory should have a possibility to be falsified (proven wrong). In other words, an acceptable scientific theory should postulate proof(s) by which it can be discarded. In case the opposite should be proven true (e.g., the prediction of a theory was correct), then the theory is said to be either confirmed or supported by such facts, depending on the extent of proposed rules. Supporting observations also give credibility to other predictions of such theories. It is striking that working on confirmation of many scientific theories over the past half a millennium has been a challenge for humankind that greatly improved human civilization and standard of living. And, it continues to be the beacon of its progress.

Therefore, we appreciate confirmed predictions of a theory as arguments for the correctness of that theory. The more confirmation, the more the theory becomes persuasive. Some theories might be better off than others for predicting natural events within certain limits of detection. For example, Newton's theory of gravity was "roughly" correct in terms of *classical mechanics*, but for finer details, when the errors began appearing between observations and predictions, Einstein's general theory of relativity (1916) could correctly predict them.

However, theory which is not falsifiable is not scientific. For example, in a potential theory in which everything and all explanations are possible, nothing can be disproved. This is important because all-inclusive descriptions of nature have no predictive power. They are not theories but beliefs, personal (subjective) impressions, descriptions, stories, or, at best, science fiction.

Many theories in physics and chemistry made their makers famous during the past century. During the same time, prominent theories in biology and biomedicine were only a few, such as those about monogenetic

The Cytokines of the Immune System
http://dx.doi.org/10.1016/B978-0-12-419998-9.00009-2

inheritance and DNA structure. Perhaps it can be said that the biological sciences are only at the stage of collecting observations on natural phenomena. Discoveries are focused on descriptions of new molecules, for example, in a cell or about new species. Only when we gather all the information about the structures in a cell, its genes and their products will we be able to move on to the theoretical understanding of their function in an organism. One of the last challenges about the function of cells is their integration and communication in a body. Pharmacologic substances that are potentially therapeutic can be designed in order to inhibit or stimulate functional features of the cell.

The complexity of such an undertaking will definitely require the help of computer programs and aids. The aim would be to create theories and to predict whether a particular drug would cause the desired therapeutic effect with the list of side effects that could be expected from each one. The credibility of such biomedical theories will then be tested empirically in various therapeutic settings (provided the drug was approved, i.e., it is a non-toxic substance that has undergone testing in experimental animals) thus having the opportunity to be falsifiable.

Why do we need theories about the function of the immune system? Basically the answer is the desire to predict the outcome of various types of vaccination or immunization and to control them. The term "immune," which is widely used and not only in immunology, is thought to mean "protected," "impossible to hurt," or "not affected." In the immune system context it assumes a shielding action of its cells and products. The earliest theory of immunity is therefore concealed in its name that simply means defense. More elaborate theories about how the defense system works aim to explain molecular and cellular events that would be kicked into action by vaccinations, which are either used in the prevention of infectious diseases, or as therapeutic vaccines for cancers. These explanations would need to be in accord with predictions of action of the immune system after transplantation of foreign antigens, or in causing autoimmune diseases and allergies.

These goals should be achieved once we gather all the knowledge about the complexity of the human genome and proteome. However, it might be enough to learn only about the genes that are important for the immune response. Without theories, scientific research might not have been focused enough on these objectives. Thus, immunological theories can accelerate the development of biomedicine and clinical immunology, resulting ultimately with greater benefits for healthcare.

The immune response to infection is comparable to the defense of a country. Although comparing such unrelated issues could be fun, these two systems are not necessarily comparable when it comes to discussing the finer details. I wish to make complex issues in immunology clearer if not simpler by such assessment. The question the immune theorists would ask resembles the following:

What "policy" do higher vertebrates (humans) use in order to defend and maintain the integrity of their bodies (or "states")?

A good defense system exploits the features of tissues that are in contact with the environment (skin and mucosa of the respiratory, digestive, and reproductive tracts) as the first defense, or as a "battlefield." The other tissues would be used for "logistics" (migration); "renewal" (proliferation); "training" (activation); and "burial" (phagocytosis) of the participants in the battle. It is the blood and lymphatic system that provides "logistics" to the defensive force. The bone marrow gives rise to all cells of the blood and immune system. "Schools" for antigen recognition are the thymus and bone marrow, while the "graveyards" are organs such as the liver and spleen. Then, the centers of "logistics" could be lymph nodes and spleen. There the initial (nonspecific) part of the defense can be turned into a specific one, if it becomes necessary. In the spleen, perhaps, the "central administration, library, or evidence depository" might reside. However, this is a description of the immune system during "war," as for example, during infection, which is a harmful invasion by microorganisms. And what would it be in peace? How would society define the status of "foreigners"? Would it be according to foreigners' usefulness to society, society's need for them, or certain laws (e.g., hidden prejudice) by which they would be judged? Do these issues have analogous (biologic, immune) mechanisms?

New theories about the workings of the immune system expand the definition of immunology in the biological field beyond the limits of inflammation and homeostasis, and actually state that defense, although important, is not the only function of the immune system (see *the Integrity model*, below).

There are several theories about the basic function of the immune system. Their goal is to present the simplest working general principle of the system in a form of a metaphor (however, newer theories try not to overdo it with simplifications, because of the increasing number of factors and the complexity of the system).

SELF–NONSELF DISCRIMINATION

According to the theory of *self–nonself discrimination* (S–NS) by Bretscher and Cohn (1970), the immune response is a specific reaction to the emergence of foreign antigen (nonself), which is usually a part of some microorganisms (viruses, bacteria), parasites, or transplanted tissue.[1] Thus, harmful or unharmful bacteria will face an equal response according to this theory.

S–NS has up to last few decades been recognized as the only theory and the most suitable to explain the function of the immune system. Newer theories (especially the danger model) seem to have slowly assumed that role. Thus, S–NS has fallen into the difficulty of explaining natural phenomena such as tolerance of commensal bacteria in the digestive tract, the appearance of novel antigens in the body during development (i.e., during puberty, when the immune system is already fully developed), as well as finding solutions to many others.

Associative Recognition of Antigen (Cohn and Langman)[2]

Since newer theories are based on S–NS theory, it is important to mention its basic settings and rules. Specific immune response would occur when the "nonself" is recognized by B or T lymphocytes. Its recognition is associated with distinct interactions and not part of a network of them, which allows the concept of the activation of a cell, which leads to division and differentiation. A requirement for activation is that the immune cells must receive two signals. According to the most recent version of the associative recognition of antigen (ARA; M. Cohn) the "signal-1" for naïve T cells is delivered by antigen presenting cells in the form of peptide/MHC ligand. The "signal-2" comes as help from an effector T-cell clone specific for the very same ligand (thus, associated recognition). This begs the question immediately, as to how was the first such effector cell created? The explanation is controversial, because it claims that each naïve T cell can slowly over time become an effector cell without the signal-2. And, the latter is in contradiction with the former proposition. Furthermore, if naïve T cells receive only signal-1, it would result in tolerance to the ligand (by clonal deletion) in the central immunologic organs as well as in the periphery of the immune system.

Definition of Self

What the immune system recognizes as *self*, has been a subject of a long-term discussion among scientists. Perhaps the ideal definition is that *self* is everything in the body that the immune system tolerates (or has learned to see as its own). Unfortunately, this is in conflict with the explanation that the immune system in certain conditions can also tolerate nonself (as, e.g., with intravenous injection of antigen). In other words, it is difficult to make the boundary between *self* and *tolerated* by such a theory.

It is believed that the classical molecules of the major histocompatibility complex (MHC) are the best examples of *self*. MHC class I and class II molecules have a central role in the immune response. They bind parts of processed antigen (peptides) and present them to T cells, which, in turn, might recognize some peptide/MHC ligands as *foreign*. The specific immune system, according to this theory, has almost unlimited ability to tell apart *self* from *foreign* protein molecules. It should have high accuracy and minimal risk of damaging its own tissues. The repertoire of recognition of nonself (its specific part) is acquired in each individual (i.e., it is not inherited, but somatically assembled and selected). The nonspecific counterpart of the repertoire has a limited ability to recognize *foreign* (and thus *a greater chance of damaging its own tissues*).

An Alternative Explanation of Problems with the S–NS Theory

Older S–NS theory (ARA) excludes the nonspecific immune system from the consideration of initiating a specific immune response. In other words, S–NS claims that the specific immune system is independent in controlling the activation of immune cells (B and T), and nonspecific immunity can only regulate the path of the activation into different types (classes) of response.

For better clarification, we will continue our previous comparison of immunity (according to S–NS theory) and the defense of an imaginary country. The army would represent the defense. For example, it should react to any illegal penetration of foreigners into the country, whether they are harmful or potentially useful for her. Political leadership of such imaginary state (i.e., nonspecific immunity) could only regulate the path of the reaction, and the people (i.e., other somatic tissues), just watch. Thus, in the organization of the imaginary state (the immune system) by S–NS theory, the army's soldiers (immune cells) control themselves (decide on their own activation, when and where), and the political leadership of the state (nonspecific immune system) can only point their (rightful?) anger to some specific location, whereas the citizens (somatic target tissues) are innocent bystanders or victims.

Because immune cells control their own actions, S–NS theory predicts that regulatory (suppressive) Treg cells with the same repertoire of recognition as *normal* T cells would not know whether to activate themselves or not upon encounter with the *foreign* or *strange*. There is no logical way out of this dilemma. Therefore, it follows that Tregs cannot exist according to the initial S–NS model, because they are not required for the simplest model. However, the growing evidence in the literature over time describing the various functions of Tregs was confusing, and that posed a theoretical contradiction. However, the only solution for this contradiction was the elevation of the complexity of the theory. The explanation implied that Tregs would serve as a negative feedback to the immune response. Thus, by introducing this explanation for Tregs, S–NS was no longer the simplest theory for describing the function of the immune system. Why? Well, by postulating that a non-required cell population is wandering around in the body haphazardly being activated (or not), only to check the ongoing response, requires an explanation as to when such negative feedback would ensue, and when not, for each infection. No wonder immunology seemed extremely complicated by such an explanation (and still appears to be, as "ghosts" of this explanation are widely present). Newer theories avoid this infinite complication. They raise the level of simplicity, however, but only by a small step. Thus, only if we reject the S–NS theory of the immune system and replace it with one from the following list, we can perhaps have a better insight into the workings of the immune system in a less complicated way. Interestingly, only one can predict the role of Treg cells and can explain their role.

THE "PATHOGEN-ASSOCIATED MOLECULAR PATTERN (PAMP) RECOGNITION" THEORY (JANEWAY)

The latest addition to the S–NS theory is "discrimination of infectious principle from a non-infectious one" (Figure 9-1). The theory proposed detection of pathogenicity by some specialized type of receptor.[3] They were discovered to be special molecular pattern-recognizing receptors in cell membranes (i.e., Toll-like receptors, TLR), or cytosol (nucleotide-binding oligomerization domain [NOD]-like receptors, NLR). These are expressed on cells of the innate system (dendritic cells and macrophages), but recently their expression was found to be more widespread than previously anticipated or predicted. According to the theory, these molecules should bind molecular patterns of infectious (pathogenic) agents and thus generate the immune rejection of invasive microorganisms by adaptive immunity. Such "pathogenic" forms are thought to be evolutionarily older (present in microorganisms and parasites) than "self" patterns (present in eukaryotic cells). The *pathogenicity* would have characteristic molecular conformations, designs, or patterns (hence the name of their receptors "*Pattern recognition receptors*"; PRR). The theory is currently popular,[4] because it follows the standard S–NS model, and can explain many features of immunity (except the problems mentioned earlier for S–NS). It is, however, different from S–NS, because *nonself* does not equal all *foreign* molecules, but has *strange* features of foreignness (i.e., only strange foreigners such as pathogens, but not commensals, provoke response). Unlike ARA hypothesis, this theory takes the APCs (B cells, macrophages, or dendritic cells) as

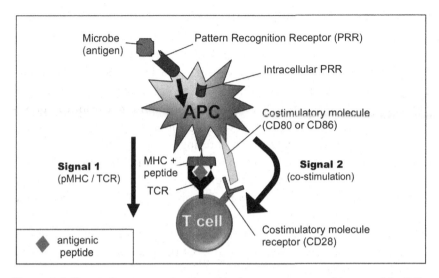

Figure 9-1 The pathogen-associated molecular pattern recognition model of the immune system function (as a variant of the Self/Nonself discrimination theory). MHC: major histocompatibility complex molecule; TCR: T-cell receptor; pMHC: peptide plus MHC (a ligand for TCR). The PRR receptor signal is sufficient for APC activation.

drivers of the immune response. APCs would provide a complete activation signal to naïve T cells, and would not require cognate (of the same clone) effector T cells for the second signal.

Arguments of the opponents of S–NS theories include the observation that "nonself" and "self" do not differ in the primary biochemical structures, but only by the frequency of some specific molecular patterns in phylogenetically distant species (bacteria and viruses). Because of that, the questions such as when, how, and why the immune cells react to microbes at all further complicate the S–NS theory. For each immune response a somewhat different explanation would be required. All together, these explanations made immunology more complicated than necessary. Sometimes, explanations are illogical or mutually incompatible. However, the complexity of the whole system can be much reduced if we choose to understand immunity as proposed in recent theories (see Sections The "Danger" Model and The "Integrity" Model below).

IDIOTYPIC NETWORKS AND SUPPRESSION (JERNE)

The theory of "*Idiotypic network*" or "*Idiotypic suppression*" (Jerne, Coutinho, Bandeira)[5–7] is based on initial Jerne's immune network theory,[8,9] but it is in essence a subspecies of the "*self-nonself discrimination*" principle. It tends to explain how the immune system works by implying it is constantly responding to self antigens, but these responses are also under constant suppression (i.e., under regulation, so that they are stopped in a hypothetical half-phase of a response). It's actually a collection of different hypotheses that have a common feature called network recognition. Here, the concept of the activated cell is quite different from the previously described model—associative recognition of antigen.

In short, infectious agents upon entering the body shift the balance of the suppressive network by creating an imbalance in it. Binding of an antigen by specific B cells frees them from suppression exerted by its idiotype specific B cell partner in the network. The absence of the suppressive clone causes the former clone to fulfill its "activation" process that results in proliferation, but not differentiation. This is a start of an immune response against the antigen that results in features of the immune response that we are already familiar with: production of antibodies that can neutralize an infectious agent and kill the infected cells.

The idiotype network model postulates that B cells have partners that cross-inhibit each other in blood as well as in somatic (immunologically) peripheral tissues by binding each other via BCRs. The BCR contact surface, called idiotype, is recognized by the partner's BCR contact surface, called anti-idiotype, and they would interact similarly as a key would fit into a keyhole.

Thus, if there were a disruption of cross-inhibition, such as the arrival of a soluble antigen, they would divide and develop differently. The B cell that can bind antigen will process and present antigenic peptides as peptide/MHC ligand to a specific T cell. T cells that could recognize the antigenic peptide/MHC ligand would be subsequently activated. Depending on the class of the MHC molecules involved in the presentation, either cytotoxic or helper T response would ensue. T helper effector cells would in turn help to differentiate B cells that had already bound the antigen to develop into plasma cells (with production of antigen-specific antibodies). On the other hand, anti-idiotypic B cells will also multiply and their number will follow the development of their counterparts (idiotypic B cells). Their fate is doomed, as they would not be able to stimulate T cells, because they have not bound, processed, and presented antigen. However, their enlarged clonal number would be able to cross-inhibit idiotypic B cells and thus keep them under control. In other words, activated specific T helper cells would outcompete anti-idiotypic B cells in the activation of idiotypic B cells, because the antigen would break the bond between networked cells (anti-Id–Id), and T–B interaction (TCR–peptide/MHC ligand) would fully activate idiotypic B cells. Thereby, the balance between activation and inhibition of the immune response would be shifted to the side of activation. When the antigen would be neutralized by (idiotypic) antibodies, phagocytosis, and (or) cytotoxic T cell activity, then the previous balance between networking B cells would be reconstituted. They should continue cross-inhibiting each other as they did before the antigen entered into the system.

Many parts of this theory were not shown to be present in experimental models. Although here and there one can find examples of anti-idiotypic antibodies, unfortunately, the idiotypic–anti-idiotypic network (as described in the previous section) was not found in the vertebrates examined so far. It is important to note the difference between rheumatoid factors (anti-antibody antibodies) from anti-idiotypic ones, because even though the former also react with other antibodies, they bind the constant (Fc) parts of immuno-globulins and not the variable segments as the latter do.

In recent years, novel hypotheses about idiotypic T-cell networks have emerged, and there are researchers who still advocate such concepts.

THE "DANGER" MODEL (MATZINGER)

The "Danger," "Morphostasis," and "Integrity" models comprise a group of theories about the function of the immune system, with "*Danger*" theory being the first to pull away from the self–nonself discrimination principle. In simple terms, the "Danger" model refutes the ARA theory, but incorporates PRR theory with slight but important changes, building new concepts on the function of immunity. All three models place nonspecific immunity in charge (control) of adaptive (specific) immunity. (The charge/control role is different from the regulation of adaptive immunity.) The most popular of them is the "*Danger*" model (Matzinger) (Figure 9-2). The "*Morphostasis*" and the "*Integrity*" models are less known, but describe a similar *alarm* principle that could warn an organism about invasion by dangerous, harmful, and damaging microorganisms of agents. The "Integrity" model claims that tissues and the immune system "feel" the break of tissue integrity and work to recover the similar "feeling" of integrity. The "*Morphostasis*" model[10] predicts that mess (infection) in tissues provokes clearance of the mess as the structures in an organism tend to be conserved (by morphostatic principle, which is unfortunately not explained beyond the metaphor, i.e., by molecular and/or cellular interactions).

The "*Danger*" model[11–13] describes the immune system as a constantly working mechanism that closely monitors and supervises the molecular

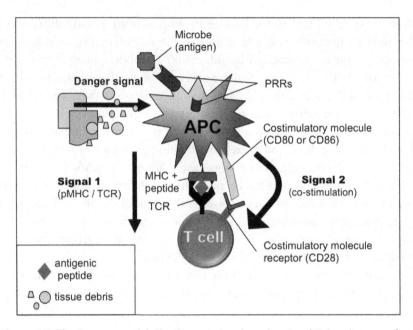

Figure 9-2 The Danger model. The Danger signal, or the signal 0 (zero), comes from outside of the APC as a consequence of necrotic cell death, tissue distress, or damage. It involves ligands for PRRs and other factors that would activate APCs and induce costimulatory molecules.

composition of our tissues and thus tolerates age, gender, and other changes that occur or develop over a lifetime. In other words, the "army" (immune cells) is "politically" controlled by those that it protects, namely, the "environment and inhabitants" (somatic tissues).

The "*Danger*" theory has added to the previously described signal (self/non-self discrimination) another signal from the microenvironment that through antigen-presenting cells induces alarm (danger, damaged integrity, or the disappearance of a conserved, hereditary form of tissue). In detail, the "Danger" model describes either exogenous or endogenous (with respect to the body) dangerous alarm that activates APCs, by which in turn T cells activate the immune response. The nature of alarm has three Ds: death (necrotic), distress, and damage (Figure 9-2). It is different from the PRR model in which the APC sends the alarm. Here, in the Danger model, APCs receive. The Danger-associated molecular patterns (DAMPs) have been suggested to represent internal cellular stress molecules leaked from cells, produced or formed during the 3 D's and sensed by a variety of receptors.

Thus, the "*Danger*" theory predicts equality of endogenous or exogenous stress signals in the activation (maturation) of dendritic cells (that can activate T cells).

THE "INTEGRITY" MODEL (DEMBIC)

In contrast to the "*Danger*" model, the "*Integrity*" model (Dembic)[14–17] stipulates that any exogenous stress has to be recognized in the context of endogenous stress. In other words, dendritic cells would be activated (and matured) only if they receive at least two such signals (endogenous + exogenous) (Figure 9-3), whereas, in the Danger model, either of them would suffice for DC activation (i.e., for kick-starting the immune response).

According to the Integrity model, the consequence of this subtle difference with the Danger theory is that the immune system could be envisaged to have more than previously anticipated functions. Namely, three main functions, regarding the defense of an organism, can be listed: (1) to reject the harmful; (2) to protect the useful; and (3) to ignore (tolerate) the rest of the harmless world in the microenvironment. For these roles, it would be necessary to use some energy to "feel" the presence of the *others*; however, most would be used to establish the first two categories. The first function predicts the existence of the known (previously described) effector cells. The second function provides for the (physiologic) existence of regulatory cells (in tolerating self-antigens, as well as commensals), and a third function predicts a variety of other forms of tolerance (anergy, chimeric, tolerance, etc.).

The mechanism by which these functions of the immune system are executed involves theoretical signals that can be steering all the cells of the immune system. To have minimally three different results (functions) one needs more than two qualitatively different signals as proposed by *S–NS discrimination* (*PRR*) or *Danger* models. The inclusion of the third signal complicates the theory, but it is necessary in order to explain the three predicted functions by the *Integrity* model. Thus, the simplest explanation of the immune system function according to Integrity hypothesis is the three-signal model (Figures 9-3 and 9-4). However, in reality, more signals (in molecular terms) might be implicated, all of which should be possible to group under these three theoretical ones. The idea behind it is to group signals that focus on the basic immune response axis (Figure 9-5), which involves:

(a) sensing the disturbance within somatic tissue (i.e., by dendritic cells [DC]);

(b) transfer of this information to the center of the immune response (i.e., lymph nodes) and informing T cells;

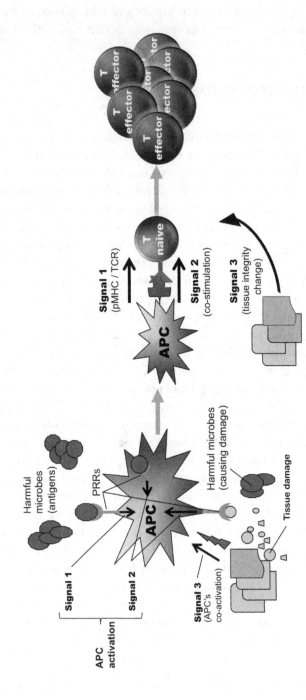

Figure 9-3 The Integrity hypothesis. The Integrity has three signals that act on both APCs and immunocytes. Signal 3 comes from the environment (tissues). This scheme shows the activation of APCs, and consecutively activation and proliferation of T cells. It is an example of the defense case, when harmful microbes invade the host.

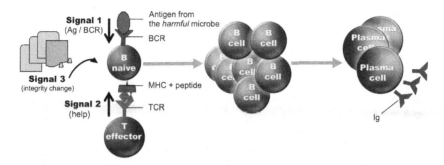

Figure 9-4 The Integrity hypothesis, part 2. This is a continuation of the defense case shown in Figure 9-3, when harmful microbes invade the host and have activated T cells making T effectors. This part shows the activation of B cells (for T-dependent antigens). Signal-3 transmits (in this case) the damage caused by harmful microbes. Ag: antigen; BCR: B-cell receptor, Ig: immunoglobulin.

(c) engagement of T-B collaboration and formation of germinal centers (with somatic mutation of BCR and Ig-isotype switch in B centroblasts);

(d) formation of effector cells (i.e., plasma cell differentiation, generation of T helper subsets, and formation of cytotoxic T cells); and finally

(e) migration of effector cells to somatic tissues to execute three proposed functions—defense (combating infections); tolerance (anergy, clonal deletion of potential autoreactive clones of immunocytes); or protection of self-tissues or commensals (suppression by Tregs).

The first type of signal includes detection of molecular patterns. This is done by the innate immune system by detecting *Integrity-associated molecular patterns* (IAMPs) or *Integrity-associated functional patterns* (IAFPs), which should detect tissue cohesiveness or its loss, in addition to microbial presence. The detection of the latter can be sorted into two vague groups based on molecular patterns predominantly characterizing certain microbes. Therefore, one pattern can represent foreign (non-self, i.e., microbial, parasitic) bearing potential pathogenic, dangerous, or potentially damaging characteristics (perhaps PAMPs or DAMPs), and the other might be self-like (i.e., eukaryotic cells) having unharmful characteristics. Here, the *Integrity* model predicts the existence of another pattern—IAMP that would give a beneficent characteristic (i.e., vitamin K in commensals) information to the immune system. These three signals would then steer the immune response axis into the three different outcomes:[16]

1. fighting harmful microbes by effector immunocytes;
2. integrating useful commensals by the regulatory cells; and

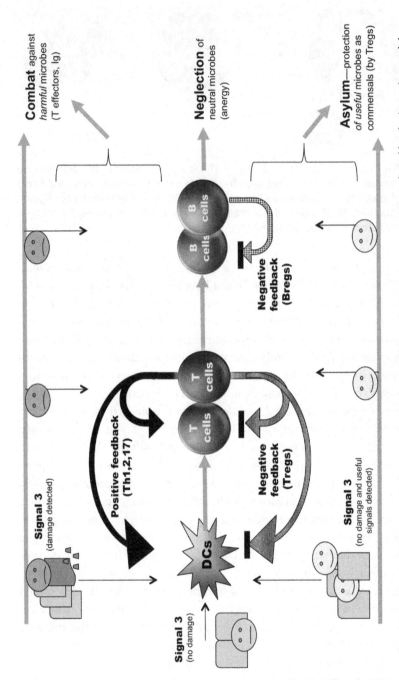

Figure 9-5 A schematic view of three outcomes (functions) of the adaptive immune system predicted by the Integrity model.

3. neglecting (but keeping notice of) the rest of the non-harmful, non-useful microbes, thus establishing vigilance.

These actions result in tissue remodeling after combating parasites and microbes, wound healing, and restoration of the tissue integrity. The enhancement of tissue functionality may come from beneficent symbiosis (i.e., between the useful commensal and mucosa) and the immune system would detect, allow, and protect such communion (the asylum function). Thus, the name—the immune system—meaning the defensive system, should be renamed by giving it a more appropriate name that includes the asylum function.

In general, according to Integrity, the immune system has three functions: (1) a *defensive* function (making effector cells capable of eliminating the intruding microbe); (2) a *vigilance* function (keeping notion and sentinel cells available for eventual combat, or regulatory action); and (3) the *integrity* function, by which cells of the immune system have a cohesive role in establishing tissue, organ, and organism homeostasis. Different failures of these functions can let cancer cells evade the immune attack, or in autoimmune diseases, disorders of the three predicted functions can be envisaged (Figure 9-6).

There are however many unanswered questions and among them are how can the T-independent responses be explained or how can different types (classes) of immune responses (i.e., Th1 – Th2 – Th17 – Th9 – Th22 – Treg) be reconciled?

The S–NS model can explain these by a difference in antigen-receptor strength (affinity affecting duration of interaction) and frequency of

Function of the immune system	Host tissue	Autoimmune disease	Infection	Cancer
Defense	Repertoire is clonally deleted in thymus and bone marrow (central tolerance)	Failure of clonal deletion in thymus or bone marrow of autoreactive clones	Combating *harmful* microbes and parasites (T and B effectors)	Mutating antigens to escape immunity, or clonally delete thymocytes
Vigilance	Peripheral tolerance (anergy) of self tissues (but keeping vigilance)	Neglection fails, anergic cells become activated	Neglection of *neutral* microbes (anergy of effectors)	Faking neutrality to anergize immune cells effectors
Integrity	Protection of self-integrity (tissues, organs) by Tregs	Tregs fail to become generated	Protection (asylum) of *useful* microbes like commensals (by Tregs)	Faking integrity signals to engage Tregs and evade immune attack

Figure 9-6 The immune system's functions (defense, vigilance, and integrity) according to the *Integrity* model, and predicted consequences for host homeostasis, autoimmunity, infection, and cancer.

interaction (i.e., molecular on–off rates) between MHC–TCR on APC and T cells, respectively, during activation. Because some Th subsets might arise even without direct influence of lineage specific cytokines, the duration, and strength of signaling are proposed to be important determinants in lineage fate.[18] Others suggest the dose of antigen as a controller of lineage commitments. Lower dose within the activation environment for T cells would generate Th2 type, whereas higher doses of antigen would lead to development of the Th1 response.[19,20]

The *Integrity* model explains T-independent responses by the ability of B cells to group signal-1 and signal-2 as a result of crosslinking BCRs during recognition and binding of antigen (however, they would still be influenced by signal-3 from the environment). The S–NS model would explain the independence of T cell help solely by the greater strength of B-cell receptor interaction with antigen (i.e., high affinity). T-dependent responses would then fall into those antigen-BCR interactions that have lower affinities. T subsets are similarly explained: Th1 would have higher avidity TCR–pMHC interaction, whereas Th2 would have lower affinity of interaction. On the other hand, according to the *Integrity* hypothesis, the T subset generation (or type of immune response) requires the additional (signal-3). It would provide a qualitative characteristic like damage-potential, harmlessness, or usefulness to guide the activation step of each T subset. The signal-3 includes in essence the epigenetic regulation of T and B cell activation.

Furthermore, if such activation turns out to be harmful for the body, or fails to focus combating the intruder at a correct location, it would have the chance of correcting the mistake, namely, it could switch to generate another T subset by influencing the generation of either Tregs (to repair the mistake, and inhibit autoreactive clones) or to engage another type of defensive effector cells (by switching T subsets in order to use the proper one) in an ideally endowed host.

In the end, the remaining question deals with the (molecular) nature of these signals. According to the *Integrity* model, the first two signals would be cell–cell interactions that would lead to transcriptional changes in responding cells. At the molecular level, signal-1 would be receptor–antigen for B, and receptor–peptide/MHC interaction for T cells. Signal-2 would be for T cells costimulation/co-inhibition (i.e., CD28-B7, CTLA4-B7, or PD1-PD1L) (Figure 9-3) and for B cell/T-cell help in germinal centers, or crosslinking BCRs (Figure 9-4). Signal-3 would be basically epigenetic control of accessibility of various genes in the genome of responding cells including most importantly those involved in T- and B-cell activation.[15] The exemplars for the latter group (IAMPs and/or IAFPs) are yet to be found.

OTHER THEORIES ABOUT IMMUNITY
The "Cytokine Burst" Model (Weigle)

Cytokines are secreted more or less by all the cells of the nonspecific (innate) and specific (adaptive) immune systems, and by almost all nucleated somatic tissue cells. Cytokines allow cell communication, facilitate activation, regulate proliferation, and promote the development of immunocompetent cells, and operate mainly in the immediate microenvironment, and rarely in distant tissues. Because of their wide range of effects, the theory according to which cytokines were responsible for initiating and controlling the immune response is called the cytokine burst. It involves regulation of the balance of cytokines. Thus, control of the immune response would not lie in the discrimination of self from nonself, but in microorganisms that can cause the sudden burst of the secretion of cytokines.[21]

The "Antigen Localization" or (the "Ignorance") Model (Zinkernagel)

According to the theory of "Ignorance," naïve (non-activated, resting) lymphocytes could not respond to antigenic challenge in somatic (peripheral) tissues, due to their unawareness.[22] The problem with this hypothesis is the definition of the unawareness, namely, the state of unawareness in itself cannot be proven by a positive result. Furthermore, all the other theories claim that naïve or resting memory lymphocytes in principle can react (to a challenge with antigen) in tissues (more precisely, they could be activated in all the tissues, provided appropriate conditions were met). According to the *Ignorance* model, under physiological conditions resting lymphocytes cannot be activated outside the lymph nodes (or in any way respond, not even with anergy or tolerance).

Compared to other models like "Danger" and "Integrity," the "Ignorance" hypothesis does not allow for the possibility that under physiological conditions lymphocytes can react in tissues, and be aware. The result, however, might be different from that in the lymph nodes, namely, the signal-2 would be lacking in somatic tissues under normal conditions. Hence, lymphocytes could receive only signal-1 and (without signal-2) undergo programmed cell death, with a consequence of creating a clonal deletion in the repertoire of immune responses.

According to the "Integrity" model, lymphocytes could additionally be able to receive signal-3 (from microenvironment, which includes stromal cell–immune cell contact and cytokines) and thus prone to either generate regulatory lymphocytes or other forms of tolerance. In conclusion, the most important difference between the Ignorance and the Danger or Integrity theories is that lymphocytes, as suggested by the latter models, would not be lame in somatic tissues.

The "Calibration" Model (Sinclair and Anderson)

A similar thought has been used in proposing the Calibration model, in which signal-2 could be calibrated and hence useful for the regulation of immunity. The "*Calibration*" model suggests that lymphocytes receive a neutral signal by antigen receptors, which can be modulated by co-stimulatory or co-inhibitory factors that would shape the immune response according to the influence of the environment.[23,24]

Summary of Discussion about Theories

It is likely that one of the above theories would provide the basis for the development of a more complete picture about the functions of the immune system in the future, especially once we learn about the structure of all the molecules involved in immune reactions. So far, we know about only some of these molecules, including the structures of Ig, BCRs, MHC molecules, T-cell receptors, peptide/MHC ligands, nonconventional MHC molecules, lipids, polysaccharides, TLRs, NLP, KIRs, KARs, signal transducers, cytokines, their receptors, adapters, and nuclear factors.

Based on recent knowledge, we can explain a large part of the workings of the immune system, but the overall vision is still missing. For example, the dominant theory of self–nonself discrimination is confusing, because we still cannot explain why some organ grafts are successfully transplanted and well received (tolerated), while others (or in another person) are not; what are the initial mechanisms of autoimmune diseases; why some people's immune systems, in rare instances, can eradicate cancer cells; and why the immune system generates regulatory cells (when theoretically unforeseen and superfluous). Particularly, for the explanation of the latter question, the paradox is that the immunizing antigen could generate two antagonistic actions: (1) the one being the rejection (of antigen) by effector cells; and (2) the inhibition of the rejection by regulatory lymphocytes. The theoretical result is a stalemate, which does not correspond to reality. The solution to this paradox lies in the influence of the tissue microenvironment in immune responses.

Continued

Summary of Discussion about Theories—cont'd

Theories that take into consideration such putative regulatory effects of the tissue microenvironment on immunocytes (B and T lymphocytes) have not yet entered mainstream use, perhaps because they have not been understood by scientists including most immunologists. It seems that the theory of reaction to *"dangerous"* (the *Danger model*) first opened the door to such considerations as it claimed that the microenvironment recognized danger by recognizing cellular distress, necrotic death, and damage, and that in turn was what controlled the adaptive immune response. However, the explanation for regulatory T cells (a satisfying one, in my opinion) is still lacking.

Subsequently, other hypotheses have tried to include the microenvironment in the explanation of immunological events such as the "Ignorance" model (lymphocytes are unaware of the antigenic world in somatic tissues, and can only be activated in the lymph nodes). Finally the "Integrity" model predicts that the microenvironment can control the adaptive (and innate) immune system, by the various cells of adaptive (and innate) immunity. The outcome is the tendency of maintaining the *status quo* (*homeostasis*) in somatic tissues (as is encoded in the genome of a species).

The *"Integrity"* model can explain anergy and the occurrence of regulatory lymphocytes in a simpler way than other models, especially the self–nonself discrimination theory and its latest *"Pathogenicity"* model that involves recognition of *"strange nonself"* by pattern recognition molecules.

REFERENCES

1. Bretscher P, Cohn M. A theory of self-nonself discrimination. *Science* 1970;**169**:1042.
2. Cohn M, Langman RE. The protection: the unit of humoral immunity selected by evolution. *Immunol Rev* Jun, 1990;**115**:11.
3. Janeway Jr C. Approaching the asymptote? Evolution and revolution in immunology. *Cold S Harb Symp Quant Biol* 1989;**54**:1.
4. Medzhitov R, Janeway Jr C. Innate immune recognition: mechanisms and pathways. *Immunol Rev* Feb, 2000;**173**:89.
5. Bandeira A. The evolutionary origins of immunoglobulins and T cell receptors. *Res Immunol* 1996;**147**:193–268.
6. Coutinho A. The network theory: 21 years later. *Scand J Immunol* Jul, 1995;**42**:3.
7. Coutinho A, Stewart J. A hundred years of immunology. Paradigms, Pardoxes and Perspectives. In: Cazenave J, Talwar GP, editors. *Immunology: Pasteur's Heritage*. New Delhi: Wiley Eastern Limited (Pb); 1991. p. 175–99.
8. Jerne NK. The somatic generation of immune recognition. *Eur J Immunol* Jan, 1971;**1**:1.
9. Jerne NK. Towards a network theory of the immune system. *Ann Immunol (Paris)* Jan, 1974;**125C**:373.
10. Cunliffe J. Morphostasis and immunity. *Med Hypotheses* Feb, 1995;**44**:89.
11. Matzinger P. Tolerance, danger, and the extended family. *Annu Rev Immunol* 1994;**12**:991.
12. Matzinger P. Friendly and dangerous signals: is the tissue in control? *Nat Immunol* 2007;**8**:11.

13. Matzinger P, Kamala T. Tissue-based class control: the other side of tolerance. *Nat Rev Immunol* Mar, 2011;**11**:221.
14. Dembic Z. Do we need integrity? *Scand J Immunol* 1996;**44**:549.
15. Dembic Z. Immune system protects integrity of tissues. *Mol Immunol* 2000;**37**:563.
16. Dembic Z. Response to Cohn: the immune system rejects the harmful, protects the useful and neglects the rest of microorganisms. *Scand J Immunol* 2004;**60**:3.
17. Dembic Z. On recognizing 'shades-of-gray' (self-nonself discrimination) or 'colour' (Integrity model) by the immune system. *Scand J Immunol* Oct, 2013;**78**:325.
18. Lanzavecchia A, Sallusto F. Dynamics of T lymphocyte responses: intermediates, effectors, and memory cells. *Science* Oct 6, 2000;**290**:92.
19. Constant S, Pfeiffer C, Woodard A, Pasqualini T, Bottomly K. Extent of T cell receptor ligation can determine the functional differentiation of naive CD4+ T cells. *J Exp Med* Nov 1, 1995;**182**:1591.
20. Hosken NA, Shibuya K, Heath AW, Murphy KM, O'Garra A. The effect of antigen dose on CD4+ T helper cell phenotype development in a T cell receptor-alpha beta-transgenic model. *J Exp Med* Nov 1, 1995;**182**:1579.
21. Weigle WO. Immunologic tolerance: development and disruption. *Hosp Pract (Off Ed)* Feb 15, 1995;**30**:81.
22. Zinkernagel RM. Immunology taught by viruses. *Science* 1996;**271**:173.
23. Sinclair NR, Anderson CC. Do lymphocytes require calibration? *Immunol Cell Biol* Dec, 1994;**72**:508.
24. Sinclair NR, Anderson CC. Co-stimulation and co-inhibition: equal partners in regulation. *Scand J Immunol* Jun, 1996;**43**:597.

INDEX

Note: Page numbers followed by "f" and "t" indicate figures and tables, respectively.

A

Activated Tregs, 120–121
Acute graft rejection, 67
Adaptive/acquired immunity, 19–20
AIRE. *See* Autoimmune regulator (AIRE)
Allograft, 66–67
Anergy, 119–120
Antibody feedback regulation, 97–98
Antigen localization model, 299–300
Anti-nuclear antibodies (ANA), 127
Autoimmune regulator (AIRE), 48–49
Autologous graft, 66–67
Autonomous immunity, 22

B

B-cell receptors (BCR), 40–42, 41f
Bcl6 nuclear factor, 78

C

Calibration model, 300–301
Cell marker profiles, 33
Cellular innate (nonspecific) immunity
  DC, 30–34, 31f
  granulocytes, 35–36
  innate type 2 cells/Is2, 39
  macrophages, 34–35
  mast cells, 36
  monocytes, 35
  natural killer cells, 36–38
    T cells, 38
Central immunity, 99
Central self-tolerance, 96
CFA. *See* Complete Freund's adjuvant
    (CFA)
Chemokines
  CCL1, 248
  CCL2, 248
  CCL3, 249
  CCL4, 249
  CCL5, 249
  CCL6, 249–250

CCL7, 250
CCL8, 250
CCL9/10, 250
CCL11, 250
CCL12, 251
CCL13, 251
CCL14, 251
CCL15, 251
CCL16, 251–252
CCL17, 252
CCL18, 252
CCL19, 252
CCL20, 252–253
CCL21, 253
CCL22, 253
CCL23, 253
CCL24, 254
CCL25, 254
CCL26, 254
CCL27, 254
CCL28, 255
CXCL1, 255
CXCL2, 255–256
CXCL3, 256
CX3CL1, 259
CXCL4, 256
CXCL5, 256
CXCL6, 256
CXCL7, 257
CXCL8, 257
CXCL9, 257
CXCL10, 258
CXCL11, 258
CXCL12, 258
CXCL13, 258
CXCL14, 259
CXCL15, 259
CXCL16, 259
definitions, 241–243, 242f–243f,
    244t–245t
features of, 260–261

Chemokines (*Continued*)
  in immune system, 246–248, 246f–247f
  XCL1, 260
  XCL2, 260
Chemotaxis, 8
Chronic inflammatory diseases, 119
Ciliary neurotrophic factor (CNTF)
  features, 274–275
  function, 274
  receptor, 274, 275f
  source, 274
  structure, 274
  therapeutic options, 275–276
Classic pathway, 26–28
Coinhibitory molecules, 105
Complete Freund's adjuvant (CFA), 24f, 25
Costimulatory molecules, 105
Cross-presentation, 70–71, 71f
Crosstalk molecules, 105
Cytokine burst model, 299
Cytokines
  biological function of, 14–16
    cells migration, 15
    growth and development, regulation
      of, 15–16
    interleukins, 15
    metabolism and ion balance, 16
    viruses and regulation, defense against,
      14–15
  division, 3
  hormones and, 11–14, 12f
    biological role, 12–13
    blood circulation, occurrence in, 13
    breadth of actions, 13
    influence, sphere of, 14
    mode of action, 14
    redundancy, 13
    sources, 12
    target cells, 12
  intracellular signal transduction, 8–11,
    9f–11f
  receptors, 6–8, 6f–8f
  structures, 3–4, 4f
Cytotoxic CD8 T lymphocytes, 104

D
Danger associated molecular patterns
    (DAMPs), 30, 295
Danger model theory, 291–293, 292f
DC. *See* Dendritic cells (DC)

Dendritic cells (DC), 30–34
Di-acyl-glycerol (DAG), 75
Differentiation profiles, 33

E
Effector CD4 T cells, 104
Endothelins, 281
Epidermal growth factor (EGF), 278
Epithelial barrier immunity, 117

F
Fibroblast growth factor (FGF), 279–280
Final immune repertoire, 95–96
Follicular dendritic cells (FDC),
    103–104
Foxp3, 79, 111, 120
Fratricide, 86–87

G
GATA-3, 78, 108–109
Genome-wide linkage analysis, 138
Granulocytes, 35–36

H
Hematopoietic cells, 17–18
Hepatocyte growth factor (HGF), 277
Heterodimeric molecule, 59
Heterotrimeric receptor, 7–8, 8f
Homodimeric ligand (IFNγ), 8
Humoral innate (nonspecific) immunity
    complement, 26–30
      alternative pathway, 28
      cascade, completion of, 28–29
      classic pathway, 26–28
      lectin pathway, 28
      regulation, 29–30
Hyperacute rejection, 66

I
Idiopathic inflammatory myopathies, 136
Idiotypic network theory, 289–291
Idiotypic suppression theory, 289–291
Immature single-positive stage (ISP), 46
Immune response, 23–24
      activation, immunocyte development
        regulation after, 105–106, 106t
      course of, 99–105, 100f–105f
      cytokines, control functions of
        B lymphocytes, effects on, 113–114, 113f
        NKT cells, generation of, 111–113

Th1-type effectors, generation of,
        106–107, 107f
Th2-type effectors, generation of,
        107–108, 108f
Th9-type effectors, generation of,
        108–109, 109f
Th17-type effectors, generation of,
        109–110, 109f
Th22-type effectors, generation of,
        110–111, 110f
Treg cells, generation of, 111, 111f
Tfh subset, 121
Th3-type and Tr1 cells , role of, 119, 119f
Th1-type, role of, 114–115, 114f
Th2-type, role of, 115–116, 116f–117f
Th9-type, role of, 116, 117f
Th17-type, role of, 116–117, 118f
Th22-type, role of, 118, 118f
Tregs, regulatory CD4 T lymphocytes,
        119–121
Immune system
    adaptive humoral (specific) immune
        system, 39–42
        antibody molecules, variable parts of,
            40–42, 41f
        immunoglobulins, 39–40, 40f
    cellular adaptive (specific) immune
        system, 42–56
        B and T lymphocytes, common
            precursor of, 43–44
        B-cell development, 51, 52f–53f
        clonal distribution, 43
        γδTXP (γδT cells), T lymphocytes
            with, 55–56
        T-cell development, 44–51, 45f
    cellular innate (nonspecific) immunity.
        See Cellular innate (nonspecific)
        immunity
    humoral innate (nonspecific) immunity,
        25–30
        complement, 26–30
        mucosal surface, factors secreted in,
            25–26
    organization of, 19–25
        antigen, 19
        immunity, classification of, 19–22,
            20f–21f, 20t
Immunization, 23–25, 104–105, 284
Immunoglobulin receptors, 58
Immunological disorders, 2–3

Immunological synapse, 72–73
Induced Treg (iTreg), 77
Inflammasomes, 99–101
Inflammatory bowel disease (IBD), 135
Innate immunity, 19–20
Insulin-like growth factor (IGF), 278–279
Integrity associated molecular patterns
        (IAMPs), 30, 292, 295
Integrity model theory, 293–299,
        294f–295f
Interferon-α
    features, 126–127
    function, 124
    receptor, 124–126
    source, 124
    structure, 124
    therapeutic options, 128–129
Interferon-γ (IFN-γ), 4
    features, 132–135, 134f
    function, 129–130
    human diseases, association with,
        135–139
    receptor, 130–132, 131f–132f
    source, 129
    structure, 129
    therapeutic options, 139–140
Interferon-λ (IFN-λ), 140
Interleukin-1
    association with diseases, 146–151
        asthma/osteoarthritis and autoimmune
            diseases, 146–148
        cancer, 149–150
        conditions and diseases, 150–151
        infections and chronic inflammations,
            148–149
        myocardial infarction and stroke, 149
    features, 145–146
    function, 143–144
    receptor, 144–145, 144f
    source, 143
    structure, 143
    therapeutic options, 151
Interleukin-2
    association with diseases, 157–159
    features, 153–155
    function, 151–152
    receptor, 152–153, 152f
    source, 151
    structure, 151
    therapeutic options, 159–160

Interleukin-3
  features, 161
  function, 160
  human diseases, associations with, 162
  receptor, 160–161, 161f
  source, 160
  structure, 160
  therapeutic options, 162
Interleukin-4
  features, 164–165
  function, 163
  human diseases, associations with, 165
  receptor, 163–164
  source, 163
  structure, 162
  therapeutic options, 166
Interleukin-5
  association with human diseases,
    167–168
  features, 167
  function, 166
  receptor, 166–167
  source, 166
  structure, 166
  therapeutic options, 168
Interleukin-6
  associations with human diseases,
    172–174
  features, 171–172
  function, 168–169
  receptor, 169–170, 169f–170f
  signal transduction, regulatory feedback
    loops in, 170
  soluble receptor, 171
  source, 168
  structure, 168
  therapeutic options, 174–175
Interleukin-7
  associated with human diseases,
    177–178
  features, 177
  function, 175
  receptor, 175–176
  source, 175
  structure, 175
  therapeutic options, 178
Interleukin-8, 178

Interleukin-9
  association with human diseases, 180
  function, 179
  receptor, 179, 180f
  source, 179
  structure, 179
Interleukin-10
  association with human diseases,
    183–184
  features, 181–182
  function, 181
  receptor, 182, 183f
  source, 181
  structure, 181
  therapeutic options, 184
Interleukin-11
  association with human diseases, 186
  features, 185–186
  function, 185
  receptor, 185, 185f
  source, 185
  structure, 184
  therapeutic options, 186
Interleukin-12
  association with human diseases,
    189–190
  features, 188–189
  functions, 187–188
  receptor, 188, 189f
  source, 187
  structure, 186–187, 187f
  therapeutic options, 190
Interleukin-13
  association with human diseases, 192
  function, 191
  receptor, 191
  source, 191
  structure, 190–191
  therapeutic options, 192
Interleukin-14, 193
Interleukin-15
  association with human diseases,
    196–197
  features, 195–196
  function, 193, 194f
  receptor, 193–195, 194f
  source, 193

structure, 193
therapeutic options, 197
Interleukin-16
  association with human diseases, 199
  features, 199
  function, 197–198
  receptor, 198, 198f
  source, 197
  structure, 197
  therapeutic options, 199
Interleukin-17
  association with diseases, 202
  features, 201–202
  function, 200
  receptor, 200–201, 201f
  source, 200
  structure, 200
  therapeutic options, 202
Interleukin-18
  association with diseases, 204–205
  features, 204
  function, 203
  receptor, 203–204, 203f
  source, 203
  structure, 202–203
  therapeutic options, 205
Interleukin-19
  alias, 205
  association with human diseases, 207
  features, 207
  function, 206
  receptor, 206–207, 206f
  source, 206
  structure, 206
Interleukin-20
  alias, 207
  association with human diseases, 209
  features, 209
  function, 208
  receptor, 208–209, 208f
  source, 208
  structure, 207–208
Interleukin-21
  association with human diseases, 211
  features, 211
  function, 210
  receptor, 210, 210f

source, 209
structure, 209
therapeutic options, 212
Interleukin-22
  alias, 212
  association with human diseases, 213–214
  features, 213
  function, 212
  receptor, 212–213
  source, 212
  structure, 212
  therapeutic options, 214
Interleukin-23
  alias, 214
  association with human diseases, 216
  features, 215
  function, 214–215
  receptor, 215, 215f
  source, 214
  structure, 214
  therapeutic options, 216
Interleukin-24
  alias, 216
  association with human diseases, 217
  features, 217
  function, 216
  receptor, 216–217, 217f
  source, 216
  structure, 216
  therapeutic options, 217–218
Interleukin-25
  association with disease, 219
  features, 219
  function, 218
  receptor, 218, 218f
  source, 218
  structure, 218
  therapeutic options, 219
Interleukin-26
  alias, 219
  association with human diseases, 221
  features, 220–221
  function, 220
  receptor, 220, 220f
  source, 220
  structure, 220
  therapeutic options, 221

Interleukin-27
  alias, 221
  association with human diseases, 223
  features, 222–223
  function, 221–222
  receptor, 222, 222f
  source, 221
  structure, 221
  therapeutic options, 223
Interleukin-28
  features, 224
  function, 224
  receptor, 224, 225f
  source, 224
  structure, 224
  therapeutic options, 224–225
Interleukin-29
  features, 224
  function, 224
  receptor, 224, 225f
  source, 224
  structure, 224
  therapeutic options, 224–225
Interleukin-30, 225
Interleukin-31
  association with human diseases, 226
  features, 226
  function, 225
  receptor, 226, 226f
  source, 225
  structure, 225
Interleukin-32
  alias, 227
  association with human diseases, 228
  features, 227–228
  function, 227
  source, 227
  structure, 227
  therapeutic options, 228
Interleukin-33
  alias, 228
  association with human diseases,
    229
  function, 228
  receptor, 229, 229f
  source, 228
  structure, 228
  therapeutic options, 229

Interleukin-34
  alias, 229
  association with disease, 230
  function, 230
  receptor, 230
  source, 230
  structure, 230
Interleukin-35
  association with disease, 231
  function, 231
  receptor, 231, 231f
  source, 230–231
  structure, 230
Interleukin-36α/β and γ
  aliases, 232
  association with diseases, 233
  effects, 233
  function, 232–233
  receptor, 232, 233f
  source, 232
  structure, 232
Interleukin-37
  alias, 233
  association with diseases, 234
  function, 234
  receptor, 234
  source, 233
  structure, 233
Interleukin-38
  alias, 234
  association with disease, 235
  function, 235
  receptor, 235
  source, 234
  structure, 234
Intracellular signal transduction, 8–11
IRF4 nuclear factor, 79
ISP. See Immature single-positive stage (ISP)
ITAM sequences, 73
iTreg. See Induced Treg (iTreg)

K
Keratinocyte growth factor (KGF), 271
KGF. See Keratinocyte growth factor (KGF)

L
Lectin pathway, 28
Leukemia inhibitory factor (LIF)

association with human diseases, 274
function, 273
receptor, 273–274, 273f
structure, 273
synonyms, 272
Ligand affinities, 7
Lipopolysaccharide (LPS), 99
Lymphokine activated killer (LAK)
cells, 38

M

Macrophages, 34–35
Major histocompatibility complex (MHC)
molecules
associations with diseases, 68–70
haplotypes and alleles
predisposing, 68–69
protecting, 69–70
non-conventional MHC molecules, 70
Mammalian target of rapamycin (mTOR),
130–132
Mast cells, 36
Master regulator T-bet, 107
Membrane phase, 29–30
Monocytes, 35, 133
Multiple sclerosis, 126–127

N

Natural killer (NK) cells, 36–38
Nerve growth factor (NGF), 280
Neural differentiation factor (NDF), 280
NF-κB, 78
Nitric oxide synthase (NOS2A), 138

O

Oncostatin M (OSM)
features, 276
function, 276
receptor, 276
source, 276
structure, 276

P

PAMPs. *See* Pathogen-associated molecular
patterns (PAMPs)
Pathogen-associated molecular pattern
(PAMP), 30, 99–101, 295
recognition theory, 288–289, 289f

PDGF. *See* Platelet derived growth factor
(PDGF)
Peripheral tolerance, 119–120
Phagocytosed antigen, 70–71
Platelet derived growth factor (PDGF), 278
Pleiotropy, 13
Polygenism, 64–65
Polymorphisms, 137
Programmed death-1 (PD-1) molecule, 80

R

Repertoire, 94
Respiratory syncytial virus (RSV), 128
RORγt, 78, 110

S

Secreted cytokine profiles, 33–34
Self-nonself discrimination theory, 25,
285–288
alternative explanation of problems,
287–288
associative recognition of antigen, 286
definition, 286–287
Signal transduction, 121
Single nucleotide polymorphisms (SNPs), 135
Soluble phase, 29
Somatic hypermutation, 59
Split tolerance, 97
Stem cell factor (SCF), 271–272
receptors, 271–272
therapeutic potential, 272
Suppressor of cytokine signaling (SOCS)
factor, 132
Supramolecular activation cluster (SMAC),
72–73
Systemic administration, 129

T

T-bet nuclear factor, 78
T-cell activation
B cell, signal transduction in, 80–81,
81f, 83f
CD4 and CD8, T cells coreceptors,
70–71, 71f
costimulation during, 71–72
effector cells, types of, 85–89
Ad 1, 85–87, 85f–86f
Ad 2, 87

T-cell activation (*Continued*)
    Ad 3, 87–89, 88f
    Ad 4, 89
  mast cells, signal transduction in, 81–83
  memory cells, 89–90
  naïve/effector and memory
      immunocytes, 90–93
  recognition, immunologic repertoire of
    negative and positive selection of,
      94–96
    species, genetic organization of, 94
  repertoire and tolerance
    immunologic tolerance, 96–97
    recognition, immunologic repertoire
      of, 94–96
    split tolerance, 97–98
  signal transduction in
    activation signal initiation, 73–75, 74f
    communication molecules, 79–80
    master regulators of differentiation,
      78–79
    phosphatidyl-inositol triphosphate
      derivatives, 75–76
    PI3K and treg cells, 76–77
    supramolecular complexes and
      immunologic synapse, 72–73, 72f
    transcription factors, 77–78
  specific recognition, 58–70
    antigen, specific receptors for, 59
    HLA complex, tissue typing and organ
      transplantation, 63–68, 63f–65f
    major histocompatibility complex
      (MHC) molecules, 59–63
  T lymphocyte homeostasis, 93–94
T-cell development, 44–51, 45f
  secondary lymphatic tissue, 51
  thymic checkpoints, 46–49, 47f
  treg cells, development of, 49–51
Terminal pathway, 28–29
T follicular helper (Tfh) subpopulation, 121

TGF-β
  receptor, 267–269, 268f
  structure, 266–267
Th1-type effectors, 106–107, 107f
Th2-type effectors, 107–108, 108f
Th9-type effectors, 108–109, 109f
Th17-type effectors, 109–110, 109f
Th22-type effectors, 110–111, 110f
Thymic stromal lymphopoetin (TSLP),
    49–50
  association with human diseases,
    270–271
  features, 270
  function, 269
  receptor, 269, 270f
  source, 269
  structure, 269
T-independent antigens, 91
TNF. *See* Tumor necrosis factor (TNF)
Toll-like receptors (TLR), 99, 100f
Transcription factors, 8–9
TSLP. *See* Thymic stromal lymphopoetin
    (TSLP)
Tumor necrosis factor (TNF), 4–5, 106t,
    136, 143, 168–169, 204, 263, 264f
Tumor necrosis factor-α/β (TNF-α/β)
  associations with disease, 266
  features, 264
  function, 263–264
  receptor, 263, 265f
  source, 263
  structure, 263, 264f
  therapeutic options, 266
Typical immune response, 95

V

Vaccination, 23–24, 284
Vascular endothelial growth factor (VEGF),
    280–281
Vertebrates, 17

Printed in the United States
By Bookmasters